The Psychiatric Guide to Pharmacotherapy

Edited by
James M. Ellison, MD

Mosby Year Book

St. Louis Baltimore Boston Chicago London Philadelphia Sydney Toronto

Copyright 1989 by Mosby–Year Book, Inc. All rights reserved. No part of this publication may be reproduced, stored in a retrieval system, or transmitted, in any form or by any means—electronic, mechanical, photocopying, recording, or otherwise—without prior written permission from the publisher. Printed in the United States of America.

A Year Book imprint of Mosby–Year Book, Inc.

Mosby–Year Book, Inc.
11830 Westline Industrial Drive
St. Louis, MO 63146

2 3 4 5 6 7 8 9 CL/MV 0 93 92 91

The Psychotherapists' guide to pharmacotherapy.

Library of Congress Cataloging-in-Publication Data

  Includes index.
  1. Mental Illness—Chemotherapy.   2. Psychotherapy.
I. Ellison, James, 1924- .
RC483.P7795   1989   616.89'18   88-34487
ISBN 0-8151-3158-5

CONTRIBUTORS

Stephen J. Bartels, MD
Assistant Professor in Psychiatry, Dartmouth Medical School
Hanover, New Hampshire

Gregory A. Clark, MD
Instructor in Psychiatry, Harvard Medical School
Director of Adult Inpatient Psychiatry, The Cambridge Hospital
Cambridge, Massachusetts

James M. Ellison, MD
Assistant Professor in Psychiatry, Harvard Medical School
Lecturer in Psychiatry, Tufts University School of Medicine
Boston, Massachusetts
Director of Somatic Therapies in Psychiatry, The Cambridge Hospital
Cambridge, Massachusetts
Director of Psychopharmacology, Metropolitan State Hospital
Waltham, Massachusetts

William E. Falk, MD
Instructor in Psychiatry, Harvard Medical School
Senior Staff Psychiatrist, Psychopharmacology Clinic, Massachusetts General Hospital
Boston, Massachusetts

Eliot Gelwan, MD
Instructor in Psychiatry, Harvard Medical School
Medical Director, Schiff Center
Staff Psychiatrist, The Cambridge Hospital
Cambridge, Massachusetts

Diane Grimaldi, RN, MS, CS
Associate Clinical Professor, Boston University School of Nursing
Instructor in Psychiatry, Harvard Medical School
Cambridge, Massachusetts

Michael L. Johnson, MD
Instructor in Psychiatry, Harvard Medical School
Staff Psychiatrist, Cambridge Center, HCHP
Cambridge, Massachusetts

Nancy Kielhofner, RN, MS, CS
Director of Nursing
Psychiatric/Chemical Dependency Services
Hinsdale Hospital
Hinsdale, Illinois

Pamela Marlink, MD
Clinical Fellow in Psychiatry, Harvard Medical School
Chief Resident, Psychopharmacology Clinic, The Cambridge Hospital
Cambridge, Massachusetts

Kerim Munir, MD, MPH
Instructor in Psychiatry, Harvard Medical School
Director, Pediatric Psychopharmacology, The Cambridge Hospital
Cambridge, Massachusetts

Susan Primm, LICSW
Clinical Instructor, Simmons College School of Social Work
Senior Staff Social Worker, Adult Psychiatry Clinic, Massachusetts General Hospital
Boston, Massachusetts

Janna M. Smith, LICSW
Staff Social Worker, The Cambridge Hospital
Cambridge, Massachusetts

Edward Yeats, PhD
Instructor in Psychology, Department of Psychiatry, Harvard Medical School
Supervising Psychologist, The Cambridge Hospital
Cambridge, Massachusetts

CONTENTS

Preface **vii**
Acknowledgments **ix**

SECTION I. COMBINING PHARMACOTHERAPY AND PSYCHOTHERAPY IN CLINICAL PRACTICE

1. Fundamentals of Combined Treatment **3**
2. Rational and Irrational Pharmacotherapeutics on the Psychiatric Inpatient Unit **22**
3. Pharmacotherapy from the Perspective of Family Ecology **51**
4. Some Dimensions of Transference in Combined Treatment **79**
5. Intertherapist Conflict in Combined Treatment **96**

SECTION II. A PSYCHOPHARMACOLOGY KNOWLEDGE BASE FOR PSYCHOTHERAPISTS

6. Medications for Mental Disorders: A Brief History and an Overview of Current Uses **119**
7. An Introduction to Psychiatric Medications **144**
8. Child and Adolescent Pharmacotherapy Comes of Age **191**
9. Organic Mental Disorder: When To Suspect Medical Illness as a Cause of Psychiatric Symptoms **205**
10. Interactions of Alcohol, Street Drugs, and Prescribed Medications **240**
11. ADHD, CEBV, FM, PMS, Etc: Controversial Syndromes at the Psychiatry/Medicine Interface **257**

Appendix: Use of the Laboratory in Pharmacotherapy **289**

Index **295**

PREFACE

This book is addressed to social workers, psychologists, and nurses who wish to learn more about the medications that are revolutionizing psychiatric treatment. This is increasingly valuable knowledge as nonmedically trained psychotherapists assume greater responsibility in the treatment of medicated patients.

For patients with major mental illness, it is now the rule rather than the exception for treatment to include concurrent medications and psychotherapy. When these treatments are provided by two clinicians, provision of medications and psychotherapy may occur in parallel, with little communication between therapists. The psychotherapist and pharmacotherapist in such an arrangement miss many opportunities to understand and appreciate each other's contributions to the treatment process. The patient may end up confused about the roles of each treatment and of each caregiver.

Training programs for psychotherapists are attempting to remedy this situation by including courses on psychopharmacology in their curricula. Postgraduate seminars, too, such as the Cambridge Hospital's "Psychopharmacology for the Non-M.D. Psychotherapist," have built bridges between the highly interrelated fields of psychotherapy and pharmacotherapy. The essays which follow are a further attempt to integrate these areas.

The first half of this book is concerned with interactions of pharmacotherapy and psychotherapy in a variety of clinical settings. The fundamentals of obtaining consultation and maintaining a relationship with a pharmacotherapist, the role of transference in combined treatment, and issues of integrating pharmacotherapy into family and inpatient psychotherapy are each considered. The goal is to increase clinicians' awareness of the interactions between concurrent treatments, and to stimulate further thinking on these important topics.

To provide a reference and a base of factual knowledge, the second half of this book reviews topics in clinical psychopharmacology. The indications for use of medication in adults and children, descriptions of the drugs of greatest value, and the interactions between prescribed and recreational drugs are discussed. In addition, because psychiatric consultation is often requested for the purpose of helping to detect the presence of organic mental disorders, there are chapters on common and difficult-to-diagnose behavioral syndromes with physical causes.

Throughout, this book emphasizes aspects of pharmacotherapy and combined treatment that are most relevant to the practicing psychotherapist. The focus is on practical issues that affect clinical work. Case examples illustrate the principles discussed. The goal is to improve psychotherapists' ability to help their patients benefit from two different but potentially synergistic treatment modalities.

ACKNOWLEDGMENTS

This book, which focuses heavily on the importance of collaboration in treatment, has also been a lesson in the benefits of collaboration in writing! For the many ways in which they have contributed, I thank each co-author of this volume. Those who have served as readers and critics as well deserve particular gratitude. Collectively, the contributors and I owe our thanks to the many patients who populate these pages as case examples. While their stories have been disguised to protect confidentiality, the ways in which these individuals have shaped our thinking remain apparent.

The germ of this book was a brief manual developed by a 1984 task force devoted to studying the integration of psychotherapy and pharmacotherapy at The Cambridge Hospital. Diane Grimaldi and Nancy Kielhofner, two valuable organizers of that committee, are represented in this volume. Ellen Sinnott, BSN, also a member, deserves appreciation for the anonymous contribution to this book made by her presence on that task force.

One recommendation of that committee was the establishment of a post-graduate, multidisciplinary educational conference. Entitled "Psychopharmacology for the Non-M.D. Psychotherapist," this has been presented annually since 1986. Judy Platt, MEd, Director of Continuing Medical Education at The Cambridge Hospital, has been instrumental in producing this conference and has helped us to test the interest and value of a broad range of topics presented there.

Invariably, each conference brought requests for reading material about pharmacotherapy and the integration of treatment modalities. Several excellent reference sources on clinical psychopharmacology are available, but writing on combined treatment has been sparse. The need for a book such as *The Psychotherapist's Guide to Pharmacotherapy* became clear, and work began. While most of the initial planners of this project are listed in the list of contributors, two others deserve special mention. Diane Mosbacher, MD, PhD, and J. Christopher Perry, MD, each wrote drafts that helpfully influenced the development of specific chapters.

Among the generous readers who reviewed early versions of this manuscript were David Adler, MD; Nancy Blum, MEd; Mona Fishbane, PhD; Leslie Fuchs, MD; Blanca Gonzalez, MA; Henry Grunebaum, MD; Judy Grunebaum, LICSW; David Kantor, PhD; Edward Khantzian, MD; Suzanne Loughlin, MS, CS; Carolyn Maltas, PhD; Nina Masters, LICSW; Linda Miller, JD, MSW; David Osser, MD; J. Christopher Perry, MD; and Matthew Warner, MA. Their thoughtful comments have improved this book in many ways, ranging from organization and content to matters of style. Finally, I wish to express my gratitude to two people whose consistent support and constructive criticism have been essential in urging this project onward to its conclusion: my colleague, Teri Hodel, and my sister, Katherine Ellison.

Section I
Combining Pharmacotherapy and Psychotherapy in Clinical Practice

1

Fundamentals of Combined Treatment

*Susan Primm
William E. Falk
Diane Grimaldi
Nancy Kielhofner
Janna M. Smith
James M. Ellison*

Combined treatment refers to the shared treatment of a patient by two clinicians, one responsible for psychotherapy and the other for pharmacotherapy. In today's mental health system, it constitutes the most common approach to treating patients with major mental illness. In a recent survey, the majority of psychologists and psychiatrists reported participating in combined treatment.[1] It is likely that the majority of social workers and nurses providing psychotherapy also share patients with pharmacotherapists.

Several factors have contributed to the growing acceptability of this treatment approach over the past 20 years. Perhaps most important has been the impact of deinstitutionalization on mental health care. Beginning in the 1960s, the large-scale discharge of chronic patients from state institutions and the growing importance of community mental health have shifted the treatment needs of outpatient populations. Social workers, psychologists, and nurses must provide treatment to individuals who function in a state of chronic psychosis or who are vulnerable to episodes of very severe behavioral disturbance. While developing new psychotherapeutic approaches to help such patients, psychotherapists have also observed firsthand that medications can effectively alleviate or prevent patients' most disruptive (if not always their most painful) symptoms.

The popularity of combined treatment has also been fostered by the development and availability of effective psychotropic medications. There are currently at least 14 antipsychotic drugs, 15 antidepressants, 14 antianxiety drugs, and 4 mood-regulating drugs from which to choose.[2] The members of each class of drugs tend to be equivalent in effectiveness, but differences among their side effect profiles allow considerable attention to an individual's needs or sensitivities.

Controlled investigations have demonstrated the usefulness of these medications in the treatment of a growing list of disorders. Thirty years ago, psychotherapists considered the use of medications most appropriate in the treatment of schizophrenia or severe mood disorders. Now medications are also known to help some people with milder depressions or mood swings, panic attacks, agoraphobia, performance anxiety, eating disorders, posttraumatic stress disorder, and certain personality disorder syndromes. In many of these conditions, medication and psychotherapy are known or believed to have complementary or synergistic effects.[3]

An educated public, too, has contributed to the popularity of combined treatment. Psychotherapy patients may ask about medications as a result of information gained via the news media or through personal experiences with relatives, friends, or neighbors. Many patient-initiated requests reflect a valid and realistic assessment of the role medication might play in their treatment. These requests, of course, also have psychological implications, some of which are discussed later in this chapter and elsewhere in this book.

Finally, an increasing number of psychiatrists have subspecialized in psychopharmacology. Working in individual or group settings, they provide accessible evaluations of medication and treatment to patients referred by their mental health colleagues. In turn, these pharmacotherapists may seek psychotherapy evaluations for patients whom they have treated primarily with medication.

When pharmacotherapy and psychotherapy occur in parallel and unintegrated, opportunities are lost for improving the quality of each treatment modality. In a combined treatment, psychotherapy and pharmacotherapy are interwoven into a larger treatment process. The patient and both caregivers pay attention not only to the therapeutic and adverse effects of medication, but also to the dynamic implications of considering medication, the decision to seek consultation, and the experience of involving a pharmacotherapist. This chapter provides guidelines for when to seek a pharmacotherapy consultation, offers suggestions for making the consultation meaningful and useful within the context of a combined treatment, and addresses issues relevant to successful collaboration between psychotherapists and pharmacotherapists.

INDICATIONS FOR CONSULTATION WITH A PHARMACOTHERAPIST

During a psychotherapy evaluation or later in treatment, consultation with a pharmacotherapist/psychiatrist is usually sought as a way to provide diagnostic clarification or pharmacotherapy evaluation. Often the psychotherapy evaluation has turned up symptoms suggesting untreated physical illness, which may be exacerbating emotional distress. Referral to a psychiatrist will facilitate identification and treatment of such illness.[4] This would be important, for example, in the treatment of an elderly depressed individual who also describes increasing memory dysfunction, which could indicate the onset of a dementing illness. Often there are no indications of physical illness or cognitive dysfunction, but the patient's symptoms are among those known to respond to medication. For example, a young adult in apparently good physical health who has gradually begun to experience increasing hallucinations, delusions, and fragmented thinking is likely to benefit from the early involvement of a pharmacotherapist.

Symptoms that suggest the need for a physical evaluation or pharmacotherapy consultation may escape an evaluator who relies too heavily on the open-ended interview style preferred by many psychotherapists. Though such a nondirective approach allows a patient greater freedom to describe his situation as he experiences and understands it, important informational gaps may result. A patient may not share information when he is unaware of its significance. A recent increase in the number of headaches, for example, may not be spontaneously mentioned, or even linked by the patient with the depressive symptoms that have prompted him to seek a psychotherapy evaluation. Information experienced as shameful, such as self-mutilation or a feeling of being ridiculed by onlookers, may also escape the leaky net of a nondirective interview. To make sure that all of the fish are caught, many psychotherapists include a directive component (direct questions about specific topics) in the initial psychotherapy evaluation. This facilitates the early recognition of chronic psychiatric disorders or physical illness presenting with mental symptoms. For most patients, the psychotherapist may defer the directive part of an evaluation until after the initial nondirective assessment. For a patient who seems more disorganized, however, it may be preferable to begin with a directive historical inquiry and an examination of the mental status.

Whether obtained through directive or nondirective evaluation, certain elements of the history suggest that a psychiatric consultation would be valuable (see Table 1-1). Chief among these are current symptoms suggesting physical illness or a medication-responsive behavioral disorder. Past occurrence of these symptoms is also relevant, as the present illness may then represent a relapse. If psychotropic drugs were ever taken, it is important to ask about their names, dosages, the duration of treatment, and (most importantly) their usefulness to the patient. The evaluator should also ask about the use of alcohol and other recreational drugs, including the ubiquitous caffeine and nicotine. Details of a patient's eating habits, including the presence of bingeing or purging, and a careful sexual history, which has become increasingly relevant as a result of the current acquired immune deficiency syndrome (AIDS) epidemic, should be obtained. Human immunodeficiency virus (HIV) infection sometimes remains obscure until the onset of neuropsychiatric symptoms.

The importance of obtaining a thorough medical history (detailed listing of past medical illnesses) cannot be overstated.

Many medical illnesses or medical treatments can produce behavioral symptoms indistinguishable from those seen in "functional" depression, anxiety, psychosis, or other disorders.[4]

It is important also to obtain a family history of psychiatric illness, since there is excellent evidence that some disorders or a vulnerability to them may be inherited. For thoroughness, the family history should include members as far back as the patient can determine. To elicit the pertinent information, the patient can be asked whether any relatives had psychiatric hospitalization, outpatient treatment, or evidence of an undiagnosed illness, as indicated by alcohol or drug abuse, fear of leaving the house, extreme mood shifts, severe anxiety, bizarre behavior, suicide, or unexplained deaths. If family members have received pharmacotherapy, the details of this treatment may shed light on the patient's genetic legacy and likelihood of treatment response.

Information on mental status, like history, tends to be collected in a nondirective manner during a psychotherapy evaluation. Many aspects of the mental status examination can be well assessed in this way, but several areas of information are likely to be missed. For this reason, a psychotherapist may supplement nondirective observations of mental status by directively seeking three types of disturbance: potentially destructive behavior, psychosis, and cognitive dysfunction. The presence of any of these may indicate a physical illness with behavioral symptoms or a medication-responsive behavioral disorder for which pharmacotherapy should be combined with psychotherapy.

Though often requested during psychotherapy evaluation, a pharmacotherapy consultation may first become appropriate at a later phase of treatment. Pertinent new information about the patient may become available; for example, a young man with unexplained chronic apathy and confusion may admit to ongoing solvent abuse. Or a shift may have occurred in the patient's daily functioning, as with a schizophrenic woman who finds her hallucinations increasingly interfering with her participation in day treatment activities. Some of the symptoms listed in Table 1-1 may develop for apparently psychodynamic reasons, in the wake of disturbing life events or the exploration of painful issues in psychotherapy. The existence of a stressor or precipitant, how-

Table 1-1
Symptoms Which Suggest Usefulness of a Psychiatric Consultation

Depression or Mania	Anxiety	Psychosis
Sleep disturbance	Panic attacks	Hallucinations
Change in eating habits	Agoraphobia	Delusions
Fatigue, loss of energy	Dissociative states	Thought disorder
Diurnal variation of mood	Performance anxiety	Violent actions
Loss of interest or pleasure	Obsessions	Homicidality
Impaired concentration	Compulsions	Suicidality
Hyperactivity, agitation	Physical restlessness	
Sexual dysfunction		
Hallucinations/delusions	Miscellaneous	
Homicidality	Bingeing	
Suicidality		
Fluctuating alertness		
Seizures or "spells"		

Organic Disorders
Confusion
Disorientation
Memory difficulty

ever, does not prove that the symptom's basis is psychological or that it should be treated through talking. In general the new appearance of one of these symptoms should prompt reconsideration of a consultative evaluation. Finally, an unexpectedly poor response to psychotherapy over an appropriate length of time may signal the need for consultation. A young man with cycling moods, for example, sought treatment for disruptive episodes of increased irritability and activity. He made little progress in psychotherapy until treatment with lithium allowed greater stability of his moods.

PREPARING FOR A PHARMACOTHERAPY CONSULTATION

Effective use of a pharmacotherapy consultation requires attention to a number of issues. The psychotherapist's own motivations for making the referral are among the first considerations. Sometimes referral is appropriate because of the patient's symptoms of anxiety, depression, or another condition amenable to drug therapy. Other times, the psychotherapist may wish for help in assessing whether a physical illness is contributing to a patient's symptoms. Or the psychotherapist may simply be seeking a second opinion about the patient's diagnosis, formulation, or response to psychotherapy. On occasion the psychotherapist may be experiencing difficult feelings of anger, boredom, or overinvolvement. Such countertransference and human reactions to patients may overtly or covertly prompt a consultation request. A referral reason, for example, which often accompanies conditions that can be helped by medication, is the wish to share the treatment of a patient whose complexity, acting-out, or suffering are difficult for the therapist to bear alone. Often a referral is multidetermined, reflecting a combination of these reasons.

When the patient has initiated the idea, the psychotherapist must assess his or her response. Is the request unexpected? Does it feel devaluing? Does it elicit anger? Does it induce relief? Does it make sense? The psychotherapist's exploration of countertransference feelings may provide a window into the patient's dynamic motivations.

When consultation is considered, its meaning to the patient should be examined. Exploring this in psychotherapy will facilitate the patient's acceptance of the referral, the new doctor, and any medicine prescribed. The potential for sabotage of the referral or noncompliance with medication instructions can be diminished by attention to the patient's fears about the consultation. Does the patient fear that the psychotherapist will abandon him to the pharmacologist? Does the patient worry that the psychotherapist feels hopeless about the treatment? Are expectations of the consultation realistic? If the patient has unrealistically high hopes about the result of the consultation, a disappointing outcome can have harmful effects. Damage can be done to the patient's willingness to take a partially effective medication, and even the working alliance with the psychotherapist can be endangered.

During discussion of the referral with an adult patient, it is especially important to bear in mind that the choice whether or not to be medicated belongs to the patient. The process of learning about alternatives and reaching an informed decision enhances the patient's self-esteem and autonomy. With this in mind, the therapist's and patient's expectations of the referral, including the hope that pharmacotherapy will facilitate participation in psychotherapy, need to be discussed. The patient may need time to consider and discuss the referral and may wish to choose the exact timing of it.

Another important area to consider and discuss with patients is how they view psychiatrists and medications in general. Does the patient experience referral to a pharmacotherapist as stigmatizing? Does it mean he or she is seriously ill, mental, or crazy? Or does the patient feel that the involvement of a medical professional means the problem is being taken more seriously? Attitudes of the patient's family or others who are important must also be considered, since the support of the patient's social system can make or break the referral or subsequent treatment. The patient's preferences or reactions to the pharmacotherapist's gender are also worth noting. As with the other issues, these will provide material for psychotherapy and aid the patient in working through the reasons for referral and expectations of its outcome.

Some patients who meet criteria for pharmacotherapy will refuse a consultation despite all attempts to help them understand or overcome their resistance. With such individuals, the psychotherapist can continue to explore feelings about the referral as tolerated and repeat the suggestion when the patient may be more accepting. Psychotherapists need to be aware that recent court proceedings have viewed failure to offer somatic therapy for certain severe mental disorders as malpractice. With this in mind, a refusal to accept medical or pharmacotherapeutic consultation should be clearly documented in the patient's record.

Many psychotherapists find it useful to prepare a patient for the consultation by anticipating the experience with them in detail. The patient is told the doctor's name, where the meeting will take place, how to set up the meetings, the number of sessions likely to be needed, the kind of questions that are likely to be asked, something about how the physician works, and the cost of the evaluation when relevant. It is helpful to add that medication may not be prescribed as a result of the consultation, and that trial and error may be required to find an effective agent and dosage. The patient's subjective responses to the medications will be important data, and something useful will be learned even if medications are not tried or are ineffective. Informed consent needs to be obtained for the caregivers to share clinical information prior to and following the consultation. In order for combined treatment to function effectively, this must be negotiated at the outset. For many patients this comes as an unwelcome surprise. It may threaten the sense of trust or safety in the psychotherapy relationship, but promises of strict secrecy can lead to great problems or promote destructive splitting of caregivers. A discussion of the patient's feelings about the sharing of information between caregivers can provide therapeutic material by invoking issues of trust, guilt, and self-esteem. It is helpful to emphasize that personal issues other than those involving the patient's safety will be raised in a general rather than a specific way with the co-therapist.

Nowhere is the issue of confidentiality and communication more important than around suicidal or homicidal feelings experienced by the patient. It must be clear that such thoughts or behaviors are important to manage safely and promptly. The psychotherapist and pharmacotherapist should agree about who makes decisions regarding hospitalization or other alterations in the treatment plan in the face of such life-threatening situations. When one caregiver notes the new appearance of suicidality or homicidality, it should not be assumed that the other is aware of the change in clinical status. On the contrary, the opposite should be assumed. The caregivers must be in touch to discuss the patient's safety and review the treatment plan.

CHOOSING A PSYCHOPHARMACOLOGY CONSULTANT

Strictly speaking, any physician is licensed to prescribe psychotropic medications. A sensitive and knowledgeable internist or surgeon can prescribe psychotropic drugs in an uncomplicated case. In some communities underserved by psychiatric specialists, such a referral may be a practical approach. Generally, however, a psychiatrist with a subspecialty in psychopharmacology is best equipped to do a full evaluation of a patient's medication needs and/or the usefulness of further medical evaluation for physical illness manifesting with behavioral symptoms. Not all psychiatrists are equally knowledgeable about or interested in keeping up with the expanding literature on medication practices. As experimental studies accumulate, the recommendations about optimal dosages have varied. New medications are frequently introduced, and new uses for older medications are being found. A physician who has not kept up with developments in the field may provide less than optimal collaboration in a combined treatment.

Beyond finding a knowledgeable physician, the therapist must attempt to choose someone with whom it is comfortable to work. This comfort requires mutual respect. Caregivers' true attitudes toward each other are often detected by patients, and can either enhance or undermine the effectiveness of combined treatment. There are numerous schools of psychotherapy and the pharmacotherapist may not be familiar with a particular treatment orientation. A lack of this information, however, does not preclude a compatible working relationship.

Since communication between clinicians is an important part of successful combined treatment, the psychotherapist should seek a pharmacotherapist with whom communication is relatively easy. This requires both accessibility and openness. In a crisis, it is valuable to have a collaborator who is responsible about returning phone calls. If life-threatening behavior occurs, effective coordination of caregivers is crucial. Even in less emergent situations, of course, communication between caregivers is important. Disability determinations or prior authorization requests for insurance reimbursement, for example, may require discussion between caregivers to determine how the appropriate forms will be handled. Such administrative aspects of treatment have both pragmatic and psychotherapeutic implications, both of which can be effectively managed in a smoothly working combined treatment.

PREPARING THE CONSULTING PHARMACOTHERAPIST

A physician who receives a request for "medication evaluation" lacks the guidance needed to provide an optimal response. A great deal of work may be wasted in an attempt to answer all possible questions, while the primary concern prompting consultation (e.g., "This patient plans to become pregnant and wishes advice on whether her medication treatment must be changed or discontinued") may be lost in the shuffle. A referral note or early discussion that includes a clearly formulated request and the information of greatest use will save the consultant, psychotherapist, and patient time and effort in the long run.

A referral note or discussion should include a *Chief Complaint*, designating the most pertinent symptoms presented by the patient. Next the *History of the Present Illness* is given. This account of the patient's difficulties focuses on the most recent episode of stress, coping, and symptoms of illness. The time course of the illness, associated symptoms, and secondary complications are important. Some comment about the presence or absence of psychosis, suicidal or homicidal behavior, self-injury, or substance abuse is usually included in the history of the present illness. Next, a *History of Past Treatment*, which includes relevant psychotherapy or pharmacotherapy, is given. A *History of Medical Illnesses*, including medication use, substance abuse, or major surgical operations, is given next, followed by a *Family History* of pertinent mental illnesses or their absence. It is extremely helpful to the pharmacologic consultant to receive some comments about the psychotherapist's direct observations of the patient's *Mental Status* during the course of evaluation or ongoing psychotherapy. A *Dynamic Formulation* of the patient's symptoms and the reason for consulting at this time in treatment will alert the consultant to pertinent psychological factors. Finally, a clearly phrased *Consultation Request* (e.g., "Please advise on the nature of this patient's anxiety symptoms and whether medication would be of help.") will focus the consultant's interview of the patient and his response. Some psychotherapists prefer to write a narrative report to the consultant, while others prefer to fill in a form designed for this purpose. Fig 1-1 demonstrates a referral request form that the authors have found useful.

THE CONSULTANT'S RESPONSE

In turn, what should the psychotherapist expect? To begin with, a skilled and sensitive consultant does not wait for a psychother-

PHARMACOTHERAPY CONSULTATION REQUEST FORM

Date of Request: _____   **Patient Name:** _____
Referring Therapist: _____   **Date of Birth:** _____
Therapist's Phone: _____   **Patient's Phone:** _____

Reason for Consultation Request:

History of Present Illness (Include target symptoms):

Current Outpatient Treatment:

___ Day treatment, ___ Aftercare, Therapy: ___ Individual, ___ Family, ___ Meds
List details:

List current medications:

Past Psychiatric History:
Past psychiatric hospitalizations (include number, dates, precipitants, locations, durations):

Medication history (include specific past and current meds, dates of treatment, effect on target sx, side effects, reason if discontinued):

Alcohol and/or drug history:

Past suicidal or homicidal behavior:

Medical History:

Known illnesses: **Caffeine intake:**

Operations: **Smoking history:**
Allergies: **Pregnancy history:**
Most recent physical examination and name of examiner:
Any recent pertinent lab tests (eg, lithium level):

Family History of Mental Illness:
___ Schizophrenia, ___ Depression, ___ Mania,
___ Alcoholism/Drug abuse, ___ Anxiety disorders,
___ Suicide, ___ Other
Details:

Figure 1-1

Current Mental Status Examination:
Appearance:

Alertness: ___ Vigilant, ___ Alert, ___ Drowsy, ___ Stuporous

Thought and Speech:
Process: ___ Logical, ___ Coherent, ___ Loose associations,
___ Pressured speech, ___ Flight of ideas, ___ Blocking,
___ Incoherence
Content: ___ Phobias, ___ Obsessions, ___ Compulsions,
___ Panic attacks, ___ Hallucinations, ___ Delusions,
___ Depersonalization/derealization

Mood and affect:
___ Appropriate, ___ Inappropriate, ___ Flat, ___ Shallow,
___ Labile, ___ Euthymic, ___ Depressed, ___ Anxious,
___ Euphoric, ___ Irritable
Details:

Insight and judgement:

Memory: ___ Can recall three words after 2 minutes
___ Can recall significance of 4 names or historical events

Orientation: ___ Person, ___ Place, ___ Time

Physical harm: ___ No suicidal or homicidal ideation,
___ No intent, ___ No plan, ___ Able and competent to contract not to act in harmful way

Diagnostic impression:

Consultant's differential diagnosis and assessment:

Recommendations regarding treatment:

Side effects of medications discussed with patient (including sedation, restrictions on driving or work, interactions of medication with alcohol or other drugs or food, extrapyramidal side effects including tardive dyskinesia, and sexual function):

___ Yes, ___ No

Follow-up plans:

Signature of consulting physician: ___   **Date:** ___

apist to learn about the consultation from the patient's report. A prompt call or written response should provide the opportunity for discussion and treatment planning between the psychotherapist and pharmacotherapist. This should include at least tentative recommendations regarding medication treatment and its rationale, the type of medication recommended, the dosage and possibly the schedule, the expected duration of treatment, and the frequency of follow-up visits. Ideally, the consultant's note includes a clear explanation of how the pertinent data from history, interview, and mental status examination led to the recommendations. When pharmacotherapy is not recommended, the reasons for this should be clearly stated.

After the pharmacotherapist has interviewed the patient, the caregivers should discuss how medication will fit in with the overall treatment plan. The consultant should explain the recommended medication's side effects; dangerousness in overdose; effects on pregnancy or breast-feeding; and interactions with other medications, foods, or drugs to which the patient may be exposed. Agreement should be reached about whom to contact in various kinds of emergencies (such as suicidal behavior), how coverage will be handled when one clinician is unavailable, how and when future communication will take place about the patient (with the patient's consent), and whether a joint meeting of the two caregivers with the patient might at some time be indicated to clarify any aspects of medication treatment.

REFERRAL FROM A PSYCHOPHARMACOLOGIST TO A PSYCHOTHERAPIST

Sometimes a psychotherapist receives a referral from a pharmacotherapist of a patient already on medication. When this occurs, it is important to learn why the patient is being referred and what the patient has been told about the referral. Just as with referral from a psychotherapist to psychopharmacologist, the meaning of the referral to all concerned is important to understand. Is the pharmacotherapist feeling confused or frustrated with a patient's lack of response? Has he noted evidence that the patient is interested in psychotherapy? Does the patient view the referral as a rejection, a preamble to the pharmacotherapist's withdrawal from his case, or is it experienced as a gift or compliment? Patients' concerns about feeling abandoned or fears that their doctor is weaning them away can have a basis in reality. Referrals may have both overt and covert reasons. Pharmacotherapists on occasion refer patients for countertransference reasons, of which they are partially or wholly unaware. Boredom, anger, or a feeling of helplessness with a patient are among the hidden motivations for such a referral. Psychotherapy may or may not be indicated. A psychotherapist can avoid disappointing a patient and alienating a pharmacotherapist by accepting referrals for evaluation with the understanding that psychotherapy may not necessarily follow. To prepare the patient, it is important to explain at the outset that he or she is being evaluated for appropriateness of psychotherapy and that a subsequent recommendation of psychotherapy is not a foregone conclusion.

When a referring pharmacotherapist plans to gradually diminish his involvement with the patient, the patient needs to be aware of this goal. The psychotherapist needs to know whether the pharmacotherapist will continue intermittent visits to assess the patient when he or she stops taking medication, a practice followed by most pharmacotherapists. The patient's feelings about giving up contact with the pharmacotherapist must be considered, since the giver of medications has often become an important person in the patient's life.

MAINTAINING THE COMBINED TREATMENT RELATIONSHIP

Combined treatment, of course, continues beyond the initial evaluation or referral of a patient. To help the patient benefit from both modes of treatment, it is valuable to maintain an open channel of communication between the caregivers. When psychotherapist and pharmacotherapist work in the same small agency, this communication occurs more easily. When the clinicians are less likely to cross paths, it is worth making the effort to remain intermittently in touch, even in the absence of a crisis situation. In a treatment complicated by factors such as concurrent medical illness, rapid shifts in mental status, or acting out, a discussion should probably occur at least monthly. A quarterly discussion may be sufficient for patients who are in a more stable condition.

If one clinician plans to be absent for an extended amount of time, clear plans need to be made regarding coverage. To avoid misunderstandings, it is important to inform the patient about these plans. In some combined treatments, the psychotherapist may ask the pharmacotherapist to provide crisis or temporary psychotherapy backup. This can provide the patient with a relatively familiar individual, and benefits the pharmacotherapist by providing an opportunity to become more deeply aware of the patient's nonmedication concerns. Such an arrangement, however, must be discussed between clinicians before it is offered to a patient.

When major changes in treatment are contemplated by either pharmacotherapist or psychotherapist, a discussion between caregivers is indicated. Sometimes, for example, one clinician will plan to terminate a patient's treatment despite the planned continuing involvement of the other clinician. The pharmacotherapist who learns first from a patient that psychotherapy has been terminated may feel justifiably miffed. Perhaps she would have been unwilling to assume the increased level of responsibility implied by the patient's loss of involvement with a psychotherapist. Similarly, a psychotherapist who becomes aware of a patient's change in medication only by noting increased symptoms has been poorly informed by the pharmacotherapist. Some factors that interfere with open communication among caregivers and some strategies for dealing with them are discussed more fully in chapter 5 of this book.

Of the two clinicians involved with a patient in combined treatment, the psychotherapist generally maintains the more intimate and frequent involvement. This places the psychotherapist in a position to facilitate the combined treatment in two important ways — by helping to assess the medication's effectiveness and by helping to educate the patient about medication treatment. Each of these functions requires an awareness of the therapeutic and adverse effects of medications, a topic covered in chapters 6 and 7. The following comments, however, address special considerations regarding the psychotherapist's role in assessment and education.

Assessing the effectiveness of medication may be difficult when a patient is concurrently receiving psychotherapy and/or other types of treatment. Ongoing life crises can make it difficult to know whether a specific component of treatment is truly helpful. Assessment is simplified by consideration of target symptoms, which characterize each medication-responsive disorder. These symptoms, chosen for their potential responsiveness to pharmacologic treatment, can be assessed by observation and inquiry. Their improvement suggests that treatment has been appropriate. When they worsen over time or fail to improve, it is necessary to reconsider the working diagnosis and treatment plan.

In the treatment of situational anxiety, for example, medications are effective if they improve a patient's ability to sleep, if they do not produce unacceptable daytime sedation, and if they reduce anxiety symptoms to the extent that occupational and social functioning are supported. Treatment of panic disorder is monitored by assessing the frequency and intensity of panic episodes. Although panic attacks may not cease entirely, there should be a very noticeable decrease in frequency and intensity if medications are effective. When agoraphobic symptoms are also present, efficacy is signalled by the patient's greater ease in leaving home, driving, or facing feared situations.

Target symptoms most responsive to antipsychotic medications include agitation, irritability, and restlessness. Sleep and appetite should improve rapidly. Thought disorder, hallucinations, and delusions tend to improve over a period of days to weeks. For some patients, antipsychotic treatment is only a qualified success, in that it reduces painful perceptual disturbances and anxiety while introducing distressing physical side effects. Symptoms such as apathy, withdrawal, and poverty of thought often fail to improve with conventional antipsychotic medications.

When medications are used to treat depression, the patient often will feel worse for about a week before feeling better, because of the initial side effects of the drugs and the lag which precedes their therapeutic effects. If by two weeks there has been no improvement in the targeted depressive symptoms, a change of dosage may be necessary to achieve response. During the period of dose adjustment, the patient may need extra encouragement and support to continue with the trial despite physical discomfort. The depressive symptoms most responsive to antidepressants are the "vegetative" symptoms of insomnia, loss of appetite, poor concentration, anhedonia, and fatigue.

Lithium and other mood regulators used in the treatment of bipolar disorder tend also to produce initial physical discomfort while requiring two or more weeks to establish a clear therapeutic effect. Improvements in sleep, appetite, judgement, and impulse control as well as decreased rate of speech, irritability, and grandiosity are all among the signs of a positive response to lithium.

In combined treatment, a patient's questions about medication and concerns about the meaning of being medicated are often first raised with the psychotherapist. Many of these concerns have psychological or transferential implications, as discussed in chapter 9. Other questions may require of the psychotherapist some factual knowledge or a willingness to point the patient in the direction of such facts by involving the pharmacotherapist.

While no nonmedical clinician is expected to be an expert on medications, psychotherapists can help their patients by remaining informed about the medications they are taking, their intended therapeutic effects, and their possible side effects. Periodically, the psychotherapist should also wonder whether new or persistent complaints, especially physical ones, may represent medication toxicity. When worsening target symptoms or adverse effects of medication are mentioned in psychotherapy, it is important to ask whether the patient has also notified the psychopharmacologist.

CONCLUSION

Judicious use of psychopharmacologic consultation and combined treatment enhances the psychotherapist's ability to treat a variety of disorders. Psychotherapists, therefore, must remain aware of current indications for consultation. A psychotherapist who maintains an ongoing collaborative relationship with a psychopharmacologist is able to offer patients a broader range of treatment options when consultation is appropriate or medication information is sought. Attention to the choice of consultant, the process of referral, and ongoing communication can prove rewarding to patient and caregivers alike.

REFERENCES

1. Chiles JA, Carlin AS, Beitman BD: A physician, a nonmedical psychotherapist, and a patient: The pharmacotherapy-psychotherapy triangle, in Beitman BD, Klerman GL (eds): *Combining Psychotherapy and Drug Therapy in Clinical Practice*. New York, Spectrum Publications, 1984, pp 89–101.
2. Baldessarini RJ: *Chemotherapy in Psychiatry*. Cambridge, Harvard University Press, 1985.
3. Karasu TB: Psychotherapy and pharmacotherapy: Toward an integrative model. *Am J Psychiatry* 1982;139:1102–1113.
4. Ellison JM: DSM-III and the diagnosis of organic mental disorders. *Ann Emerg Med* 1984;13:521–528.

2

Rational and Irrational Pharmacotherapeutics on the Psychiatric Inpatient Unit

Gregory A. Clark

It is by now a commonplace in our field to note that every form of human enterprise is beset by a significant and seemingly inevitable measure of irrationality. The prescription and the management of psychotropic medications are not exceptions to this rule. Despite clinical pharmacology's century-long dream of a scientifically based rational therapeutics, this ideal is rarely attained in actual practice. Nonrational forces such as transference, countertransference, conflict, and competition interact with our reasoning about medications and can compromise clinical judgment. At our best, we are alert to such influences and can rise above them to act in the best interests of our patients; at our worst, we succumb to them and practice irrationally.

Other contributors to this volume describe the various ways in which nonrational factors can affect practice in outpatient combined treatment and family therapy. Although each of these discussions is relevant to inpatient practice, there is more to the matter. Hospital treatment involves increased numbers and types of caregivers, groups of patients in severely dysfunctional states, and multiple contacts with families and outside caregivers. The logistics and dynamics of this complex network of relationships challenge our most able and insightful management efforts. The result is a vulnerability to irrational action which often exceeds that seen in outpatient combined treatment. At the same time, the presence of multiple points of view can provide checks and balances on clinical judgment and built-in consultation to enhance rationality. In all, these factors combine to generate unique opportunities for psychiatric practice and unique temptations to irrationality. In what follows, I will explore the special features that distinguish inpatient treatment from treatment in other clinical settings and I will follow their effects and implications for combined treatment through the sequence of a typical hospital course.

THE INPATIENT UNIT

The contemporary psychiatric unit is one of the most exciting settings available for the study of lives and the treatment of mental disorders. Its comprehensiveness and rich resources are unparalleled. Staff members from a wide range of disciplines and backgrounds work together to generate a multidimensional understanding of their patients. Close availability of the clinical laboratory, consultation with physicians from other medical specialties, and input from psychological testing enhance the power and depth of the diagnostic evaluation. The multidisciplinary treatment team fosters professional growth through ongoing opportunities for collaboration and peer consultation. Because the patients are in residence on the unit, they are available for round-the-clock observation and intervention in a variety of interactive contexts. The unit's capacity for surveillance and containment permits the study and treatment of patients who are too dysfunctional or disorganized for outpatient treatment. Furthermore, because most patients are in crisis when they are admitted, there is the opportunity to gain meaningful clinical leverage on their treatment and the possibility of dramatic change and recompensation during the course of the hospitalization. Because of the severity of the disorders treated on an inpatient unit, psychotropic medications are a key treatment component.

At first glance, the inpatient unit would seem to be an ideal setting for rational psychiatric practice. Nonetheless, it is common to find both inpatient staff members and outside therapists caught up in some of psychiatry's most concentrated experiences in therapeutic irrationality. The origin of this paradoxic vulnerability lies in the fact that the unit's strengths of comprehensiveness, intensity, and multiple perspectives can also pose obstacles to the effective delivery of combined treatment. Coordination of the unit's rich staffing resources around the tasks of observation, interpretation, and intervention presents special problems in logistics and communications. In hospital treatment, the therapeutic relationship is not confined to the classic dyad or even to the triad of most outpatient combined therapies. Instead it is distributed across a complex system of staff members representing different roles and disciplines. In this distributed treatment relationship, the team may include one or more therapists, mental health workers, and trainees. Separate team members may work on complementary or overlapping aspects of a case and therapists of all disciplines may provide individual or group treatment on the unit. The diversity of staff roles and personnel means that each patient works with a relatively large number of caregivers during any given hospital episode.

Hospital treatment, then, is group therapy of a very particular sort: each patient is treated by a group of staff members. In this arrangement the problems and pitfalls of coordinating any combined treatment are significantly multiplied. The staff must somehow organize itself around the basic tasks of collecting data, formulating diagnoses, planning treatment, and implementing the treatment plan. For the team to work in concert from a consistent therapeutic stance, team members' roles and responsibilities must be adequately defined and differentiated and also grounded in a shared understanding of the patient and the treatment plan. The situation is facilitated by the fact that the staff works together closely over time in a single setting and can develop organizational routines and channels of communication. Nevertheless, the management of information and communication remains a basic problem on the inpatient unit.

The difficulty of managing the flow of information and activity related to planning and implementing a medication trial illustrates the magnitude of this issue. The inpatient staff typically collects data about a patient's condition from the patient, the family, outside caregivers, and old records during encounters that are spread out over time and space. The data collected must then be sifted, focused, and fed back to the team, where it is integrated and interpreted. Target symptoms must be identified and a medication chosen. The team's reasoning and the choice of medication must then be communicated back to the staff at large, the patient, and the involved family. Medication must be obtained and dispensed accurately. The behavioral and medical status of the patient must be monitored during the trial. Relevant observations of progress must be fed back to the team so that any needed adjustments can be made. All of this must be coordinated with the outpatient treatment team.

Despite the use of routine verbal and written reports, a chain with so many links is liable to suffer occasional breaks. Staff members or outpatient therapists may then find themselves in the irrational position of acting on the basis of inaccurate or incomplete information supplemented by assumptions, suppositions, or fantasies.

Another consequence of the distributed treatment relationship is the engagement of staff's and patients' unconscious defenses by intense group dynamics. Freud,[1] Bion,[2] and others[3-5] have noted with both fascination and alarm how readily the members of human groups may collude to sacrifice their grip on reality in the service of fending off the awareness of painful or threatening experience. This process is analogous to the use of intrapsychic defense mechanisms by individuals in that painful realities are sidestepped, transformed, or flatly ignored in the interests of conscious comfort or short-term coping. In group life, individuals may collaborate unconsciously to reinforce each other's use of defenses when the parties share a wish to avoid certain painful realizations. Indeed, the collective use of splitting, projection, stereotyping, scapegoating, primitive idealization, and magical thinking appears to be a basic human characteristic. As such, it naturally affects the courses of individual and combined therapies in all settings.

Within the unit's comprehensive envelope of 24-hour care and frequent interactions, however, collective defense can become particularly problematic. For instance, Main[6] pointed out that those of us who enter the helping professions prefer to see ourselves as helpful, competent, and benign in our transactions with our clients. Consequently, when conflict, uncertainty, and helplessness arise, as they often do in the treatment of severely distressed patients, helpers may seek respite by locating the sources elsewhere than in themselves. In this reallocation of blame and responsibility, the unit's complicated organizational connections can break down. Real or perceived differences in discipline, ideology, status, authority, affiliation, and gender become potential lines of cleavage along which the coordination of care can become split or fragmented. When we perceive our colleagues or patients as supportive and understanding, they may become willing conspirators in our efforts to alleviate our pain. When we perceive them as hostile, incompetent, or uncooperative, they may become the unwitting recipients of our ejected distress. Medication decisions are likely to be affected by these splits.

Problems in logistics and group dynamics are common to all organizations, but they are intensified on the inpatient unit because it is a setting where patients are thrown into prolonged, direct contact with the vicissitudes of their caregivers' administrative and professional lives. Dislocated from their usual contexts and supports, patients live among staff on the ward and are open to the influence of the staff's dynamics. By the same token, the emotional burden of their illnesses can pose a threat to the maintenance of the unit's organizational integrity and the rationality of its practice. Every inpatient unit sustains a steady influx of individuals in profound states of distress and dysfunction. As these individuals take up membership in ward society, they may disrupt or disequilibrate established relationships and routines. Staff members' efforts to make empathic contact with patients may entangle them in difficult countertransferences and evoked responses.[7] The continuous importation of confusion and distress into the group life of the unit generates tremendous pressures for certainty and action. When treatment is optimally managed, the staff is able to contain and transform these pressures in the work of psychotherapy and discovery, as described by Bion[8] and Winnicott.[9] Patients improve and painful tensions are relieved. However, these patients soon leave and are replaced by others in more acute states. When containment fails, even the sturdiest staff may fall back on the use of collective defenses with renewed fervor. As in other areas of psychotherapeutic practice, the provision of rational inpatient care requires a vigilant effort to acknowledge and interpret the powerful nonrational forces that influence all of us.

Imperfect communications, collective defenses, and high levels of emotional stress are constant features of the inpatient setting. They affect all aspects of care, including the use of medications. In the complex drama of inpatient treatment, medications may take on a variety of meanings and roles above and beyond their specific pharmacologic actions. They may appear as saviours or villains, as sources of relief or distress. They may be a battleground where warring caregivers struggle for control, or a currency through which caring or conflict is conveyed. What follows is more an essay on the decisions and dynamics surrounding use of medication in the hospital than a treatise on the pills themselves.

THE PHASES OF HOSPITALIZATION

When Lewis Carroll's Alice crawls through the mirror into Looking-Glass House, she enters a world dramatically different from the world of her everyday life. It is filled with new characters, unfamiliar demands, strange alliances, and bizarre shifts of perception and language. A journey into the world of psychiatric hospitalization can be just as unfamiliar and jarring. Just as Alice's journey through the looking-glass moves across the ranked squares of a chessboard, the typical hospitalization develops through a series of phases, each with its own tasks and challenges. The hospital course can be conceptualized as having three main phases: (1) an initial phase involving intake and stabilization, (2) a middle phase involving evaluation and the implementation of specific treatments, and (3) a terminal phase involving preparation for discharge and the transition to outpatient care. A study of actual hospitalizations shows that these phases may overlap and blend into one another but they are all present in even the briefest hospital stay. Each phase ushers in its own set of dilemmas regarding the coordination of medication use and other therapies.

The Initial Phase

The initial phase of hospitalization begins with the patient's admission to the inpatient unit. It continues through the beginning stages of stabilization of the patient's mental status and membership in the ward community. It typically lasts from one to five days. Like Alice's transition it is a dramatic dislocation of context in which the patient leaves the familiar surroundings of daily life to come and live in the hospital. In accepting the asylum of the hospital, patients and their families also experience major changes in their previous roles and options. The patient gives up freedom and autonomy as the unit staff assumes responsibility for monitoring daily schedule and care. Previously used medications are turned over to the nursing staff who will keep them and dispense them for the duration of the hospitalization. Family members become visitors. Outpatient caregivers lose control and jurisdiction over treatment decisions unless they are on the hospital staff. These dislocations and role shifts carry with them risks of loss of containment and continuity of care. The central tasks of the initial phase of hospitalization are to maintain continuity of care and to establish containment of the patient in the new caretaking environment.

To maintain continuity of care as much as possible across this abrupt transition, inpatient and outpatient caregivers should be in contact early in the admission period. Critical information about the patient's history and treatment course prior to hospitalization and about the unit's routine and approach to care should be exchanged. Early contact and ongoing communication between outpatient and inpatient caregivers can save time and effort for all concerned and will typically result in a more focused hospitalization and a shorter length of stay. The concept here is one of establishing a system of care in which the inpatient unit is one component of a coordinated network of caregivers. For patients whose long-term care involves repeated hospitalization, this model can lead to effective and rewarding use of the hospital:

> Case 1. A 28-year-old woman with diagnoses of post-traumatic stress disorder and borderline personality disorder was followed in the outpatient clinic and day hospital of a community mental health center. Over several years of treatment she had multiple hospitalizations characterized by prolonged regressions, ineffective changes in medication, and extended lengths of stay. Dismayed by the apparent lack of benefit of these hospitalizations, her caregivers met to plan for future hospital stays. They agreed to use hospitalization only for containment during acute crises and to hold the length of stay to a three-week maximum. Treatment in

the hospital would focus only on the crisis at hand and avoid longer term issues. To maintain continuity in an aspect of care not involving acute crisis but vulnerable to unproductive manipulation, inpatient and outpatient caregivers agreed not to change medications during hospitalization.

Use of this plan clearly defined the hospital's role in the patient's overall treatment plan. Over the next two years, caregivers noted a decreased total hospital time and general improvement in the patient's other therapies.

Family members may also hold important information regarding medications or other aspects of history. They should be contacted early in the admission process. Like outside caregivers, they may be sensitive to feeling disempowered as the inpatient team takes up the work.

Case 2. A 48-year-old divorced woman with a history of recurrent paranoid psychosis, analgesic abuse, and anxiety attacks was admitted in a panicked paranoid state following the arrest of her teenage son. Her medications on admission were perphenazine, 32 mg/day, and diazepam, 20 mg/day. When interviewed by the unit social worker, the patient's mother declared that her daughter was drug dependent and should be on no medications at all. Hospital staff and the outpatient team thought the patient clearly needed antipsychotic medication. Given the patient's high level of anxiety, they did not believe it wise to change the diazepam dose. The dose of perphenazine was raised gradually to 128 mg/day over the next six weeks, with observable but limited improvement. Analgesic use was strictly limited.

After eight weeks of hospitalization, the patient fled the unit in a panicked state and was returned to the hospital by her mother and son. When the hospital psychiatrist met with the patient and her family to review the incident, the mother reiterated her frustration about the fact that her daughter was on drugs and expressed a particular concern about diazepam, which she felt had been harmful to her daughter in the past. Subsequent contact with a former prescribing psychiatrist confirmed the mother's observation and a decision was made to withdraw the diazepam. Weeks later, following a long and difficult withdrawal, the patient appeared much improved. One day she announced that she had woken up from her confused, psychotic state. She was successfully discharged a few weeks later.

More extensive contact with this patient's family and with previous caregivers in the first days of the admission might have saved two months of hospitalization and a compromised relationship with the family.

Attention to continuity of care and contact among caregivers can also foster containment. Admissions usually take place in times of crisis when feelings are running high. Caregivers as well as patients may feel out of control. The outpatient team may feel stretched and desperate by the time the admission takes place and may be sensitive to criticism. It is not unusual for hospitalization or medication trials to be viewed as a somewhat magical intervention to which unrealistic hopes may be attached. On the other hand, the inpatient team may feel intruded upon by the acuteness of the patient's mental status or by other features of the case. These feelings may exacerbate the outpatient team's sense of vulnerability and, in the context of poor communications, may slow the progress of the case:

> Case 3. A 29-year-old chronically psychotic man was admitted for treatment of a symptomatic exacerbation precipitated by the recent loss of his girlfriend of five years. He was noted by the inpatient staff to be particularly needy and demanding. Review of his medications revealed a complicated regimen combining an antipsychotic, an anticonvulsant, two anxiolytics, and an antidepressant. The inpatient team quickly concluded that the outpatient caregivers had succumbed to the patient's relentless demands by providing pills rather than understanding. This attitude was readily perceived by the outpatient team who became hostile and defensive, though they remained involved with the patient through phone contacts and visits. The patient remained regressed and decompensated. Only when the outpatient caregivers attended a team meeting on the unit and carefully reviewed the patient's course of treatment and the rationale and effectiveness of each of his medications did the inpatient team concede the appropriateness of an unusual regimen for this patient. Relations among the caregivers improved and the patient subsequently compensated into a depressed state in which he was more able to grieve the loss of his girlfriend.

As containment is being established, attention to the course of the patient's transition into the ward community can yield important data pertinent to decisions concerning medication. Hospitalization is a powerful intervention and typically has a marked effect on the patient's mental status. Hastily made plans to medicate because of symptoms present on admission may miss the fact that acute disturbances often improve spontaneously over the first few days of hospitalization. This improvement occurs in part because the patient is insulated from outside stressors. In addition, as Kernberg[10] and Pinderhughes and colleagues[11] noted, the hospital provides a new cast of characters with whom patients may engage in relationships which complement intrapsychic structures and enhance stability. As this occurs, apparently biological syndromes present on admission may resolve without need for medication:

Case 4. A 33-year-old accountant with a wife and three children was admitted in a severely depressed, agitated state with symptoms of insomnia, poor appetite, anhedonia, pessimism, and suicidal ruminations of several weeks' duration. Several months prior to admission a favorite aunt, who had cared for him following his mother's death when he was eight, died. He had managed her death with appropriate grief but was soon caught up in a busy time at his job. He found his concentration poor as he tried to keep up and was then passed over for a desired promotion.

Despite the severity of his mental status on admission, he quickly involved himself with others on the milieu and soon found himself one of the more able members of the hospital community. Insulated from the demands of his job, he recovered his sleep and appetite. Psychotherapy sessions focused on issues surrounding his grief and his experience of himself at work. He recovered fully without a need for antidepressant medication.

Case 5. A 75-year-old widow who was in a confused, tearful state and who complained of a variety of bizarre somatic symptoms was admitted. Her behavior at home had been disorganized and frightening to her family. Her decompensation was apparently precipitated by a family feud in which her youngest and most favored daughter had grown more distant. She had previously spent much of her time babysitting for this daughter's children, who were now older and less in need of her attention. Given the bizarreness of her complaints and the intensity of her agitation, an attempt was made to medicate her on the first hospital day with oral haloperidol, 1 mg, as needed up to several times per day, based on her degree of agitation. After one dose, she complained bitterly that the medicine made her hand burn. She became even more agitated, refused further medication, and was managed psychosocially. Over the next three days staff noted a remarkable improvement in her symptoms as she befriended several younger female patients and began to mother them, thus recreating on the unit the lost relationship with her own daughter. Family therapy became the focus for the rest of the admission. The discharge diagnosis was hysterical psychosis.

Though no longer feasible on many private psychiatric units that are under pressure to discharge patients quickly, it is still preferable when possible to commit the first few days of hospitalization to observation, without making major changes in established regimens or starting new medications. The information gained through this observation can be invaluable in helping to focus the overall treatment effort and in avoiding unnecessary medication trials.

There are several exceptions to the guideline of deferring medication changes beyond the initial period of hospitalization. When discontinuation of a previously effective regimen is among the precipitants for the admission, it is best to restart the regimen promptly, once this has been discussed with outpatient caregivers. In adjusting antipsychotic drugs to achieve restabilization, the best guideline is to use doses that restabilized the patient during a previous admission.

Another circumstance when medication should be started promptly is when a patient is too psychotic or agitated to maintain behavorial control on the unit. In such a case, doses of antipsychotic or anxiolytic agents must be titrated to the patient's mental status over the first several days after admission. This is most often done with a combination of standing and prn (or as needed) doses and requires close monitoring both to achieve optimal medication levels and to avoid tension on the inpatient team.

The major caveat to the use of prn medication during the period of acute stabilization is inattention to timely adjustment of dosage. The total daily dose should be reviewed every 24 hours and prn doses converted into standing doses as the patient's optimal medication level becomes known. Failure to do this leaves the dosing schedule too dependent on the staff's anxiety level, which can result in the patient being medicated only when he or she is agitated. Such a program may lead to oversedation or may undershoot the level needed to achieve full stabilization, resulting in a stuttering course and a prolonged initial phase. For similar reasons, chronic use of prn doses can be undesirable.

There is also a psychosocial dimension to the use of prn doses in the initial phase. The safe management of the unit from shift to shift is entrusted to nursing staff who are present around the clock and spend the most time on the floor. Patients with overt or impending behavioral problems can threaten to disrupt the unit's safe functioning. In these situations, nursing staff will often request the availability of prn medication to offset a patient's unpredictability. Physicians sometimes resent the request and refer to it derogatorily as "treating the nurses." In fact, it is a sound practice both pharmacologically and administratively. Pharmacologically, it allows doses to be flexibly tailored to the patient's mental status in an ad hoc fashion. Administratively, it allows nursing staff to feel prepared to contain a patient's behavior whether or not prn doses are actually administered.

Understanding the meanings of patients' medications can be important in establishing continuity and containment. Many patients who are already on medications at the time of admission may be attached to their medications as transitional objects, as discussed in chapter 4. Altering these patients' medications without first establishing relationships with them and their outpatient caregivers can lead to increased distress and mistrust of the hospital. In addition, some patients will test the availability of the inpatient team through struggles about the type and availability of their medications. Failure of the inpatient team to adhere to these patients' accustomed regimens is regarded as evidence of lack of understanding or caring. Patients who are subject to acute anxiety states or chronic pain syndromes can be especially invested in this type of testing. As much as possible, early identification of the issue and clarification of what can be expected during the hospitalization may help to avoid painful and unprofitable struggles:

> Case 6. A 42-year-old woman with a history of atypical facial pain and dependent personality disorder was admitted in suicidal crisis following the breakup of a romantic relationship. Though her pain had been well controlled with non-opiate analgesics for several months prior to the admission, it flared on the second hospital day following an appointment in which she cried bitterly over her lost lover. Mindful of this apparent precipitant to the pain and of the patient's past history of substance abuse, the inpatient staff refused her requests for opiates. After several disruptive episodes around the patient's escalating requests, she signed out of the hospital. Four days later, her outpatient therapist requested readmission because the patient remained unstable.

This time admission was preceded by telephone contacts among her therapist, her neurologist, and the inpatient psychiatrist. Together they worked out a regimen for treating the acute exacerbations of her pain with relaxation and limited doses of opiates. The plan was presented to the patient by her outpatient therapist prior to the admission and was also approved by the inpatient team. Following admission, the patient's pain flared several times in the first three days and was managed successfully with the agreed-upon regimen. She then entered a period when the pain was relatively quiescent and she was able to focus on the loss of her lover in psychotherapy.

A last phenomenon observed during the initial phase of hospitalization is the discovery of covert noncompliance with the outpatient medication regimen. This occurs because the nursing staff becomes responsible for the dispensing of medications and accountable for every dose. Poorly compliant patients who are ashamed or embarrassed to admit to their poor compliance may now find themselves receiving substantially increased doses with attendant side effects. Cases of oversedation or toxicity may result as serum levels rise rapidly to new peaks.

Case 7. A 59-year-old self-employed store owner with known bipolar illness was admitted to the inpatient unit in a hypomanic state, apparently precipitated by an economic fluctuation that threatened the integrity of his business. On admission, he informed the unit staff that he was maintained on 1500 mg/per day of lithium carbonate, and produced his prescription as further evidence. His serum lithium level on admission was 1.0 meq/L. His hospital psychiatrist continued the lithium at this dosage and added an antipsychotic to aid recompensation. Six days after admission the patient complained of gastric distress and diarrhea and was noted by nursing staff to be mildly ataxic and tremulous. The lithium level measured at this time was 1.3 meq/L. Upon closer questioning, the patient revealed that he had been erratic in dosing himself for months. Preoccupied with his business, he would often forget doses though he did go to have his level checked. Ashamed of his noncompliance, he hid the information from his outpatient physician. Convinced that it had been the cause of his decompensation, he had hidden it from the hospital staff until his subterfuge was exposed by his toxicity. His dose was subsequently adjusted downward. He was educated about the relationship between dose and level and encouraged to maintain more honest communications with his outpatient team.

In summary, the initial phase of hospitalization is a time for the establishment of continuity of care and psychosocial containment through the linking of relationships with the patient, the family, and the outpatient team and through the judicious use of medications when it is indicated. Although some tensions in this phase may arise among unit staff, the primary focus is on the unit's relationship with the outside. This focus becomes more internal as the middle phase begins.

The Middle Phase

The middle phase of hospitalization begins as the patient stabilizes in the ward community and lasts until planning for discharge is engaged. Its boundaries are often poorly defined and typically overlap with both the initial and the terminal phase, especially in the current climate of abbreviated hospital stays. The tasks of the middle phase center on the achievement of a comprehensive evaluation of the patient's condition, the determination of the causes of hospitalization, and the design and implementation of a specific treatment program. It is around these tasks that the difficulties of managing the distributed treatment relationship trouble the provision of rational care. Just as Alice's journey through Looking-Glass World became more complex and entangled as she moved through it, so does the average hospitalization become more vulnerable to irrationality as its course proceeds. The tasks of the middle phase will be reviewed with attention to some common problems and recommendations for their management.

The need for hospitalization in itself warrants a comprehensive evaluation of the patient's condition and a reassessment of the outpatient treatment plan, where one exists. The evaluation must include a systematic review of possible sources of distress and dysfunction on biological, behavioral, psychodynamic, and psychosocial levels. Most psychiatric hospitalizations have complex determinants and it is more productive to start with a broad range of diagnostic hypotheses and narrow it down than to focus too narrowly on one formulation at the outset.

Collection of the data base for the evaluation typically begins at the time the intake process is initiated and should ultimately include coverage of the areas listed in Table 2-1.

Table 2-1
Elements of Inpatient Psychiatric Evaluation

1) Admission anamnesis
    History of present illness
    Past psychiatric history
    Family history
    Personal and developmental history
    Medication history
    Substance use history (drug and alcohol)
    Mental status examination
2) Complete medical history and physical examination
3) Family assessment
4) Functional assessment
5) Interviews with outpatient caregivers (as described above)
6) Records of previous hospitalizations and treatments
7) Observations of the patient in the hospital setting

In history taking as in most things the ideal is hard to reach. Nonetheless, the effort should be made and will typically involve several team members working on different fronts. The task of obtaining a thorough and accurate medication history should not be viewed as solely the responsibility of the team's psychiatrist, as each inpatient team member can contribute valuable information.

In taking the medication history of a newly admitted patient it is good to push for details. Changes in medications often precede hospitalization either because of lapses in the patient's compliance or because of adjustments in the regimen made in an attempt to avoid admission. Dates, doses, and effects are important in piecing together the prehospital course. When patients have discontinued or tapered doses of antipsychotic medications prior to admission, it is important to screen them for signs of tardive or withdrawal dyskinesias before resuming the increased dose.

On the basis of the collected information, the team must arrive at an understanding of the patient and the hospitalization and design a treatment plan. The treatment plan will often include one or more medication trials or a trial period off of medication. In either case, specific target symptoms should be chosen and tracked to avoid confusing global improvement or deterioration with the specific drug effect. As noted already, patients may improve or worsen in the hospital for a variety of reasons. The choice of medication should be discussed with the outpatient team. They may have information about past drug trials and will be responsible for continuing the medication after discharge. Early consideration should also be given to the economics and practicality of a given regimen for a given patient. Some patients cannot afford the cost of newer patented medications and some cannot bear adequate responsibility for maintaining a complex regimen. When these facts are discovered late in the hospitalization, discharge may be delayed.

Before a medication trial is begun, the rationale should be documented and communicated to the patient and unit staff. On an inpatient unit, this is particularly important because of the nature of the distributed treatment relationship. In the outpatient setting, a medication trial is initiated by discussing the change and giving the prescription to the patient who may then react and ask questions as needed. On the hospital unit, this communication does not always occur. The trial is initiated when the physician writes a medication order. The order is then taken by a nurse who calls the hospital pharmacy, obtains the pill, and dispenses it to the patient. Both the nurse and the patient may be uninformed as to the reasoning behind the trial or change and the resulting confusion or resentment may hamper the trial's success.

Medication trials must be monitored and coordinated with other treatment interventions. This can be straightforward or complicated. As transferences thicken during the middle phase of hospitalization, team tensions and treatment crises can create painful medication-management dilemmas, such as the following:

> Case 8. A 29-year-old man with a history of chronic psychosis was admitted reluctantly to an open unit. He was in a psychotic suicidal state precipitated by a mugging in which he was seriously injured. Although he had benefited from antipsychotic medication in the past, he now refused it. He displayed disorganized, bizarre, and often violent thoughts, which made the staff anxious. Perphenazine and lorazepam were prescribed in prn doses and he was encouraged to use them. He generally refused both, though he showed some preference for the lorazepam. Medication appeared to help but his overall dose level was too low to yield sustained improvement. He was ambivalent about the hospitalization in general, resenting the "regimentation" of the inpatient unit.

As hospitalization progressed into its second week, a pattern developed. In individual sessions with his psychiatrist, the patient was focused and affectively contained. He showed insight into the impact of the mugging and its resonance with his history of childhood abuse. On the unit at large, he remained bizarre, provocative, and disorganized. The psychiatrist thought he was overstimulated and would benefit from a looser approach to management, while the nursing staff believed he should be restricted to the unit with strict limits around his disorganized behavior. Everyone agreed he should be on regular medication but felt helpless in the face of his refusal to take it. Meanwhile, the patient developed a strong attachment to the psychiatrist who "really understands me" and reviled the nursing staff as "gestapo."

A compromise plan was implemented. Firm limits were set and compliance was rewarded with increased time out. The increased time out was typically followed by clinical deterioration, resulting in reinstitution of restrictions and renewed staff conflict. All agreed that the hospitalization was going poorly and the team began to debate the relative merits of outright discharge versus commitment to a locked unit. At this point, the patient eloped from the unit and refused to return. On a follow-up visit to the emergency room he was judged to be unimproved but not commitable. He resumed his outpatient treatment.

This case illustrates several of the themes that have been noted previously. The patient's ambivalence about hospitalization was externalized into the treatment environment as a split in the staff's perception of and management of the case. To the extent that the patient stabilized on the unit, it was through externalization of unresolved intrapsychic conflict. As a consequence, medication was not effectively prescribed, containment was never achieved, and the patient remained unstable throughout the hospitalization. While it is possible that a clearer formulation of the patient's ambivalence and resolution of the staff split might have made the unit a more effective container, it seems equally likely that this patient could not have been treated successfully on any open unit without the stabilizing effect of an antipsychotic medication in appropriate dosage. The inpatient unit is a busy place and can be profoundly disorganizing for psychotic patients who have little ability to screen out stimulation. Antipsychotic medication and a structured schedule including quiet time can be crucial to management. In the case just described, the team might have done better had it taken a more forceful stand on the need for medication. Consistent confrontation around the patient's resistance and a refusal to proceed further until the issue was settled might have resulted in a more contained hospitalization or a negotiated discharge with treatment issues in focus.

The close interlock between case formulation, team effort, and medication regimen is illustrated also by the following case:

Case 9. A 44-year-old woman who was separated from her husband and who had a history of borderline personality disorder and recurrent migraine headaches was admitted. She was in a state of severe depression precipitated by her husband's petition for divorce and the second anniversary of her mother's unmourned death. Her migraines had worsened with her depression and by the time of admission she was on a complex regimen of opiate and non-opiate analgesics and anxiolytic medication. She considered this regimen absolutely essential to her welfare and expressed suicidal ideation at the thought of relinquishing it. She was followed in the hospital by her outpatient psychiatrist, who found her an appealing and deeply sympathetic character. In contrast, her husband was infuriated with her and refused to meet with the unit's social worker.

Difficulties began soon after admission, when the patient requested increasing amounts of medication for her near-continuous headaches. Nursing staff observed a correlation between her anxiety level and her use of medication and expressed concern that the unit was supporting a pattern of entrenched substance abuse. They found it difficult to talk with the patient because she was "doped up." The psychiatrist conceded the existence of the patient's current addiction to opiates but thought this was less pressing than the stresses of her mother's death and her impending divorce. He believed that the focus of the current admission should be exclusively on working out the grief and that the issues of the patient's chronic pain and substance abuse could not be approached until further grieving took place.

As the hospitalization progressed, the split deepened. The unit nurses could not hide their feelings when dispensing medication and the patient began to experience the unit as a hostile and rejecting place. The psychiatrist became less communicative as he tired of endlessly having to defend his position. He too came to experience the unit as hostile and rejecting and in turn the unit experienced him as having been hopelessly seduced by his manipulative and drug-addicted patient. Disempowered by the husband's refusal to participate in the admission, the social worker sided with the unit staff. Communications dwindled, polarization deepened, and the patient increased her medication use and threatened to leave.

As the situation reached crisis proportions, the team sought consultation from a senior colleague. In a well-attended team meeting the case was reviewed and reformulated. The consultant urged the team to see the patient's grief, chronic pain, substance abuse, and primitive character structure as interacting components of a complex disorder. She suggested that while the patient appeared unwilling to give up her medication, excessive opiate use was impairing her capacity to use psychotherapy. Both the psychiatrist's perception of the patient's need to grieve and the staff's perception of her substance abuse were validated.

A staged plan was developed. The first stage consisted of capping the medication use to avoid oversedation while focusing actively on the losses. Medication orders would only be changed in team meetings. The patient was told her medication use was problematic and would need attention before the hospitalization was over. As she stabilized and her grief abated, a second stage would be activated in which the focus shifted to her headaches and medication use with a goal of helping her to work toward discharge to a specialty unit treating chronic pain.

Although the hospitalization remained a difficult one, the integrated formulation and plan enabled the team to work together more effectively and the patient was eventually able to accept the referral to the specialty unit.

It is not uncommon for staff on a general psychiatric unit to feel out of their element in working with patients who have substance use problems and these cases often become polarized. This case illustrates the difficulties which arise when reductionistic formulations of a complex case go to war. The patient's problem was neither purely dynamic (grief) nor biologic (addiction). Failure to achieve an adequately complex formulation prior to the consultant's arrival left the team divided. Failure to prioritize and sequence interventions resulted in a feeling that if everything was not being done at once, nothing was being done at all.

Even when the case is adequately formulated and the team is not split there is still room for irrationality around the heartache of bearing the severity of some patients' illnesses:

Case 10. A 24-year-old man with diagnoses of schizoaffective disorder and mixed episodic substance abuse was admitted. He was in paranoid decompensation following a period of cocaine abuse during which he lost his housing. Although followed by a therapist and medication doctor in a day hospital program, he had been recurrently hospitalized over the two years preceding admission, after being discharged from a halfway house for nonpayment of rent. He was maintained on trifluoperazine and carbamazepine with only partial remission of his psychosis.

Following admission, he quickly settled into the unit routine. The staff found him an engaging person. A history of profound childhood neglect and abuse heightened staff's sympathy for him. Although he was initially admitted for a brief stay, it soon became clear that without a monitored living arrangement he would continue his pattern of frequent decompensations. The patient had applied for supervised housing but would be ineligible until he had been cocaine-free for six months. Short of continuous hospitalization, this goal seemed unattainable and the team grew more despondent and hopeless. The outpatient therapist shared the team's sense of pessimism.

The case was presented to a visiting psychopharmacologist in hopes that a thorough review might uncover a new approach or a new medication regimen. Staff who attended the conference were deeply affected by the tragedy of the patient's life history and were heartened when the consultant suggested that an untreated depressive component to the patient's illness had prompted the patient to "self-medicate" with cocaine. An MAO (monoamine oxidase) inhibitor was recommended on the grounds that as an activating antidepressant it might both relieve the patient's depression and obviate his need for cocaine.

The patient was informed of the recommendation and staff began instructing him on the risks of the medication and the need for a special diet. The potential lethality of mixing cocaine and an MAO inhibitor was well known to the team but was apparently minimized around the hope that the MAO inhibitor would remove once and for all the patient's desire for cocaine. Despite the renewed atmosphere of hope, the case ground to a halt when the outpatient psychiatrist developed reservations about maintaining the patient on a medication that could prove lethal. Disgruntled, the team called for a joint conference with the unit director to deal with the outpatient psychiatrist's "obstructionism."

In the conference, the director pointed out the patient's long record of impulsivity and sporadic drug use during times of interpersonal stress. The expectation that he would never use cocaine again was seen to be clearly unrealistic no matter how effective the MAO inhibitor might prove to be. It could only be safe if it were foolproof, which it could not be. The team was able to see how its attachment to the patient and its sense of helplessness had affected its judgment, and to agree upon a trial of imipramine which had previously been rejected as a "second best" agent despite its greater safety in the event of recurrent cocaine abuse.

In this case the team's hopelessness drove it toward an unrealistic plan in which medication and the psychopharmacologist were viewed as having a kind of magic which could solve the problems of homelessness, depression, psychosis, and drug abuse in one stroke. Because of its concreteness and its association with the power of science and technology, medication is vulnerable to being perceived in this way when cases become overwhelming to staff. This kind of reductionism rarely serves patients well and may pose a danger. In this case the team's capacity to maintain a complex vision of its patient collapsed as it felt more helpless. It was only restored through consultation with an outside party who was less contaminated by the staff's sense of helplessness.

The cases reviewed here are difficult ones even by inpatient standards. Nevertheless, they illustrate well the recurrent vulnerability of the inpatient team to reductionism, splits, misperceptions of patients and other staff, magical thinking, and plain oversight. In each case, treatment bogged down in the middle phase around painful and complicated dilemmas involving the coordination of medication and dynamic therapies.

There is no way to completely avoid such difficulties but there are ways to minimize them through the use of biopsychosocial formulations, participatory management, clearly defined treatment plans, and case consultants. Routine use of biopsychosocial formulation serves as an antidote to the pitfalls of reductionism. This approach, pioneered by Engel[12,13] and others,[14-16] hypothesizes that no cases are simply biological, psychological, or psychosocial in nature. Instead, every case is seen as containing a unique combination of factors on these various system levels. The task of formulation is to identify the factors operating on each level and to specify their interaction. To be sure, certain factors may be more dominant in a particular presentation, but they never appear in isolation. If the diagnostic search routinely addresses each level, the likelihood of significant omission is greatly reduced. Once the components are identified, a comprehensive course of treatment can be designed to address them, whether simultaneously or sequentially.

Just as the case formulation is critical to containing and organizing the complexity of the team's vision in conceptual space, a clearly defined treatment plan is critical to containing and organizing the complexity of the team's treatment activity over time. Properly specified, the plan assigns the role and tasks of each team member and integrates the distributed treatment relationship into a unified effort. By sequencing interventions, team members can feel assured that important issues which must wait will not be lost. Together, the formulation and the plan can coordinate pharmacotherapy with other interventions in a given patient's care while minimizing reductionism or oversight.

Both the formulation and the treatment plan are most effective in containing the team's emotional dynamics when they are constructed and managed in a fully participatory team meeting. In this model, each team member is responsible for regularly reporting on his or her observations and work on the case and for actively contributing to the design of the overall treatment. Tension on the team is seen as reflecting the complexity of the case and the team is charged with the responsibility of achieving consensus around the design of the plan. As noted previously, it is important for continuity's sake and for avoidance of inpatient-outpatient splits that the outpatient team be included early in the team's work. Regular meetings in which the formulation and plan are reviewed and updated by the team are essential to providing optimal management as a case unfolds. The team's approach to the patient is then known and "owned" by each member of the team and there is a reduced risk of fragmentation and acting-out of team conflict. When the team reaches an impasse, an outside consultant can often be helpful.

The Terminal Phase

At the end of *Through the Looking Glass*, Alice pops out of Looking-Glass World to find herself back at home with her Kitty in hand and little idea of how to make sense out of her recent adventures or how to link them to her everyday life. Likewise, when inadequate attention is paid to the terminal phase of hospitalization, discharged patients may find themselves with prescription in hand but confused about what to make of their hospital stay. Like the initial phase, the terminal phase of hospitalization is a phase of transition. It begins whenever the issue of discharge is engaged and continues through the discharge itself. Its tasks are preparation of the case for discharge and management of the outward transition. It is a time of major psychosocial change as the locus of containment shifts and the patient and outpatient caregivers disengage from the hospital team and prepare to resume full responsibility for the ongoing course of treatment.

In terms of pharmacotherapy, the work of preparation includes simplifying the regimen, educating the patient and family about the medication, and reengaging the outpatient team. Anticipation of impending changes is the key to each of these tasks.

In the context of the unit's sophisticated system for dispensing and monitoring medication doses, it can be easy for caregivers to overlook the fact that the patient has been placed on a regimen that is unnecessarily complex. The facts that the doctor prescribes but does not dispense, that the nurses who dispense rotate from shift to shift, and that the patient generally bears little responsibility for dosing may combine to obscure the presence of an overly complicated regimen until it is time to write discharge prescriptions. In general it is wise to review the regimen as discharge is planned to be sure that it will fit into the patient's life after discharge. Both the prescribing physician and the hospital therapist can be involved in this review and the patient should also be actively included. The earlier this is done in the course of hospitalization, the more stable and routine the regimen will be by the time of discharge.

In simplifying the regimen, it is best to avoid the use of prn doses. Prn doses are harder to monitor in the outpatient setting and may risk operantly conditioning the patient to turn to medication in times of stress. When the use of ongoing prn doses appears necessary, it should be monitored carefully both by the prescribing physician and by the psychotherapist so that the use is controlled and the dynamics of the use can be explored.

In preparation for discharge, clues to noncompliance must be heeded:

> Case 11. A 32-year-old chronic schizophrenic patient was admitted with an exacerbation of psychotic symptoms in the wake of the death of the maternal aunt with whom he lived. He was restabilized on a slightly increased dose of antipsychotic medication and discharged to live with his cousin. He looked so well at

discharge that the staff was surprised when he presented for readmission a few weeks later. Under close questioning, he acknowledged that he had never filled his discharge prescription and had taken only sporadic doses of medication from a former supply. He further revealed that for years his aunt had taken charge of his medicine and reminded him when doses were due. In the light of this information, the hospital staff now recalled that he had needed consistent reminders to come for doses during the previous hospitalization and had almost forgotten to take his prescription with him at discharge. During the second hospitalization a program was designed to make the patient more responsible for reporting for doses and to educate him to the importance of the medication for his stability. Further work was done to get him to grieve the loss of the aunt and her caretaking function, and the cousin was brought in and informed of the problem as were the outpatient therapist and medication doctor.

In general, patients who regularly forget to come on time for medication doses in the hospital may be presumed to be at risk for noncompliance after discharge and should be confronted and made more responsible for their medication.

Education of patients and their families about the role of medication in treatment is another important part of preparation for discharge. Review of target symptoms, side effects, and perceived therapeutic efficacy can help them to learn on a practical level. Cautions and warnings regarding specific agents should be reiterated and the future course of drug therapy can be anticipated. Besides improving the likelihood of compliance, an educational discussion facilitates the patient's informed consent to treatment.

Reengagement of the outpatient team is a third preparatory task during the terminal phase. This is greatly simplified in cases where the outpatient team has been routinely informed of the course of hospitalization and involved in treatment planning during the initial and middle phases as recommended previously. Occasionally this will not have happened either due to geographical or scheduling constraints or due to the fact that the outpatient team has been newly recruited through referral as a result of the hospitalization. In any case, the outpatient team should be involved actively in the terminal phase of hospitalization to assure continuity of care during the outward transition. Plans and recommendations should be clearly communicated prior to discharge and documented in the hospital discharge summary. There should be an accurate statement of the discharge regimen and any specific recommendations regarding its monitoring or future revision. Inclusion of the outpatient team in planning toward discharge will reduce surprises and conflicts during this phase.

It is also helpful to plan contact between the patient and the outpatient caregivers prior to discharge, preferably in the outpatient setting. Such a contact gives the patient and the outpatient team the opportunity to review current status and anticipated plans directly rather than as mediated by the outpatient staff.

Both patients and staff members may be affected by the emotional stresses of loss and separation that attend the transition out of the hospital. Many patients will become increasingly symptomatic in the face of discharge and may begin to doubt the soundness of the plan. This is usually a natural response to the loss of the hospital context and can provide an occasion for psychotherapeutic work around separation issues. It may also, however, tempt both patient and caregivers to add medications or increase doses of an existing regimen in an attempt to alleviate distress. While occasionally necessary, as for example an increase in antipsychotic medication for an actively hallucinating schizophrenic patient, the addition of medications during the week preceding discharge is generally undesirable. A marked increase in symptoms may be more related to a perceived inadequacy of the psychosocial part of the outpatient plan than to the adequacy of the drug regimen. Holding firm about medications may allow other important material to emerge, as in the following case:

> Case 12. A 29-year-old single woman with a dependent personality disorder and a history of recurrent depressions, anxiety episodes, and hysterical auditory hallucinations was preparing for discharge after a lengthy hospitalization occasioned by her outpatient psychotherapist's prolonged paternity leave. She was quite attached to her medications and at admission had been on a complicated regimen, which had been gradually simplified during the hospitalization with her begrudging consent. Despite the effort to keep things simple, her antipsychotic medication had been changed several times at her request, each time with reasonable indications based on side effects.
> Several times during the hospitalization she had announced

her intention not to return to her volunteer job but to apply to a day hospital instead. The staff perceived this as a regressive move but chose to defer struggling over the issue until after discharge. With the therapist back from leave, discharge was planned. The patient's application to day hospital was pending and no other outpatient supports were in place. In this context, she became increasingly distressed and threatened that unless her medicines were restored to their prehospital levels she could not be responsible for her behavior. The team and the outpatient therapist reviewed her status and decided not to alter her medications. She was informed that her discharge would take place as scheduled and that she should return to the familiarity and structure of her volunteer job. She became tearful on confrontation and revealed that the actual precipitant to her hospitalization had been an episode of sexual harassment in the vicinity of her volunteer job. In her therapist's absence she had felt overwhelmed and ashamed to confide the episode to anyone, out of fear that she would be blamed for bringing it on herself. She had hoped that a transfer to the day hospital would restore her sense of safety without need for disclosure. In light of this new information, the patient's discharge was postponed to allow time to process the episode and restructure the discharge plan. She was eventually discharged without change in her medications.

The caveat about adding new medications around the transition out of the hospital extends to tapering or discontinuing medications. Inpatient staff sometimes feel under pressure to reduce patients' doses to maintenance levels before discharge as though there were no outpatient team to continue the work after the patient leaves. When this occurs, falling drug levels in the blood and clinical or subclinical withdrawal syndromes can confuse interpretation of the clinical picture as discharge approaches. Furthermore, patients who are losing the support and structure of the hospital may feel additionally bereft by the loss of medication and its associated function as a transitional object.

SUMMARY

Over the past four decades our knowledge of psychotropic agents and their effects has mushroomed. Never before in history have we been at such an advantage in being able to make sound and rational decisions about the use of medications in the treatment of mental disorders. Yet for all of the rationality of our scientific methods, there remains a residue of irrationality in the ways we sometimes use medications in actual practice. Anxieties, transference binds, and conflicts can distort our perception of the proper role of medication for a given patient and bias our judgment toward prescribing in the service of nonrational agendas. Both the pharmacologic effects of medications and their psychosocial meanings in our culture leave them vulnerable to being used in irrational ways. It is a part of our responsibility as clinicians to use our skills and our knowledge of human nature to minimize the impact of these processes on the quality of care we provide to our patients.

The practice of combined treatment on the psychiatric inpatient unit presents special challenges to rational pharmacotherapeutics. These stem from the emotional intensity of the inpatient setting and from the difficulties of managing the logistics and dynamics of the distributed treatment relationship. For each specific patient, pharmacotherapeutic issues unfold around the tasks of the phases of hospitalization. In the initial phase, these tasks are the establishment of containment and continuity of care. In the middle phase, they are evaluation and treatment. In the terminal phase, they are preparation for discharge and transition out of the hospital. Both the initial and the terminal phase are times of transition in which tensions arise around the patient's movement across the boundary between the unit and the outer world. The middle phase is a time of deepening focus of the work on the unit and the transferences which attend it. Here tensions may arise around the dynamics of the unit's organization and the staff's relationships with the patient, involved family, and outpatient team. Examples have illustrated the ways in which the particular issues of each phase can affect the decisions and dynamics of prescribing psychotropic medications on the unit.

Nonrational influences on human action cannot be eliminated but they can be recognized and managed. In fact, it is an ongoing goal of psychotherapeutic practice of all types to minimize irrational action by acknowledging and interpreting the presence of the nonrational in all of us. This goal is fostered in inpatient combined treatment by paying careful ongoing attention to the interaction between the psychopharmacologic and the psychosocial dimensions of each case. Knowledge of the tasks and psychodynamics of each phase of hospitalization can aid in the timely identification and correction of irrational trends. Routine use of an integrated biopsychosocial framewok for case formulation can help to avoid the pitfalls of reductionism. Full participation of the membership of the multidisciplinary treatment team in case formulation and treatment planning can undercut splitting and fragmentation in the delivery of care. Linking of the outpatient and inpatient teams early in the hospitalization enhances continuity of care and minimizes the potential for inpatient-outpatient splitting. Maintenance of the inpatient-outpatient relationship throughout the hospitalization can smooth the way toward discharge.

The Alice of *Through the Looking Glass* is a more composed and experienced traveler than the Alice who fell down the rabbit's hole into Wonderland. Mindful of her previous experience, she is more poised and effective as she manages the new but somehow familiar irrationalities of Looking-Glass World. With vigilance, experience, and humility, we too can learn better to manage the pitfalls of nonrational influences on combined treatment and to provide safer and more productive journeys to the patients who travel through our psychiatric hospitals.

REFERENCES

1. Freud S: Group psychology and the analysis of the ego, in *Standard Edition*. London, Hogarth Press, 1955, vol 18.
2. Bion WR: *Experiences in Groups*. New York, Basic Books, 1961.
3. Colman AD, Bexton WH (eds): *Group Relations Reader 1*. Washington, DC The A.K. Rice Institute, 1985.
4. Colman AD, Geller MH (eds): *Group Relations Reader 2*. Washington, DC The A.K. Rice Institute, 1985.
5. Krantz J (ed): *Irrationality in Social and Organizational Life: Proceedings of the 8th A.K. Rice Scientific Meeting*. Washington, DC, The A.K. Rice Institute, 1987.
6. Main TF: The ailment. *Br J Med Psychol* 1957;30:129–145.
7. Sandler J: Countertransference and role-responsiveness. *Int Rev Psychoanal* 1976;3:143–147.
8. Bion WR: Elements of psychoanalysis, in *Seven Servants: Four Works by Wilfred Bion*. New York, Jason Aronson, 1977.
9. Winnicott DW: The use of an object and relating through identifications, in *Playing and Reality*. London, Tavistock, 1971, pp 86–94.

10. Kernberg OF: Toward an integrative theory of hospital treatment, in *Object Relations Theory and Clinical Psychoanalysis*. New York, Jason Aronson, 1976, pp 241–275.
11. Pinderhughes CA, Goodglass H, Mayo C, et al: A study of childhood origins of patients' ward relationships. *J Nerv Ment Disord* 1966;142:140–147.
12. Engel GL: The need for a new medical model: A challenge for biomedicine. *Science* 1977;196:129–135.
13. Engel GL: The clinical application of the biopsychosocial model. *Am J Psychiatry* 1980;137:535–544.
14. Nurcombe B, Gallagher RM: *The Clinical Process in Psychiatry*. New York, Cambridge University Press, 1986.
15. Parsons T: The relation between biological and sociocultural theory, in *Social Systems and the Evolution of Action Theory*. New York, Free Press, 1982, pp 118–121.
16. Parsons T: A paradigm of the human condition, in *Action Theory and the Human Condition*. New York, Free Press, 1978, pp 352–433.

3

Pharmacotherapy from the Perspective of Family Ecology

Edward Yeats

Every psychotherapist who makes use of psychopharmacologic consultation must be at least a biologist, an analyst, and a diplomat. As a biologist, she or he must be educated about the uses and effects of psychotropic medications. Like an analyst, she or he has to be aware of the intrapsychic meaning of medication as an "object" to the patient and of the transference and countertransference issues raised in psychotherapy by drug treatment. And as a diplomat, she or he must be observant and responsive in managing the relationship dynamics in the combined treatment triad of psychotherapist, pharmacotherapist, and patient.

To be fully empowered in integrating pharmacotherapy into a patient's treatment, a therapist must also act as an ecologist. Nearly every patient referred for pharmacotherapy, after all, is a family member whose treatment impacts upon a family environment. The family ecologist's point of view includes those of the biologist, the analyst, and the diplomat. It adds the important dimension of family context to assessment and treatment. It is not necessary to be a family therapist or to use family therapy techniques in treatment to benefit from this perspective.

The aim of this chapter is to show how the conceptual framework of family ecology can help a psychotherapist to understand what happens in families whose members are treated with psychotropic medications. Guidelines for the referral of patients for psychopharmacology consultation are offered, and the interactions between pharmacotherapy and ongoing individual or family psychotherapy are addressed.

INTEGRATION VERSUS CLINICAL IDEOLOGY

Therapists and therapies can be tyrannized and limited by adherence to one or another theoretical perspective. Each of the three major perspectives relevant to this exploration has an inherent bias, which inclines the therapist to reductionistically ignore aspects of the available clinical data. The *biological* perspective, with its disease orientation and its focus on symptom relief, tends to de-emphasize the dynamic meaning and purpose of symptoms. The *psychoanalytic* model, in which intrapsychic dynamics are the central features, predisposes the clinician to give less attention to biological factors and family dynamics. The *family systems* approach, with its emphasis on the factors in the family context that influence symptoms in family members, may lead the clinician to disregard both biological and intrapsychic levels of information.

The purpose of conceptual models should be to organize the clinical data, not to limit or deny valuable information. An integrative perspective that deliberately includes consideration of the biological, intrapsychic, and interpersonal levels of data leads to the most informed formulation and responsible intervention. It is my intention to maintain such a *biopsychosocial* point of view while highlighting the family perspective.

A LOOK AT THE LITERATURE

Outcome studies have shown family therapy to be effective in many patients of the same diagnostic categories for which treatment typically involves drugs.[1] Good results have been achieved for symptoms of depression, agoraphobia, and childhood psychosomatic disorders, especially anorexia nervosa.[1-3] There are, as yet, few controlled studies of the interactive effects of pharmacotherapy and family therapy, and I could find no quantitative studies comparing the effectiveness of the two modalities. Some aspects of the interaction of family therapy and medication have been addressed, however, in studies of schizophrenia and mood disorders.

Relapse in Schizophrenia

Studies of relapse in major mental illness have shown pharmacotherapy and family therapy to be powerful allies. This is most evident in published studies of schizophrenia and major mood disorders. Vaughn and Leff found, for example, that the single best predictor of relapse in both patients with schizophrenia and those with depression was the expressed emotion (EE) of family members toward the patient: "A high degree of emotion expressed by a relative at the time of key admission is the best single predictor of relapse during the nine months following discharge."[4]

Expressed emotion, in this research, was defined as the number of hostile or critical comments and/or overinvolvement of a relative interviewed at the time of the index admission. This and related studies, now popularly known as EE research, demonstrated the extent to which family environment could affect the rate of relapse in patients with schizophrenia.[5-8] When patients from homes with a high index of expressed emotion had more than 35 hours per week of face-to-face contact with family members; for example, they were much more likely to relapse than those who spent less time with their families. This effect occurred even when medication was prescribed and compliance carefully controlled, leading Vaughn and colleagues to conclude that: "Clinicians should look to the emotional atmosphere in the home for explanations of medication failure."[8]

These findings led to a very enlightening study of the effects of family therapy intervention on schizophrenic patients. Strang and colleagues reported that patients from homes with a high index of expressed emotion relapsed less frequently if they were: (1) taking medication, (2) limiting face-to-face contact with family members, and (3) participating in family therapy.[9] Goldstein and colleagues confirmed that family therapy along with medication significantly reduced the frequency of relapse.[10]

In a study linking family therapy to improved compliance in taking medication, Faloon and colleagues found that family therapy actually reduced the overall dose of medication required. Compliance was significantly better in patients receiving family therapy, as measured by the number of missed appointments, tablet counts, blood levels of the medication and number of patients switched to intramuscular administration.[7]

The psychoeducational approach to family intervention employed in these studies derived from social learning theory and emphasized education about major mental illness and coping skills.[11] Training in structured problem solving and communications was included. The therapy setting was the patient's home.

Mood Disorders

Investigating depression, psychotherapy, and the use of antidepressant medication in women, Rounsaville and colleagues observed that "depressed women with marital disputes have a generally poorer treatment outcome than women who are single or in supportive relationships." Presenting data showing the negative effect of marital trouble on the successful treatment of depression in women, they concluded:

> The findings of this study point to the inadequacy of individual maintenance psychotherapy or antidepressant medication for the depressed patient with long-standing neurotic maladaptations and marital problems. Conjoint marital therapy may have been the more appropriate treatment.[12]

Trying to treat depression without treating the marital distress is like trying to treat hayfever when the patient works in a flower shop.

In contrast to the studies of expressed emotion in the families of schizophrenics, the literature for mood disorders is generally more anecdotal and less conclusive. Two themes emerge quite clearly, however: that treatment with lithium, antidepressants, and individual psychotherapy is much less successful when there are marital problems; and that serious marital problems are usually present, especially when the patient has been manic.

Marital compatibility, as measured by self and other ratings, has been reported to improve somewhat when the manic patient is stabilized on lithium. In one study, spouses reported fewer undesirable traits in their lithium-treated partners, while the patient's ratings of his or her spouse did not change significantly with treatment.[13] Improvement with lithium, however, has also been noted to produce some difficulties for spouses.[14-16] Fitzgerald noted, for example, that "the spouse can become anxious or severely depressed in response to the unfamiliar normality in the patient on lithium."[14] He compared this to observations of the seemingly paradoxical intolerance for a partner's sobriety noted in spouses of alcoholics.[17] He recommended that the clinician treat the spouse's depression as a response to loss.

In an inquiry that considered medications, psychotherapy, and the couple relationship when one spouse was diagnosed with Primary Affective Disorder (PAD), Greene and colleagues expressed concern that the spouse's distress could have a negative effect on the patient's compliance with medication treatment. They reported that: "Frequently the non-PAD partner will express a desire that his spouse stop medication and be his 'own self'."[18]

These writers have speculated on the dynamics involved when improvement while the patient is taking medication seems to increase marital stress. Some suggest that power and control struggles play a prominent role in these couples' relationships.[15] Others point to the outrageous, destructive actions of the patient during a manic episode (eg, spending sprees or sexual acting out) and see the inability to forgive the now stabilized spouse as the basis for increased marital distress.[16]

Whatever the dynamics, most authors have stressed the usefulness of an intervention that actively addresses couples issues. Davenport and colleagues, for example, cite the occurrence of lower rates of divorce and rehospitalization when manic patients and their spouses were treated in a couples group.[19]

The Spouse Literature and the Seesaw Effect

Many couples are greatly helped by one spouse's improvement while taking medication. One issue raised by studies of depressed and manic patients, however, is whether there can be adverse side effects of successful treatment. Put another way, can successful individual psychotherapy or pharmacotherapy place another family member at risk for psychiatric symptoms? While there is no quantitative study of this domino effect, there is enough clinical folklore to suggest that any family's potential for adverse reactions to treatment should be assessed as part of the evaluation and referral process.

In what has become a classic paper, "Pathologic Reactions of Marital Partners to Improvement of Patients," Kohl details how spouses can attempt to sabotage treatment and/or become symptomatic themselves at just the point when the patient is showing strong improvement. He suggests, also, that the denial of marital conflict "constitutes an indication for early inclusion of the marital partner in the total plan of treatment." He makes a case for the ethical obligation of the therapist who treats one member of a couple to "give due consideration to his responsibility for the well-being of the untreated partner also," stating:

> Treatment of the marital partner as well as the patient is indicated when the former reacts to the patient's obvious progress by resisting his improvement or by development of a clinical illness. In such cases the well-being of one partner appears to be directly related to the illness of the other and it is not uncommon to find that the less sick marital partner is the first to seek treatment voluntarily.[20]

Hurvitz, reflecting on the prevalence of male therapists treating female clients, detailed the hazards inherent when a male therapist treats another man's wife in individual psychoanalytic psychotherapy. To avoid increased marital stress, alienation, and potential symptoms in the spouse, as well as sabotage of the therapy, he urges that "the other spouse, as the significant other, should be involved in the therapy from the outset."[21] Other authors also persuasively encourage therapists to be aware of the consequences of treating only one member of a couple.[22-24]

Each of these authors refers to a power dynamic in couples who become unbalanced by one spouse's psychotherapy. The notion of a seesaw effect, in which one spouse's "up" can mean the other spouse's "down," has been linked to the issues of dominance and homeostasis.[20] Other family therapists (D. Kantor, personal communication, 1988) have witnessed a kind of hot-potato effect among the siblings in a family, especially when psychosomatic symptoms are prevalent.[21] Movement of overt symptoms from parents to children and vice versa is not uncommonly observed. Some further implications of the potential systemic effects of individual treatment, including drug treatment, will be explored later. First, though, it would be useful to lay a conceptual foundation.

UNDERSTANDING THE FAMILY DYNAMICS OF SYMPTOMS AND CURES

The Identified Patient

The family systems model grew out of a certain frustration with the limitations of the psychoanalytic and biological-behavioral approaches to symptoms. In emphasizing the role of context in symptom formation, there was a reaction against the prevailing diagnostic labels, which were derived from individual and biological models. By using the term *identified patient*, the early family therapists, perhaps too identified with the patient (as a victim of the system), took the position that the presenting symptom reflected a family problem rather than an individual intrapsychic or biological problem.

One of the first goals, then, was to help the family redefine the situation as a family problem rather than as a problem in one member only. Indeed, there was a time in the early days of family therapy when whole families would be hospitalized if one member presented with schizophrenic symptoms.[25]

From this perspective symptoms are seen as reflecting difficulties in relationships between members rather than as reflecting a problem inside one member. Family therapists speak of working actively to "think systems," and are wary of individual psychodynamic formulations, viewing the narrowing of scope to the individual level to be an indication of the therapist's being inducted into the family's internal reality.

The clinician who sees the patient's symptom exclusively in systems terms can become as tyrannized by his or her theory as the intrapsychic or biologically biased practitioner. Failing at least to assess the role of context in the symptom's emergence and maintenance, however, denies the patient a powerful therapeutic resource.

From Problem Member to Family Problem

Frequently the early part of family therapy involves helping a family to explore the structures and dynamic issues of relationships that may underlie a presenting problem or symptom. Theoretically, the symptom, if it is only a reflection of the real problem, will become unnecessary once the family's structure changes or the symptom's meaning is truly understood. This was dramatically demonstrated, for example, in Minuchin's luncheon interview of a family with an anorectic daughter, as reported by Aponte and Hoffman.[26] By the end of the interview the daughter, who had previously refused to eat, munched away at her sandwich while Minuchin spoke with her parents about issues in their relationship. What had been considered the central problem became an almost unnoticed background detail, while the adults discussed more crucial matters. The problem had been redefined: it was not anorexia *in* the daughter, but rather the marital power struggle played out *around* the daughter's eating that was now the problem.

The clinician faced with a family member receiving pharmacotherapy faces a double challenge. There is a tendency to err either by stressing family dynamics and failing to support psychopharmacologic treatment, or by relying on pharmaceuticals to the exclusion of vital family dynamics. Working with the relationship problems without blaming the family, at the same time as validating the need for medication without reifying the patient's position as the ill member, requires skill and grace on the part of the therapist.

Structure and Development

To understand the family level of a symptom or a cure, one must place the ill person, or identified patient, within both the current family structure and the family's developmental process. These are referred to by family therapists as the vertical (space) and horizontal (time) dimensions.[27]

Family Structure

Minuchin developed a useful language and a graphic method for describing how current structural forces in a family may lead to symptoms.[2] He divides the family into *sub-systems* along generational lines and examines the *boundaries* between them. Boundaries can be clear, diffuse, or rigid. He attends to the age *hierarchy* among the children, and to *alliances* between members. What emerges is a diagnostic snapshot, an x-ray image of the skeletal structure of the family, which can be schematically diagrammed. In this framework, for example, the configuration of a family with a school-phobic child might show an overly close alliance between mother and child (a diffuse boundary between them), while father remained distant and underinvolved with both mother and child (a rigid boundary):

Mother	r	
	i	
....	g	Father
(diffuse)	i	
Child	d	

Maintenance, Growth, and Development

A family's structure has to be maintained. There are concepts in family systems theory that attempt to describe how this is accomplished. One early concept, borrowed from biology[28] and general system theory,[29] is that of *family homeostasis*. Demonstrating this concept, Jackson gives the example of a patient who becomes tangential as soon as emotionally laden material comes up in the family meeting:

> Thus, if the norm in the family is that there be no disagreement, when trouble begins to brew, we might observe general uneasiness, a sudden tangentialization or change of topic, or even

symptomatic behavior on the part of an identified patient, who may act out, talk crazy, or even become physically ill when family members begin to argue. The family is distracted and brought into coalition (frequently against the patient) and the norm holds until the next time.[30]

Like individual personality structure, family structure is maintained by defense mechanisms. Deviations from family rules[31] and roles are corrected through "negative feedback loops."[32] That is, when behavior exceeds the set point or range of tolerance, forces are set in motion to restore the original state. One analogy used to illustrate this concept is that of a household thermostat.

Most recent writers, viewing the concept of homeostasis as too machinelike and inadequate to describe the constant change and flux in real family relationships, have coined terms such as evolutionary feedback[33] and order through fluctuation[34] to replace homeostasis. Whatever the term, *maintenance* of a relatively stable structure is one aspect of the family's functioning as a system.

Growth, in contrast to maintenance, is characterized by deviations from the status quo and by structural change. Growth must be contained enough to sustain relative stability, and this contained growth is what we call development. Including a new member by conception, pregnancy, and birth, for example, involves changes in roles (husband and wife to mother and father), rules (division of labor in caretaking), and boundaries (including grandparents, now three generations). The accomplishment of this transition without endangering stability requires the same kind of flexibility and tolerance for stress that makes the birth process itself physically possible.

Family Development

Symptomatic family members typically tend to present for treatment at critical points in the family life-cycle. Hodley and colleagues, for example, present community clinic data linking the presentation of one member for psychiatric services with a "family developmental crisis."[35] A number of other writers have presented epigenetic stage theories of family development.[26,35,36]

The family life-cycle breaks down roughly into eight phases:
1. Individual adulthood
2. Coupling
3. Birth of the first child
4. Birth of a sibling
5. Latency family
6. Family with adolescents
7. Launching
8. Empty nest or aging

With the high prevalence of divorce and the expanding range of possibilities for the timing of childbearing, this is not intended as an exhaustive summary of normal phases, but rather as a rough guideline.

These phases build on each other, as do the phases of individual development described by Erikson.[38] How well the young adult has established a differentiated self[39] impacts on the development of a marital partnership. The marital partnership, the trunk of the family tree, must be firmly rooted to stay healthy and balanced through the fragile, tender years of infancy and the storms of adolescence.

The Symptom in Context

It follows from the concepts of structure, maintenance, and development that symptoms in a family member may be considered the consequence of at least one of three conditions: (1) *developmental impasse*, conceptualized as the collision between growth and maintenance forces within the family; (2) *structural deficit*, which includes the biologically based major mental illness of individual family members; and (3) *traumatic stress*, disruptive life events such as serious illness, death, divorce, dislocation, and so on. A therapeutic intervention with an individual (including but not limited to pharmacotherapy) should assess both the family side effects and the potential family resistances to the treatment of one member. Pharmacotherapists and individual psychotherapists seem too rarely to consider this. Family therapists, on the other hand, tend to miss opportunities to employ pharmacotherapy, when relieving symptoms could enhance a family's capacity to resolve their relationship problems.

Developmental Impasse

When the situation is one of developmental impasse, a successful pharmacotherapeutic intervention is one that reduces the identified patient's suffering, facilitating the developmental change which is stuck or blocked. One might consider treatment to be a palliative for "growing pains" or a form of structural "training wheels" that help the patient through a developmental transition. Antianxiety agents, antidepressants, or antipsychotic medications may play important roles in this type of difficulty.

When the developmental impasse is more serious, the presenting symptom typically takes the form of a metaphorical statement about the family's relationship problems. The exacerbation of asthma symptoms in a family member whose home is pervaded by a suffocating, heavy atmosphere of unspoken anger, for example, or the propensity for gastric distress in families in which more direct bellyaching is not tolerated, illustrate this idea.

The symptom both states the problem analogically or metaphorically and diverts the family's attention away from an interpersonal conflict of interests and onto the patient and his or her symptom. In this way the patient becomes a sacrificial container for the family's suffering, which is then isolated in one member. Consider in the following example:

> Case 1. In one family, the oldest son had been a heroic overachiever. Beset with severe marital problems and alcoholism, the family had placed their hopes for the future in him. This proved too much of a burden for him to carry. After leaving college in disgrace, to his parents' deep disappointment, he became acutely psychotic, presenting with the delusion that he had "destroyed the world."

A purely pharmacologic intervention may spell trouble in this kind of situation. This is not to say that pharmacotherapy is the wrong treatment, just that a purely biological intervention may be resisted and can possibly make things worse. There are two important mechanisms by which emphasis on pharmacotherapy of an identified patient may backfire:

First, by officially sharing the family's definition of the patient as the problem without exploring the contextual meaning of the illness, the isolation of the suffering in one member is reinforced as social reality and backed up by a medical authority. Next, as Haley has described, if the illness is serving a homeostatic function for the family by forestalling developmental change because of some threat to the system's stability, the family may unwittingly be threatened by a successful intervention. They could resist or even sabotage efforts at treatment.[40] Certain loyalty conflicts, in which one parent favors and the other opposes some form of treatment, may reflect this phenomenon. It is important to emphasize, of course, that this is not a conscious or intentional process. Family members usually experience themselves as caring and responsible. The tendency of mental health professionals, including family therapists, to blame their patients' families derives in part from an unfortunate misuse and misunderstanding of systems theory (H. Grunebaum, personal communication, 1988).

Structural Deficit

As with deficits in individual personality structure,[41] deficits in family structure can manifest themselves as symptoms. Like individuals with narcissistic or borderline personalities, families with structural deficits often show a failure of regulation of affect and action, resulting in poor boundary and role maintenance. The systems concept for this is the runaway process.[42,43] Examples of this type of structural deficit include chronic physical or emotional disability of a member, recurrent comings and goings of a parent, and the absence of a member whose function cannot otherwise be fulfilled. These situations may result in chronically limited or disrupted functioning, which may appear impossible to change. Carefully crafted therapeutic bolstering of the structure is analogous to supporting the sagging beams of an old house with reinforcing posts.

A specific kind of structural deficit occurs when major mental illness impairs a family member's capacity to fulfill his or her role within the family structure. Pharmacotherapy can be a crucially important intervention under these circumstances. Maintaining a manic patient on medication, for example, can reinforce and sustain a family's structure by allowing the patient to resume responsibilities and be more reliable interpersonally. In this way, symptoms in other family members may actually be prevented by someone else's medication treatment. It can be enlightening to track the patient's exacerbations with family dynamics in mind. Relapses are likely to be meaningful and possibly preventable.

> Case 2. A family consultation in which the 7-year-old daughter was the identified patient revealed that the father was rendered immobilized by his rage attacks. When he would try to set limits with any of his three children, he would become unable to control his anger. The family had adapted by developing rigid and harsh rules enforced by the mother alone. After a medication consultant initiated pharmacotherapy, the father's rage attacks came under much better control. It was then possible to work productively in family therapy with the consequences of his rages, without having to fear that he would again lose control. Gradually he was able to reclaim his role in the family limit setting, and the daughter's presenting symptoms of bed-wetting, stomach aches, and nightmares declined.

When pharmacotherapy helps to acutely stabilize a family, attention must nonetheless be given to whether this will be helpful or potentially destructive over the long run. Surely there are many situations in which an appropriate treatment goal is the sustaining of a limited but tolerable adaptation. When symptoms with meaning and structural purpose are improved in a limited way with medication, however, this may serve to delay confrontation with an underlying developmental impasse. Here the medication can partially mask a serious systemic problem, as other drugs can mask serious physical disease. Clues that this may be the case include minimal improvement during pharmacotherapy, inconsistent compliance with treatment, or frequent symptomatic relapses. For example, when an anxious or depressed spouse is marginally maintained by medication and serious marital conflict is unaddressed, the medication can serve to make life more tolerable in the short run despite episodic eruptions of symptoms. Years later, however, symptoms of more serious proportion might show up in the now adolescent children. These may be contributed to by the parents' years of marital life in parallel grooves, which have left them ill-prepared to face the empty nest. The aim of the psychotherapist in making a pharmacotherapy referral, therefore, is to advocate for relief and stability in the short term while keeping long-term developmental goals in mind.

Traumatic Stress and the Cost of Adaptation

Psychiatric symptoms or other severe illness in one member always require adaptation in the family context. Typically this adaptation is reflected in *reallocation of responsibility*, and shifts in the unspoken *rules of communication*.

When a family suffers a major stress (including the psychiatric illness of one member) its boundary structure may also change. In the case of an ill member, for example, the patient may need supervision and may need to be functionally replaced. Sometimes help is imported from outside the household, as when a member of the extended family is brought in to care for the children while their mother is in the hospital. A more costly adaptation can be reflected in a shift in the burden of responsibility to an over-responsible spouse or child.

The most striking example of this type of adaptation is parentification, the process by which a child fills in for an absent, abdicating, or disabled parent, thereby assuming responsibility and power beyond what can be seen as helpful or age appropriate.[44] One aftereffect of parentification is the bench-warmer syndrome. In sports, when a player is injured, it is not uncommon for the replacement player to resist giving up his place in the starting lineup. The coach may stick with a lineup that is winning, even though the injured player may be ready to resume play. In families, too, the tendency to stay with the status quo complicates the return from a structural adaptation to stress.

Changes that derive from the illness itself may also have secondary gain properties. The family which has adapted to having their agoraphobic mother in the house 24 hours a day, for example, may miss the security of always having someone at home (to answer the phone, to care for a sick child, etc.) if the medication trial proves successful in controlling her panic attacks.

Changes in the rules of communication may result in either an increase or a decrease of overt conflict. New rules about noise, for example, may come as a result of father's headaches. There may also be changes in the content of conversation in deference to one member's illness. In an intensely competitive family, for example, the oldest son's chronic psychotic episodes put a stop to overt discussion of academic or social successes among the brothers and sisters.

Both types of adaptation (changes in responsibility and communication) have the paradoxical effect of maintaining the family's equilibrium with the symptom, and surrounding the symptom in a way that actually makes change more difficult. Thus the changes in "who talks to whom about what" in the family of a paranoid patient may end up maintaining his or her isolation in much the same way that the tensed posture adopted by someone with back pain actually makes it worse.

It becomes clear how the treatment of an illness can actually cause new problems of adaptation. An assessment of the patient's family context can alert the clinician to what *else* has to change for an intervention to be successful. With a context-sensitive approach, compliance is likely to be increased, and the potential for environmental side effects reduced.

PHARMACOTHERAPY THROUGH THE FAMILY LIFE-CYCLE

When the psychotherapist is working with people at different phases of the family life-cycle, she or he faces a variety of issues pertinent to combined treatment. In this next section, relevant themes will be examined, with illustrative case examples. Issues for evaluation as well as for ongoing treatment will be considered.

The Young Adult

Even when the young adult is being treated in individual psychotherapy, one needs to consider the family implications of psychopharmacology referral:

> Case 3. A 20-year-old college student was referred for psychotherapy because he was having serious difficulty with his academic work. Although he had been a nationally recognized honor student in high school, his college career had ground to a halt. He had lost his motivation, and it soon became clear that he

was quite depressed. As part of the initial evaluation, the therapist suggested a pharmacotherapy evaluation.

The father, a corporate executive, urged the patient to try antidepressants. The mother, herself chronically depressed, expressed her worries about toxic side effects to the patient and sent him a newspaper clipping on the dangers of irresponsibly prescribed drugs. This left the patient immobilized and confused, even though the psychotherapist insisted that a consultation could be purely informational.

An exploration of the family issues revealed that the patient's father had always been overly invested in his son's achievements, even to the point of choosing his college and his major. The father felt that he had crafted the best path for his son to take. If medication was necessary to continue on that path, what was the problem?

The patient began to recognize that he was having trouble academically because he could no longer follow the path his father had chosen for him. His symptoms arose from a family developmental impasse around separation. While he was at a loss for what he wanted to do about his future, he knew he did not like the idea of taking medicine in order to function, and he made the choice not to consult a pharmacotherapist. This choice was an important step in his developing autonomy.

At the psychotherapist's suggestion, there followed a series of family meetings. In these meetings the patient was able to negotiate his parents' approval of a leave of absence from college and support for his psychotherapy.

The individual therapist of the young adult should consider the patient's role in the larger family system. There are usually themes having to do with separation and pulls to return to a more adolescent position in the family. When the issue of pharmacotherapy comes up, it always pays to attend to the parents' (and siblings') attitudes and the advice they give your patient. Important loyalty issues may complicate the patient's treatment choices.

In more urgent circumstances, the therapist may have to support parents' efforts to contain an out-of-control adult child. Such decisions by parents to act on the need for medication and hospitalization are extraordinarily painful and yet crucial for the future of relationships in the family. The therapist wants to encourage the parents to be firm and nonpunitive, to use the least possible force, and to be deliberate in stating how the patient can show them when and how they can take less responsibility.

Frequently, a family worries that the patient is or will be sick just like somebody else in their history. With these often unspoken worries comes the fear that the patient will have the same fate. The more a therapist knows about this, the better. In some families this topic is a guarded one — it is as if speaking of it would make it true.

Getting a sense of the state of the parents' marriage is also very helpful. This tells you how much of a struggle it will be for the patient to separate and how much pressure it will place on the parents and siblings if an intervention is successful. These issues are equally relevant when the patient is not living in his parents' household.

With these kinds of considerations in mind, it may be possible to anticipate noncompliance with pharmacotherapy and to be more understanding when it occurs:

> Case 4. A 21-year-old acutely psychotic woman was admitted to the inpatient unit. Her mother visited her daily, sometimes twice a day, and repeatedly engaged in arguments with the resident and the nursing staff about the philosophy of drug treatment. She argued that her daughter's medication "kept her from expressing her feelings." The resident reasoned that the pharmacotherapy was medically indicated, and told her he felt that discussing it further would be inappropriate, since the patient was of age to decide this for herself. The mother soon developed a reputation on the ward for being overprotective. Simultaneously, the patient began refusing medication.
>
> When the mother's concerns were addressed in a family meeting, she spoke tearfully of her guilt and shame over a psychotic sister whom the family had exiled to the state hospital when she was an adolescent. The same brand of antipsychotic medication used to treat the mother's sister was now being prescribed for her daughter.
>
> While compliance issues continued to be an ongoing problem in this case, a deeper look at this mother's concerns helped to resolve, temporarily, the power struggle between staff and patient around medications.

The Married Couple

Earlier we reviewed the hazards of treating one member of a couple in individual psychotherapy. The central conclusion was that it is perilous to treat one spouse without actively engaging the other spouse at least in an evaluation and potentially in the therapeutic work. The importance of assessing and involving the spouse is valid whether the patient is receiving psychotherapy or pharmacotherapy.

When one member of a couple presents with symptoms, the clinician should actively assess the possibility that serious current marital issues underlie the symptoms. Then, if treatment is pursued, the impact of the treatment on the marriage and the marriage on the treatment can be anticipated. The clinician should try to predict whether pharmacotherapy will help to reduce unproductive suffering, to ease the distress of a productive crisis, to maintain a limited but optimal status quo, to put off an inevitable disaster, or to tip a precarious balance. None of these possibilities can be fully addressed unless the clinician actively assesses the patient's marriage.

Case 5. A 20-year-old married woman came into the clinic complaining of panic attacks. She had seen a television talk show about panic disorder and hoped that medication would help her. In addition to complying with her request for a pharmacotherapy consultation, the intake worker inquired about the current circumstances of her life. She had noticed, for example, that the patient listed no phone number and had called several times from a pay phone to arrange the appointment. The patient explained that she and her husband had recently moved to the area from their home town in the mid-west so that her husband could find work. They were under great financial strain. Her husband was working many hours of overtime, and they could not afford a telephone. Confined to their apartment by her panic attacks, she was very lonely, brooding over how she missed her extended family. She was the oldest daughter and her mother had depended on her for help with a troublesome younger sister. She began to cry about how guilty she felt for leaving home, and what a burden she felt she was on her husband. Maybe she should let him off the hook and move back home. Maybe if she got pregnant, her symptoms would go away.

The clinician proposed both a couples meeting and a pharmacotherapy consultation. At this meeting it became clear that both spouses were having adjustment problems, although they had until then focused only on the wife's symptoms. The wife was relieved to find that she was not "just a needy female" and the husband appreciated getting some understanding of his difficulties. There followed a brief course of medication for the panic attacks and a short-term couples intervention.

This case illustrates the value of a family perspective in prevention as well as treatment of the target symptom. By including the husband in the intervention, the clinician had an impact on several other people including the husband and the child not yet conceived. A purely individual or biological approach would also have had an impact on those others, but a less ecologically considered impact.

Just as a therapist inevitably becomes part of a marital triangle, pharmacotherapy will play some role in a couple's relationship struggles. Consider some familiar patterns:

Sometimes a spouse will ignore the medication the same way she or he ignored the patient's suffering in the first place. Then perhaps the medicine bottle will be placed on the kitchen table in plain view so that "someone will notice," or, worse, the psychopharmacologist will be spoken of as "the only one who cares." That same comforting bottle might become lethal during a marital fight while the idealized psychopharmacologist is on vacation.

Worried, possibly intrusive spouses read the *Physician's Desk Reference*, warily monitor side effects, or question the doctor's choice of medication or dosage. Irritated spouses will tell their pouting, argumentative partners to "go take a pill." Subtly undermining mates, eager to be in the driver's seat, suggest that they should "take the wheel" (both concretely and metaphorically) from their medicated spouses. Others see the need for medication as a weakness and question the necessity of each dose.

All of these are understandable and expectable transactions, which are much better worked with and contained when explicitly brought into the treatment. Asking the patient about his or her spouse's attitude toward the medication can yield much valuable information.

The Family with Young Children

The profound wish to relieve children of suffering and the desire to protect them from any unnecessary chemotherapy are values strongly held by both clinicians and parents. The sometimes conflicting pressures of these two values have made the question of medicating children one of the most controversial in our field. Taking into account the recent advances in pediatric pharmacotherapy, each clinician must develop his or her own criteria for when to make a referral and when to question treatment in progress. In evaluating a child's symptoms, one rule of thumb might be: *when a child is the patient, assess the possibility that serious current family dynamics form a context for the symptoms.* It is important to keep in mind, however, that the parents of a sick child need support, not criticism or blame. To ally with parents sympathetically in an effort to understand stresses in the family (including that which results from the child's symptoms) is the aim of the ecology-minded clinician.

>Case 6. A 10-year-old girl complaining of stomach pain was brought to her pediatrician. The pediatrician examined the girl, found no organic problem, and suggested psychotherapy. When the mother called to make an appointment for her daughter, the clinician asked to see the whole family, including the 10-year-old daughter's three siblings.
>When this family came in, it became clear that each member had somatic symptoms. The oldest son had chronic asthma, the 12-year-old daughter complained of headaches which she got while compulsively cleaning the house, and the youngest son had severe joint pain when he slept, waking unable to bend his knees.
>As their story unfolded, it became clear that these children had banded together during a brutal battle and divorce between their parents during which two of the children, including the original identified patient, had been physically abused by their father. Now that the safety crisis was over, they were like shell-shocked war survivors. Fearful that bellyaching would lead to more casualties, each had a different affliction with its own biology.

The sequence of events in the treatment of this case is instructive as well. Each child's acute physical symptoms declined substantially in the first two months of family meetings, which were focused around the divorce. There followed a period during which the mother became acutely agitated and depressed, for which she was successfully treated with pharmacotherapy and individual psychotherapy.

This illustrates how the domino effect just discussed can be observed between children and parents. *When symptoms travel between generations, the psychotherapist's aim is that they travel upward in the hierarchy, so that children are relieved of relationship burdens for which they are not equipped.* When the distress is borne by the adults, they may temporarily become symptomatic. The relationship issues, however, become more accessible and amenable to therapeutic work. It is not uncommon, for example, that the parents' marriage becomes the focus of work in a therapy that began with a child's symptom. Correspondingly, the children's symptoms may improve when parents begin to take active responsibility for their own distress.

Adolescence

In contemporary culture, the greatest family developmental stresses occur when the children are adolescent. Modern expectations of successful separation, independence, and geographical mobility are extraordinary, compared to earlier times when tribal status structures were clear and rites of passage ritually enacted the transitions. In our culture, the tasks of adolescence and launching of a young adult into the world fall almost entirely to the nuclear family itself to accomplish. Great pressure is thus placed on young adults and on their parents' marriages.

When an adolescent patient is evaluated for pharmacotherapy, the clinician's considerations are much the same as when treating younger children. One important difference, however, is the greater likelihood that power and control struggles will be played out around any drugs that are prescribed. Further, since issues of identity and self-esteem are so central, adolescents are more likely to have strong emotional reactions to taking medications. Some will be very resistant to being "a person who has to take medication." Others will embrace an identity as a "mental patient" much more readily than we might wish.

Since the recreational use of drugs is today such a pervasive and charged issue, the use of prescribed psychotropic drugs with adolescents is potentially fraught with misunderstanding and confused attitudes. Educating the patient and his or her family about the actual medical use, effects, and meaning of medications is essential. Facts alone may not be heard, however, unless the clinician is sensitized to the relationship meaning of the symptoms, and the family's attitudes toward the medicine.

Launching, the Empty Nest, and Aging

At the stage of launching, the life-cycle of the family comes full circle. The children are now young adults, whose task it is to establish independent households and new families. The parents now face aging together. Clearly, there are many variations in the ages of parents and the age range of children. There are also wide cultural variations in what defines independence and adulthood. These variations make it perilous to generalize, and the clinician is best advised to work at understanding and respecting the goals and values of the families she or he sees.

Earlier I described some of the systems issues involved in treating the young adult. Emphasis was on the themes of separation and independence. The therapist was advised to assess the state of the parents' marriage and the young adult patient's role in maintaining the family equilibrium. When a parent in this phase of family development presents with symptoms, it is a mistake for the clinician to assume that relations with grown children are not implicated and also potentially at some risk. College counselors have long observed the difficulties students have personally and academically when there is trouble at home. It is helpful, in some instances, for grown children to be viewed as resources and potential allies in the treatment of aging parents in this context. Indeed, grown children often derive unexpected therapeutic gain from becoming involved in their parents' treatment.

Case 7. A 27-year-old man was worried about his father, aged 67 years, who had retired from his professional firm the previous year. Dad seemed depressed, even morbid, saying how he felt he had completed his work and was ready if God wished to take him. He also had a tremor, like someone with Parkinson's disease. As was typical in this family, nobody spoke directly of this, but each of the grown children was concerned, privately speculating on what was wrong and worrying that he was going to give up and die.

The parents' marriage had always had problems. Since junior high, when the family moved from the city to the small town where the patient finished high school, his father had kept an apartment in the city and came home every weekend. Even though this was officially a practical matter, everyone knew the distance kept the bickering and fighting to a minimum. Now that dad was retired, he was home all day, with no kids at home. Nobody expected the parents' relationship to change, and the idea of couples therapy was so alien that the patient knew there was no point in bringing it up. Efforts to interest the father in part-time work or local politics just fell on deaf ears.

The patient decided to get more directly involved after his father returned from a visit to the family doctor with a prescription for an antidepressant. His sister, who was a mental health professional, said she knew a good family-sensitive pharmacotherapist, and they agreed together to make sure their father had a consultation.

It is rare for siblings to be so equitable in distributing responsibility for aging parents. It is much more common for there to be one or more who take the most responsibility, followed either by criticism from the others or by resentment of the unfair burden. Not infrequently these issues are played out in disputes over the parents' will and estate and can be a turning point in the history of a family.

This case raises a number of other issues related to this developmental phase. There are often complicated differential diagnostic questions — as illnesses, other medications, and physical changes associated with aging combine with emotional responses resulting from inevitable losses. Also, older people are less likely to be referred for either psychotherapy or pharmacotherapy consultations. Frequently they are treated with psychotropic medications by their internists or by physicians from other specialties. Their needs may thus come to the clinician's attention indirectly, as in the case example.

When a confused or disabled elderly person receives pharmacotherapy, family members are often called on to help with appointments and compliance. Issues of passivity and responsibility arise, as the ostensibly helping relative sometimes appears to be taking over in a way that encourages the patient to take less and less care of himself or herself, thereby increasing the patient's dependence on others.

Older couples, having lived together for as long as 20 years, rely on long-established patterns of adaptation. Depression may occur in the spouses of people whose major physical illnesses (such as strokes, heart attacks, or cancer) have disrupted long-term patterns of interaction and mutual care. Depression in response to the untimely misfortunes of children and grandchildren is also common.

Anxiety disorders and paranoid reactions in response to the loss of cognitive or physical function can be frustrating to caretaking family members. A psychoeducational approach, in which family members are helped to understand their elderly relative's medical-emotional situation, can be of great help. When symptoms are better understood, family members are less likely to view the patient as stubborn, mistrustful, or passive aggressive.

Treating people in this phase of family development poses some special problems for the clinician. As Simon has noted, the therapist's position in his or her own family life-cycle interacts with the developmental position of the family in treatment.[45] When treating a patient who is the age of the therapist's parents, the therapist may have more difficulty sustaining a systems perspective; this, in turn, tends to make the authority and scientific status of pharmacotherapy more appealing. As a result, therapists may underestimate both the patient's strengths and their own capacity to intervene effectively.

CONCLUSION

Psychotropic medications, used properly, can reduce unnecessary suffering, help to maintain stability, and greatly enhance progress in psychotherapy. They can also potentially have disruptive side effects on the equilibrium of the pharmacotherapy patient's family. When integrated into a treatment program that includes awareness of systems issues, positive medication effects and compliance can be enhanced, while environmental side effects are prevented or contained. The family ecological perspective presented here can guide the clinician through the many complex decisions that must be made when pharmacotherapy consultation or treatment is considered.

The psychotherapist should take into account the patient's place in the family's structure, the family developmental themes, the family's adaptation to the patient's symptoms, and the attitudes of family members toward medication. Then, if a pharmacotherapy referral is made, the clinician is better equipped to enhance medication compliance and to improve the likelihood of a successful intervention. The psychotherapist who brings these considerations to a combined treatment can help the family to cope with the patient's illness when it is chronic, readapt when there is improvement, and consider the implications of the symptoms and the treatment for their enduring relationships.

REFERENCES

1. Gurman AS, Kniskern DP: Family therapy outcome research: Knowns and unknowns, in Gurman AS, Kniskern DP (eds): *Handbook of Family Therapy*. New York, Brunner/Mazel, 1981, pp 742–775.
2. Minuchin S: *Families and Family Therapy*. Cambridge, Harvard University Press, 1974.
3. Minuchin S, Rosman BO, Baker L: *Psychosomatic Families*. Cambridge, Harvard University Press, 1978.
4. Vaughn CE, Leff JP: The influence of family and social factors on the course of psychiatric illness. *Br J Psychiatry* 1976;129:125–137.
5. Brown GW, Birley JL, Wing JK: Influence of family life on the course of schizophrenic disorders: A replication. *Br J Psychiatry* 1972;121:241–258.
6. Faloon IR, Boyd JL, McGill CW, et al: Family management in the prevention of exacerbations of schizophrenia: A controlled study. *N Engl J Med* 1982;306(24):1437–1440.
7. Faloon IR, Boyd JL, McGill CW, et al: Family management in the prevention of morbidity of schizophrenia. *Arch Gen Psychiatry* 1985;42:887–896.
8. Vaughn CE, Snyder KS, Jones S, et al: Factors in schizophrenic relapse. *Arch Gen Psychiatry* 1984;41:1169–1177.
9. Strang JS, Faloon IR, Moss HB, et al: Effects of family therapy on treatment compliance in schizophrenia. *Psychopharmacol Bull* 1981; 17(3):87–88.
10. Goldstein MJ, Rodnick EH, Evans JR, et al: Drug and family therapy in the aftercare of acute schizophrenics. *Arch Gen Psychiatry* 1978;35:1169–1177.
11. Hogarty GE, Anderson CM, Reiss DJ: Family psychoeducation, social skills training, and medication in schizophrenia: The long and short of it. *Psychopharmacol Bull* 1987;23(1):12–13.
12. Rounsaville BJ, Weissman MM, Prusoff BA, et al: Marital disputes and treatment outcome in depressed women. *Compr Psychiatry* 1979; 20(5):483–490.

13. Demers RG, Davis LS: The influence of prophylactic lithium treatment on marital adjustment. *Compr Psychiatry* 1971;12(4):348–363.
14. Fitzgerald R: Mania as a message: Treatment with family therapy and lithium carbonate. *Am J Psychother* 1972;26:547–555.
15. Ablon SL, Davenport YB, Gershon ES, et al: The married manic. *Am J Orthopsychiatry* 1975;45(5):854–866.
16. Mayo JA: Marital therapy with manic-depressive patients treated with lithium. *Compr Psychiatry* 1979;20(5):419–426.
17. Meeks DE, Kelly C: Family therapy with families of recovering alcoholics. *Q J Study Alcohol* 1970;31:399–413.
18. Greene BL, Lustig N, Lee RR: Marital therapy when one spouse has a primary affective disorder. *Am J Psychiatry* 1976;133(7):827–830.
19. Davenport YB, Ebert MH, Adland ML, et al: Couples group therapy as an adjunct to lithium maintenance of the manic patient. *Am J of Orthopsychiatry* 1977;47(3):495–502.
20. Kohl RN: Pathologic reactions of marital partners to improvement of patients. *Am J Psychiatry* 1962;118:1036–1041.
21. Hurvitz N: Marital problems following psychotherapy with one spouse. *J Consult Psychol* 1967;31(1):38–47.
22. Fox RE: The effect of psychotherapy on the spouse. *Fam Process* 1968;7(7):7–16.
23. Goldner V: Feminism and family therapy. *Fam Process* 1985;24(1):31–45.
24. Kaplan AG: Female or male therapists for women patients: New formulations. *Psychiatry* 1985;48(5):111–121.
25. Napier A, Whitaker C: *The Family Crucible.* New York, Harper and Row, 1978.
26. Aponte H, Hoffman L: The open door: A structural approach to a family with an anorectic child. *Fam Process* 1973;12(1):1–44.
27. Carter EA, McGoldrick M: *The Family Life Cycle.* New York, Gardner Press, 1980.
28. Cannon W: *The Wisdom of the Body.* New York, WW Norton and Company, 1939.
29. von Bertalanffy L: General systems theory. *Gen Systems* 1956;1:1–10.
30. Jackson DD: The study of the family. *Fam Process* 1964;4:1–20.
31. Bateson G: *Steps to an Ecology of Mind.* New York, Ballantine Books, 1972.
32. Weiner N: *Cybernetics.* New York, Wiley, 1948.
33. Dell P, Goolishian H: Order through fluctuation: An evolutionary epistemology for human systems. Paper presented at the Annual Scientific Meeting of the A.K. Rice Institute, Houston, Texas, March 1979.
34. Hoffman L: The family life cycle and discontinuous change, in Carter EA, McGoldrick M (eds): *The Family Life Cycle.* New York, Gardner Press, 1980.

35. Hodley T, Jacob T, Milliones J, et al: The relationship between family developmental crisis and the appearance of symptoms in a family member. *Fam Process* 1974;13(2):207–214.
36. Solomon M: A developmental conceptual premise for family therapy. *Fam Process* 1973;12(2):179–188.
37. Shapiro E: Toward a theory of family development. Unpublished Comprehensives Paper, University of Massachusetts, Amherst, Massachusetts, 1977.
38. Erikson E: *Childhood and Society*. New York, WW Norton and Company, 1950.
39. Bowen M (anonymous): Toward the differentiation of a self in one's own family, in Framo JL (ed): *Family Interaction*. New York, Springer Publishing Company, 1972, pp 111–173.
40. Haley J: *Strategies of Psychotherapy*. New York, Grune and Stratton, 1963.
41. Kohut H: *The Restoration of the Self*. New York, International Universities Press, 1977.
42. Maruyama M: The second cybernetics: Deviation amplifying mutual causal processes, in Buckley W (ed): *Modern Systems Research for the Behavioral Sciences: A Sourcebook*. Chicago, Adline Publishing Co, 1968.
43. Hoffman L: Deviation amplifying processes in natural groups, in Haley J (ed): *Changing Families*. New York, Grune and Stratton, 1971.
44. Boszormenyi-Nagy I, Spark G: *Invisible Loyalties*. New York, Harper and Row, 1973.
45. Simon RM: Family life cycle issues in the therapy system, in Carter EA, McGoldrick M (eds): *The Family Life Cycle*. New York, Gardner Press, 1980.

4

Some Dimensions of Transference in Combined Treatment

Janna M. Smith

This chapter discusses some aspects of transference as they relate to psychopharmacology and combined treatment. Even in the most straightforward medical situation, the prescribing of medication by a physician to a patient is an act that has an emotional dimension. In treatments that attempt to affect people's psychological states, the emotional dimensions of prescribing medication are complex. We know, for example, that psychoactive medications alter mental functioning through pharmacologic effects that are helpful or toxic. But we have also come to understand that mental states can affect responses to medications. In a combined treatment, the caregivers and patient's feelings toward the medication and toward each other affect treatment in ways that are important to consider.

When Freud spoke about transference in the *Introductory Lectures on Psychoanalysis*, he described how in analytic treatment patients would often experience, in their relationship to the doctor, feelings which did not "arise from the present situation" and did not "apply to the person of the doctor" but which were repeating something that had happened to the patient at an earlier time.[1] Freud recognized that analyzing these feelings would provide one important avenue toward untangling patients' emotional difficulties. Moreover, he learned through hard experi-

79

ence that not analyzing transference could lead to undesirable consequences like aborted treatments or proposals of marriage. What Freud did not say is that in contemporary treatment situations that include a patient, a therapist, a pharmacotherapist, and a pill, the transference issues can become more complex than the landing patterns of airplanes at an overcrowded airport. The patient can experience transference feelings toward the pharmacotherapist, toward the therapist, and toward the pill itself; the psychotherapist might have transference feelings about the pharmacotherapist while the pharmacotherapist has them about the psychotherapist, and both pharmacotherapist and therapist are likely to have different transference feelings about medication. Additionally, each party involved will have impressions of the others which are not transferential, but which at moments are hard to distinguish from transference. For example, a patient could accurately perceive something about his psychotherapist's reluctance to have him take medication and complain about it to the pharmacotherapist, who would then have to attempt to tease apart the transference issues from the reality.

In other words, it is impressive that with so many different reactions crossing paths the situation can be monitored at all. Fortunately, much of the time some of these phenomena are peripheral. The multiple transferences can be held in perspective. Nevertheless, as with the air traffic controller, to ignore the screen is to invite disaster.

In this chapter I focus on some of the different transference situations that typically arise in combined treatment and discuss how they influence the clinical work of the nonprescribing therapist. But before I proceed, I want to mention an important point. Transference is one of those words, like "dream," or "love," or "life," that refers to a continent so vast and diverse that the kind of abstract reference I make to some of its dimensions will continually fail to do justice to it in its entirety.

I start by looking at the patient's relationship to the pharmacotherapist. A patient seeing a psychotherapist may have a preexisting relationship with a pharmacotherapist, may start both treatments simultaneously, or may be referred to the pharmacotherapist after a period in psychotherapy. While the temporal juxtaposition of treatments will have its impact on transference issues, the first point is that when there are two therapists involved there are two psychotherapeutic relationships. As Goldhamer pointed out, "a psychotherapeutic relationship is created whenever a patient presents to a physician in emotional distress and the physician prescribes a drug".[2] We know from inpatient and from day treatment experience that patients can manage simultaneous treatment relationships, but what is created here is often more and less than just a second relationship. It is *more* because our collective idealization of medicine and the power of doctors, combined with their real capacity to offer dramatic cures, is such that in many instances the relationship will evoke significant feelings particularly with regard to the doctor's authority, and the patient's transference to that authority. (As Gutheil pointed out, this situation is heightened by the fact that psychiatrists are inclined to become much more authoritarian when they are functioning in their roles as pharmacotherapists than they would ever dream of being when they practice psychotherapy.[3])

The relationship is *less* because in many instances the visits to the pharmacotherapist can be brief, infrequent, and largely focused on symptomatology. Ironically, these qualities of the relationship can further enhance the intensity of the transference because the temporal constraints leave the patient less opportunity to alter a distorted appraisal of the pharmacotherapist.

THE PATIENT'S TRANSFERENCE TO THE PHARMACOTHERAPIST

Each patient's transference to the pharmacotherapist as an authority figure is ultimately unique because of its basis in the individual's experience; affectively each will fall somewhere on the spectrum of very positive to very negative. If the patient trusts the pharmacotherapist, and she experiences that caregiver either as trying to be helpful or as actually being helpful (ie, giving a drug which provides symptomatic relief), or if she feels that medication legitimizes her sense that she is ill, the patient is likely to experience some degree of *positive transference*. If, on the other hand, the patient experiences the pharmacotherapist as being untrustworthy, indifferent, callous, or unconcerned; or if the medication produces unpleasant side effects; or if taking medicine at all aggravates a sense of personal imperfection and narcissistic injury, she is likely to experience some degree of *negative transference*.

These of course are generalizations, and it must be clear that an enormous number of variables are involved in determining where on the spectrum the transference will fall. Among them are the patient's personal history, current dynamics and character structure, the pharmacotherapist's style and character, the nature of the original referral, the transference issues with other therapists, and the characteristics of the medicine. Furthermore, transference is like a jellyfish or a sponge, one of those animate creatures that is in fact a constantly evolving colony of other creatures. If, for example, a patient says that she likes the pharmacotherapist because he reminds her of her father, it seems like a simple, straightforward statement. But to which father is she referring? The pre-oedipal one? The father of adolescence? The aging one? In a fairly well-integrated patient there is perhaps a benign composite father transference which comes forward and does good service in a low-key relationship, but as the relationship deepens different fathers come into ascendancy and can totally alter the affective cast of the word. Furthermore, a sicker patient or one who has been more traumatized often does not experience an integrated sense of father at all. The point I would like to make here is that any patient who is undergoing dynamically oriented psychotherapy is likely to experience periods of unconscious turbulence that will impact on other treatment relationships.

Nevertheless, let me make some generalizations. First of all, if the patient has a basically positive transference to the pharmacotherapist (and especially if it is coupled with a good alliance with her therapist), it is likely to enhance her willingness to comply with treatment: to follow through on a drug trial or to pursue several drug trials until a useful medication is found. The phenomenon of the placebo effect suggests that the efficacy of the drug might even be increased in the instance of a positive transference, something I will explore in greater detail when I examine patients' transferences to the medication itself.

A negative transference is more likely to result in noncompliance, though exceptions occur in situations in which the medicine is so attractive on its own terms (as benzodiazepines might be to some people for relief of anxiety, or tricyclics might be to a sleep-deprived person) as to override the effect of a negative transference. Exceptions can also occur when the negative transference solves other dynamic difficulties. For instance, if a patient experiences a sense of disloyalty to a psychotherapist by seeking medication from a pharmacotherapist, one resolution to the conflict might be to form a negative transference to the medicating doctor, but still take the medicine. Or another example occurs in a situation in which a patient experiences his need for medicine as a narcissistic injury but gains relief from the medicine and so attempts to restitute his self-esteem by devaluing the pharmacotherapist.

HOW DOES THE PATIENT'S TRANSFERENCE TO THE PHARMACOTHERAPIST AFFECT THE PSYCHOTHERAPY?

Basically, there are as many answers to this question as there are combined treatments. To begin with, it is important to remember that the psychotherapy itself is often deeply affected when a patient takes medication. As Beitman pointed out, medicines that reduce anxiety or relieve depression can allow patients to begin a therapy when it otherwise might seem too overwhelming.[4] So too, in an ongoing therapy, antipsychotic medication can allow a schizophrenic, who might otherwise be too disorganized to be coherent, to speak. Properly chosen medications can relieve the experiences of flooding in post-traumatic stress syndrome and help a patient to manage the working through of particularly horrid events. Thus, there are some instances when the therapeutic process could not begin, or could not continue, without medication. It would be intolerably painful. On the most concrete level I am suggesting that sometimes the use of medication is necessary to allow psychotherapy to proceed. While in many many instances, medication compliance is heightened by first having a working relationship with a psychotherapist, in other instances, the patient's positive transference to the medicating doctor is what allows him to take medicine and thus make himself available to treatment. A corollary here is that many patients who refuse to seek psychotherapy will visit a medical doctor or a pharmacotherapist, feeling that taking medicine is less shameful than talking to a "shrink." A patient who comes to feel a positive transference toward the physician (and the medicine) will become more likely to accept a referral for psychotherapy.

A positive transference to a pharmacotherapist can enhance a psychotherapy by increasing a patient's overall sense of well-being. If the patient experiences both therapists positively most of the time, she can feel cared about and safe, and her sense of empowerment and healing can be significantly heightened.

> Case 1. A woman in her forties with severe bipolar affective disorder had been hospitalized at least once a year during the preceding ten years. After one hospitalization, the patient's pharmacotherapist, whom she liked, referred her to a psychotherapist in a public clinic with whom the patient developed a solid alliance and basically a positive transference. I say "basically" because the patient was severely ill, and frequently had intense feelings of rage about the injustice, abuse, and deprivation she had suffered, and during those times would devalue each therapist directly, and one to the other. But neither therapist joined the devaluation of the other, and both continued to behave supportively toward her. Furthermore, her psychotherapist used the vacillations in the transference as a basis for hypothesizing and analyzing some of the patient's familial loyalty conflicts, and the patient improved. She stayed on her medication, stopped needing hospitalization, and started working part-time after 20 years of unemployment. She also ended an ungratifying relationship and started one that proved to be more gratifying. During the years of treatment, the patient would often say to the therapist, "I know you and Dr G both really care about me, and you know I love you like a sister and I love him too. And they told my husband when I was first hospitalized that I would be there forever so he left me, but they were wrong, that doesn't have to be. I can get better." The patient's positive feelings toward two therapists increased her hope, and increased her capacity to manage the anxiety of attempting to rebuild her life.

A patient's positive transference to the pharmacotherapist can sometimes help her to ride out rough times in her relationship with her psychotherapist. If she views the two therapists as working together for her treatment, she is likely to be more reticent about totally rejecting one part of a team. In some instances, the patient will allow the pharmacotherapist to encourage her to work out her difficulties partly because it reflects her own ambivalence, but partly because she experiences him positively and is thus more likely to let herself trust his perspective.

One of the most common difficulties for the psychotherapist of the patient's positive transference to the pharmacotherapist is feeling oneself as the recipient of the transference to the devalued object. Typically in these instances, a therapist is seen as the depressed and powerless person, beside whom the pharmacotherapist is viewed as powerful and efficacious. While with many patients these feelings can be productively explored, with some it is difficult. Here is a case example:

Case 2. A woman who had suffered from a psychotic illness since childhood was receiving psychotherapy from a social worker and medications from a psychiatrist. When the psychotherapist went on vacation, the pharmacotherapist covered the patient and met with her several times. He monitored her medicine and talked with her about current concerns and symptomatology. When the psychotherapist returned, the patient was angry at her. She said she wanted to see the pharmacotherapist exclusively since he was able both to help her with medication and to talk to her. Initially, the patient's reaction seemed to relate exclusively to the psychotherapist's vacation. The feelings, though, were slow to resolve in spite of consistent attention to them in their current and historic manifestations. It became clear that the patient was reliving her familial experience of viewing her father as omnipotent but unwilling to share his magic with her. It was very difficult to help the patient gain perspective on these feelings, and the psychotherapist experienced an increasing sense of helplessness and hopelessness about the treatment.

As I have suggested earlier, the patient's negative transference to the pharmacotherapist will sometimes make it more difficult for the patient to sustain a drug trial, or to experience a positive sense of the drug. At times, the patient's negative transference can disrupt a psychotherapy.

Case 3. A man in psychotherapy for a severe narcissistic disorder was referred to a pharmacotherapist for treatment of occasional psychotic symptoms. Immediately, the patient decided that his new caregiver was extremely authoritarian and insensitive. These were the words he had also used to describe his hated stepfather. The psychotherapist experienced a sudden change in the patient's feelings toward her. The patient had newly cast her in the role of his remarried mother, and experienced her as disloyal in the extreme for not joining him in renouncing the pharmacotherapist. The psychotherapist was caught off guard by the vehemence of the patient's emotions, which were a departure from his previous behavior. In time, she realized that she was reenacting the mother's historical role of a pacifying go-between rather than effectively helping the man to gain perspective on his transferential feelings.

The point I wish to make here is that the referral to a pharmacotherapist disrupted the psychotherapy by suddenly involving the psychotherapist in a transference very different from the previous transference. The therapist initially felt unsure how to understand the new feelings toward her. While the patient's reaction to the pharmacotherapist illustrated so vividly a triangular dilemma that had had a strong impact on the patient, the therapist felt less prepared to work with it because it was such a sudden and strong reaction to a colleague, which seemed to come out of nowhere, and because the patient immediately involved the therapist in a ready-made role that was different from the transference in the individual treatment during the time leading up to the referral. While this particular treatment was able to continue, there are some in which the disruption of the referral can be so significant as to prematurely end the psychotherapy.

As indicated in these examples, the patient's transference to the pharmacotherapist provides both clinical difficulties and invaluable material for the psychotherapeutic work. First of all, it can provide a second reference point for the therapist about the nature of the patient's transference issues. So, for a simple example, if a patient experiences the therapist as alternately cold and intrusive, and experiences the pharmacotherapist the same way, the therapist will be clearer that the transference is just that. Sometimes it is especially useful when the two therapists are of different genders for it can allow the therapist to know more about the patient's transference issues with people of the opposite sex.

While psychotherapists who are not practicing combined treatment successfully explore these transference issues alone, what is helpful in combined treatment is that if the therapist and the pharmacotherapist know each other, the therapist has her own sense of the pharmacotherapist against which to weigh the patient's presentation and thus can have an easier time separating reality from transference. Of course, the therapist must remain open to the possibility that the physician treats the patient differently from the way he treats his colleagues, and she must not casually dismiss the patient's perspective as transferential.

Second, because the patient knows that there is at least a symbolic connection between the pharmacotherapist and the therapist, the pharmacotherapist can become a useful object on whom difficult transference feelings may be displaced. This phenomenon allows the therapist the opportunity to work with these feelings in a way which, particularly with more disturbed patients, can be tolerated. For example, in an instance when the pharmacotherapist was about to leave on vacation, a patient felt free to rage openly about the hardship that the vacation entailed for him. While it is likely that he was primarily describing his reaction to the therapist's longer and often, for him, more difficult vacation, he could do so without having to feel as vulnerable or as aggressive. In turn, the therapist could explore the material without feeling so much guilt or anger.

Many people who have serious character disorders, or who tend to develop intense transferences, or who are particularly afraid of the intensity of some of their feelings, will experience relief at being able at times to explore these feelings first in the less intense relationships. An example is of a patient who felt deeply enraged at her therapist when the therapist became pregnant. Part of her feeling seemed to stem from her memory of the way her mother used to abandon her during childhood to care for her alcoholic father, but the patient could not tell the therapist directly about her feelings because she felt extremely guilty about being angry at a pregnant woman, and also because she feared that she could magically damage the unborn baby. She told her pharmacotherapist about her rage, and then, feeling relieved, was able to tell her therapist about what she had said to the doctor.

THE TRANSFERENCES BETWEEN THE PSYCHOTHERAPIST AND THE PHARMACOTHERAPIST

As I have noted earlier, the involvement of two caregivers creates two psychotherapeutic relationships. And it seems clear that these relationships are not separate even if the caregivers do not know each other and do not speak together. For even in this situation they are linked in the patient's conscious and unconscious by a multitude of complex pathways relating to the way that the particular patient experiences relationships and manages feeling. The two therapists are further linked by their own relationship and by their transference feelings toward each other. At times, these transferences impact on the patient's treatment.

By and large, these two groups of professionals have not been notably adept at working out their cooperative efforts. Thus the transferential field is often framed by mutual biases. The psychotherapist may feel suspicious of pharmacotherapists and view them as people who do not value psychotherapy, who are overbearing and authoritarian, and who wield undue power. The pharmacotherapist may feel that psychotherapists are hostile to his expertise, or conversely that they have magical and unrealistic expectations of the effect that the doctor and the medicine can have, or that they wish to burden doctors with the medical responsibility for difficult patients. Each can feel displaced or threatened by the other, and both can feel competitive wishes to be the more talented, more valued caretaker to the patient. If, for example, either or both therapists possesses a strong and rivalrous sibling transference toward the other, the patient can become the object of that competitive wish — an experience that, while sometimes narcissistically gratifying, is often disruptive and overwhelming.

Positive feelings can bring their own jeopardy when they become the bases for a transference where either or both therapists idealize the other, seeing the other as the repository of their missing virtues or as a partner mirroring their own strengths. In such instances legitimate conflict and disagreement are repressed or ignored, and separate opinions are not sanctioned.

These transferential feelings are most harmful to the patient when the therapists are either unconscious of them or unquestioning of their own perspective. For while the therapists are busy not examining them, the patients will be, and will quickly — often unconsciously — pick up the subliminal attitudes, which will influence their own attitudes and their overall drug experience.

Case 4. A number of years ago, I shared a patient who had schizoaffective disorder with a psychiatric resident who prescribed his medications. I was just out of school, and felt that the amount of authority and income that residents garnered compared with social workers was unjust, and I was quick to feel slighted if I felt that one was playing doctor at my expense. The particular resident seemed high-handed to me, and immediately fell heir to all of my negative transference toward doctors. The patient, a man, liked the doctor, whom he felt was an easy-going likeable guy. In this instance the patient, who was very disturbed and prone to distort relationships, probably had a less distorted view of the situation than I did. Furthermore, because he liked this doctor, the patient was complying well in taking his medicine. Nevertheless, one day the patient had a disagreement with the doctor, which made him angry and which he reported to me in great, perhaps even inflated detail. I sat and nodded judiciously, saying little, but still conveying to the patient the rather smug idea that I had known about the doctor's limitations and was glad that the patient was finally seeing reality. You can imagine how harmful such a stance by a therapist can be for a patient. Had my own feelings been more objective, I might have realized that the patient, whose parents had continually triangulated him into their many battles, was sensing a replication in his contemporary situation. My acting out led to guilt feelings and loyalty conflicts for him about his medication, which he handled alternately by not speaking with me about his good feelings toward the doctor and by not taking the medicine and spending more time psychotic.

Of course, this kind of acting out does not just go in one direction. Who has not had a patient return from a drug consultation reporting that the pharmacotherapist said psychotherapy is pointless for the ailment, or that treatment is more efficacious when the prescribing and talking are done by the same person? Another common problem occurs when the pharmacotherapist opens up a dynamic issue which is unrelated to the medication but which intensifies the patient's positive transference to the extent that the patient returns to psychotherapy complaining that "Dr. X understands me better". Such comments, irritating though they may be, are good grist for the therapeutic mill. The psychotherapist must avoid responding to them, however, as if they were statements of fact. If the psychotherapist is aware of his own transference to the prescribing doctor, it is much easier to use such material in the psychotherapy.

Patients are acutely sensitive to any idealization between their therapists, and will comment on it, often bitterly, to the degree to which it negates their capacity for a fair hearing. They will also be tremendously interested in doping out who really is the boss between the collaborators, and will quickly pick up on situations where there are authority conflicts, untoward competitiveness, or covert agendas.

Another instance when my own transference feelings to a pharmacotherapist interfered with patient care occurred in a situation when I had been referred a psychotic patient by a psychiatrist who had only recently stopped supervising me. He was to do the prescribing and I would do the treatment. The psychiatrist had been a kindly supervisor, and I admired him. I thus felt receptive to his formulations about our patient's dynamics. One of the patient's problems was that he was constantly insisting on new treatments because he wanted magically to have situations changed so that he would not have to work out discord, or face limitations. Consequently, the psychiatrist believed that it was important to take a hard line with the patient when he demanded treatment changes of any kind. This position was reasonable, but it became problematic on several occasions when the patient was not acting out, but actually expressing legitimate distress with real problems. Knowing that our policy was to interpret complaints, I had a harder time listening objectively to the patient when he tried to convey the reality of his situation. On the other hand, if I began to agree with him that, for example, he ought to try a new medication, the psychiatrist would remind me of the formulation, and I, because I overvalued the psychiatrist's opinion and enjoyed not taking full clinical responsibility, would fail to disagree with him or help to distinguish between those times when the formulation was the more important variable, and those when the patient legitimately was pointing to a real problem about which he needed support and assistance. I might add that I was helped through this situation by the patient, who found some psychotic and some not so psychotic ways of commenting on my transference.

THE MEANING OF THE MEDICINE

Years ago the Rolling Stones wrote a song called "Mother's Little Helper," in which they commented sardonically on the importance of "a little yellow pill" to mother, "though she isn't really ill". The Jefferson Airplane, during the same era, sang about the pills that Alice swallowed which made her grow alternately tiny and very large. Both songs offer commentary on the Pill, capital P, as it exists within contemporary culture as a symbol of magical alterations and enhanced capacities, or conversely of covert addictions and grotesque transformations, a manifestation of our collective transference hopes and fears.

Medication is the object of many strong conscious and unconscious feelings, and our relationship to it collectively or individually tends to be complex, so much so that it is not possible to do justice to the subject in the little space that I have here. I will do my best to offer a brief overview and will focus on describing some of the transference feelings that patients, pharmacotherapists, and psychotherapists bring to medications.

First let me note that medication includes both the substance itself and the process by which it is obtained by a patient, usually from a doctor or a nurse in the form of a prescription, though sometimes as actual pills or as an injection. When we speak of transference to medication, we are not completely correct insofar as transference properly applies to feelings toward people. Feelings about medication are better conceptualized as akin to transitional phenomena, as part objects or as nonhuman recipients of transference displacements.

In his paper on medication and transitional phenomena, Robert Hausner noted that "medication giving comprises one of the few phenomena in which a concrete object related to the therapist is possessed by the patient; it is the only one in which the object is actually ingested by the patient. This situation may immediately be recognized as an implicit repetition of the early maternal dyad: something is received from the mother and becomes part of the infant, thus satisfying an inchoate need."[5] Because of these qualities, Hausner suggested, medication can function on an other than pharmacological level to soothe patients, ward off unpleasant affects, allow the management of separations, and otherwise modulate internal states. A common example of this dimension of medication is an instance when a therapist is about to go on vacation, and a patient requests a prescription, "just in case." Furthermore, the placebo effect, the documented observation that sugar pills can sometimes make people better, probably draws some of its efficacy from the transitional object dimension of medication.

The transitional object role is but one of the functions of medication, and it is important to note here that a complete equation of the two is inaccurate in that unlike a typical inanimate transitional object, medication often initiates complex physiological activity. Nevertheless, it is an important one to comprehend in that unwitting therapists can often be disruptive by not understanding the transitional dimension of the medicine. Gutheil offers an example of the new resident who precipitates a decompensation of a patient by changing all of the medications from those prescribed by the departed doctor to whom the patient was attached.[3] Or as one schizophrenic woman said to her new pharmacotherapist, "I don't like your Cogentin, I want the kind my last doctor gave me." Therapists who are against the patient's continuing with a medication can make the same mistake, even if they are clinically correct about a particular contraindication. It is worth noting that in many instances, though the pharmacotherapist has prescribed the medication, it can be equally or more imbued with feelings about the psychotherapist. On the other hand, sometimes the nonprescribing therapist feels out in the cold — like the father of a new baby who wishes he could nurse the child.

Pills also become the recipients of displaced feelings about other people in the patient's life. These displacements provide much of the dynamic basis of noncompliance. A patient who gets mad at a parent, for example, might stop taking pills in an effort to punish his parent. He may have little insight into his motives, noting only that at times (of anger) the taste of the medication is physically revolting. A paranoid patient may experience a pill as the concrete manifestation of an authority's wish to do him harm. So, too, the medication can sometimes become the vehicle of a patient's transference hate toward either caregiver. When this occurs, an attempted or completed suicide can be the tragic result. As Howard Book noted, a patient in remission can see medication as the hated symbol of his chronic illness.[6] And as Havens pointed out, the pill may represent for the patient the return to an unbearable status quo in his life from which only psychosis temporarily frees him.[7] This last point deserves to be underscored, as so often in combined treatment we attempt to help patients by relieving symptoms that might have meanings we do not understand. Certainly letting a patient suffer unnecessarily while we explore the dynamic implications of symptoms is cruel. To allow ourselves to avoid the painful process of understanding the meaning to a patient of his condition, however, would be a serious error.

The pharmacotherapist and the psychotherapist may experience medication as a transitional object at times. When a patient is having a difficult time, for example, the therapists may soothe themselves by imagining the containment the medication will provide. As Hausner pointed out, sometimes the mother can become too reliant on the transitional object, because it is easier to have the child attached to it than to her.[5] It strikes me that this dilemma is experienced by many therapists. How often, when a patient appears more anxious or depressed, does the psychotherapist make a referral to a pharmacotherapist or does a pharmacotherapist reach for his prescription pad? If the therapist is overanxious about the patient's affect, he may attempt inappropriately to deflect the feeling from himself onto the drug. We should be warned that along this route can lie fetishism and other addictive processes. In other words, it is all too easy to communicate to a patient the message that his feelings cannot be borne within a relationship. This is a message many patients have already received in earlier situations, and it is often harmful to the psychotherapeutic process. When a medication is used in this way, a therapist can confirm a patient's fear that it is impossible to make use of other people to help feelings become manageable. Conversely, a therapist can confirm a patient's hopelessness, or anger a patient by ignoring legitimate requests for an examination of the biological component of his illness. Recently a patient who came to our clinic was seeking out a new psychotherapist because he was convinced that there was a biological component to his mood swings and his therapist did not believe in psychotropic medications. In this instance, the psychotherapist's immoderate negative transference to medication ended a therapy.

The pharmacotherapist can have an additional transference toward medication. He can see it as a physical representation of his expertise and his wish to help. He may thus feel unduly disturbed when the patient is noncompliant. In these situations some pharmacotherapists may mistakenly fall back on lecturing patients rather than understanding them. In part, this could well be a response to feelings of being rejected or disobeyed as well as concern that the patient receive treatment as prescribed.

CONCLUSION

Let me end by reiterating that it is simply not possible for any therapist to understand all of the transference issues in a combined treatment at a given time. Nevertheless, it is clear that the pharmacotherapist and the psychotherapist will have a better working relationship, and one that is more useful to the patient, if they make the effort to understand the transference dimensions of their common endeavor. Furthermore, such an understanding is likely to improve the patient's medication compliance (or at least to offer a more useful understanding of the failure of compliance), and it is likely to contribute to the patient's sense of well-being and his recovery process.

REFERENCES

1. Freud S: Transference (Lecture XXVID, in Introductory Lectures on Psychoanalysis, in Strachey JS (ed): *The Standard Edition of the*

Complete Psychological Works of Sigmund Freud, XIV. London, The Hogarth Press, 1963, pp 431–447.
2. Goldhamer PM: Psychotherapy and pharmacotherapy: The challenge of integration. *Can J Psychiatry* 1983;28:173–177.
3. Gutheil TG: The psychology of psychopharmacology. *Bull Menninger Clin* 1982;46:321–330.
4. Beitman BD: Pharmacotherapy as an intervention during the stages of psychotherapy. *Am J Psychother* 1981;35:115–117.
5. Hausner R: Medication and transitional phenomena. *Int J Psychoanal Psychother* 1985–6;11:375–407.
6. Book HE: Some psychodynamics of non-compliance. *Can J Psychiatry* 1987;32:206–213.
7. Havens LL: Some difficulties in giving schizophrenic and borderline patients medication. *Psychiatry* 1968;31:44–50.

5

Intertherapist Conflict in Combined Treatment

James M. Ellison
Janna M. Smith

Whenever two professionals from different disciplines work together, some clashing of viewpoints is likely to occur. In a collaboration between a psychotherapist and a pharmacotherapist, these clashes can diminish a patient's gains and aggravate both clinicians. Seemingly incompatible theoretical viewpoints, different priorities for treatment, personality factors, and issues of competence can lead to exasperating intertherapist conflicts in combined treatment.

Collaboration, nonetheless, is often valuable and increasingly widespread. In a recent survey, nearly 80% of psychologists and more than 60% of psychiatrists reported participating in combined treatment.[1] This chapter will explore some of the reasons why psychotherapists and pharmacotherapists choose to collaborate. It will also explore some of the roots of conflict among caregivers and offer suggestions for its prevention or resolution.

COMBINED TREATMENT'S BENEFITS ARE NOT WITHOUT RISK

Mounting evidence from clinical research supports the advisability of combining medication with psychotherapy in the treatment of mood disorders,[2] schizophrenia,[3] and panic disorder with agoraphobia.[4] The addition of medication to psychotherapy may also aid in the treatment of patients who were once considered accessible only to psychological approaches, including those with post-traumatic stress disorder,[5] bulimia,[6] and even certain personality disorders which feature transient psychotic, explosive, or dissociative states.[7] Pharmacotherapy and psychotherapy often address different aspects of a disorder, allowing synergistic treatment benefits.

In spite of these advantages, a patient may dislike some aspects of combined treatment. The involvement of a second clinician in a previously dyadic treatment relationship, for example, may seem less intimate or less private. The addition of a second clinician is likely to cost more money. A patient's interactions with two clinicians will increase the opportunities for miscommunication or acting out on the parts of all concerned. When caregivers' messages differ, the patient may wonder whose word to take, whose suggestions to follow, and where to place responsibility during a crisis.

The psychotherapist who engages in combined treatment can reap a number of rewards. She or he is able to offer a patient more comprehensive care. The involvement of a clinician with a contrasting point of view may facilitate a deeper understanding of the patient's difficulties. In addition, the psychotherapist gains an opportunity to learn how the patient relates to a known person, the other clinician. This knowledge can fill out the material obtained through the transference and explicate dynamics surrounding issues of sexuality, oral needs, control struggles, splitting, and the sense of being understood or misunderstood.

Disadvantages to the psychotherapist, however, cannot be overlooked. They include ambiguity about who is in charge, a need to yield power on occasion, a vulnerability of one's work to the scrutiny and sometimes unilateral decision making of another clinician, and the irritating need to determine who will assume responsibility for specific aspects of treatment or coverage (N. Atwood, unpublished data, 1986). In a crisis, the need to include input from a pharmacotherapist may require precious time and effort.

Advantages for the pharmacotherapist participating in

combined treatment include opportunities to make use of the specialized skills of a psychotherapist, to serve more patients as a pharmacotherapist, and to succeed professionally by building a practice and referral network in a subspecialty where there is a great need for skilled clinicians. Psychiatrists who specialize in pharmacotherapy and combined treatment acquire expertise in their field by treating a large number and variety of patients.

Disadvantages to the pharmacotherapist, however, are also present. Sharing clinical responsibility may increase medicolegal risk. Pharmacotherapists also may regret giving up the deeper involvement with a patient's inner world that develops in a psychotherapy relationship. Some psychiatrists feel undesirably constricted by the role of pharmacotherapist.[8]

SOURCES OF CONFLICT IN COMBINED TREATMENT

Ideologic conflict, arising from differing approaches to the formulation of a patient's problem, is probably the most frequent source of misunderstanding and disagreement between providers of combined treatment. Psychotherapists are often trained to understand their patients' difficulties within a psychological framework. Whether specifically guided by psychoanalytic, self-psychology, cognitive, or behavioral theory, each psychological approach shares certain features. The patient's distress is conceptualized as arising from the individual's psychological structure, interpersonal experiences, or learning; the technique of treatment relies on talking; and the vehicle for this talk is an interpersonal relationship in which openness, reflection, and self-awareness are fostered. In each individual psychological approach, the patient's mind is viewed as the locus of the problem. Change is ostensibly accomplished through communication, support, insight, and practicing of skills acquired within the therapeutic relationship.

The psychoanalytic/psychodynamic model, for example, stresses the importance of unconscious conflicts within the mind, which lead to distress. The psychotherapist may assume the role of a supportive guide who helps the patient to explore fantasies and memories as well as current experience, in an attempt to bring these conflicts into consciousness for examination. Psychodynamically trained psychotherapists also treat patients who find a deeply exploratory psychotherapy too painful or regressive and yet are significantly helped by a psychodynamically guided supportive therapy, which bolsters the patient's highest level of functioning. Self-psychology, a contrasting approach, stresses the usefulness of noncritical empathic listening in an attempt to heal long-standing deficits that impair a patient's capacity to maintain self-esteem or soothe discomfort. Proponents of cognitive psychology emphasize the destructive power of negative beliefs about oneself, which the psychotherapist helps to explore and revise. Finally, the behavioral approach examines maladaptive learned responses, which may be changed through a reeducative process in which the psychotherapist serves as a kind of teacher.

In contrast to these, the formulation and treatment planning done by a pharmacotherapist are based on a medical model which emphasizes biological aspects of mental illness.[9] Precise descriptive diagnosis is of great importance because it guides the choice of treatment. A medication, rather than talk, is the most important treatment component, and the relationship between patient and pharmacotherapist exists primarily to foster medication compliance and educate the patient about the illness. The exploration of feelings, thoughts, and experiences may be valued primarily as it aids the process of diagnosis and medication compliance. While the psychodynamic therapist may strive to increase a patient's sense of ownership and control over his or her problems, the biologically oriented clinician often works toward a seemingly incompatible goal, that of helping the patient feel less blameworthy about bearing a disease whose basis is physical, not moral. Thus differences arise between psychological and biological approaches in the conceptualization of behavioral disorders, in the role of the therapist, in the choice of therapeutic agent, and in the role of the relationship between clinician and patient.[10]

The disparity between these models and the degree to which they may divide their followers are not to be underestimated, since impasses in combined treatment often result from the inability of psychological and biological clinicians to appreciate each other's perspectives. Consider for example the following cases.

Case 1. A young woman complaining of depression, impulsive self-destructive behavior, and poor interpersonal relationships sought treatment with a very biologically oriented pharmacotherapist. He instructed her about the biogenetic origins of her depression, prescribed medication for her depression and migraine headaches, and saw her at monthly intervals for follow-up appointments.

Despite some improvement in her depression, the patient requested the addition of psychotherapy to her treatment program. Her pharmacotherapist expressed surprise and refused to make this referral. Psychotherapy, he explained, would have limited value for her and might expose her to dangerous risks such as the regression likely to occur if an intense transference developed. The patient disagreed and argued that a previous therapy had been stabilizing and helpful, ending only when her former psychotherapist relocated. The pharmacotherapist would not reconsider and the patient subsequently selected a psychotherapist without his help.

The psychotherapist, who viewed the patient's difficulties within a psychodynamic framework, was very concerned by what she considered a pattern of chronic suicidal behavior and severe poly-drug abuse. The patient confided that she was currently abusing the narcotic prescribed by her pharmacotherapist for treatment of migraine. She had not discussed this with him directly because she feared he would be disappointed and angrily terminate her treatment. She initially forbade her psychotherapist to contact the pharmacotherapist but eventually agreed that communication could take place. The psychotherapist phoned the pharmacotherapist to share her concerns about the patient's drug abuse, poor impulse control, and suicidal ideation. The pharmacotherapist, who viewed the patient's difficulties as an expression of a biologically based mood disorder, dismissed the the psychotherapist's concerns. He believed that the patient was behaviorally regressed as a result of beginning psychotherapy. This, he explained, was why she had recently worsened and why she had told her psychotherapist information she kept from him.

Communication between the pharmacotherapist and psychotherapist ultimately reached an angry impasse. Outside consultation was refused by the pharmacotherapist, and the psychotherapist thought it wiser to withdraw from her treatment role, despite concerns about the patient's safety and the appropriateness of her treatment.

This case illustrates an ideological difference which remained unnegotiated, bringing about an end to the combined treatment. Although such conflicts are often resolvable, in this case the therapists reached an impasse and the patient suffered a loss. Of major importance here were the non-negotiable differences between the caregivers' conceptualizations of the patient's problem. Though both clinicians would have diagnosed the patient as depressed, the psychotherapist understood the depression as being secondary to a personality disorder and as requiring a treatment that would offer a mixture of insight, confrontation, limit-setting, and support. She viewed the pharmacotherapist's treatment as providing excessive drugs to a patient who was unable to abstain from abuse and dependence. In contrast, the pharmacotherapist viewed the patient's depression as a biologically determined mood disorder, which only secondarily caused interpersonal and employment difficulties. He believed the migraine headaches required analgesic treatment. When the psychotherapist made explicit the clinicians' inability to reach a consensus about the nature of the patient's problems and indicated treatment, no compromise could be reached. The patient's anxiety was greatly increased by receiving contradictory directions from her caregivers. In this case, the least harmful solution was to dissolve the combined treatment. The patient was unable to benefit fully from either psychotherapy or pharmacotherapy in this conflicted triangle.

Case 2. A young man, considered to have a personality disorder, was hospitalized for acute suicidal urges. During his evaluation on the ward, he showed a capacity to explore complex and painful feelings in the safe environment of the inpatient unit. He spoke insightfully to his inpatient psychotherapist of his fears of closeness, which conflicted so painfully with his longings for greater interpersonal support and intimacy.

Prior to admission, an outpatient pharmacotherapist had treated him with lithium and supportive psychotherapy. She believed that a biologically based mood instability was at the center of this patient's difficulties. She was surprised when the inpatient psychotherapist communicated to her the opinion of the ward team, that "lithium, of course, has no pharmacologic benefit for this patient, but he needs to have a physical object to hold onto from you, so that he can feel less abandoned." This psychodynamic assessment of the medication's role (viewing it as a transitional object rather than as a pharmacologically active treatment) was taken up by the patient, who after discharge began to take lithium on an "as needed" basis when he felt alone.

The patient's inconsistent use of lithium and the resulting reduction in serum level seemed associated with an increased frequency of self-destructive depressive moods. The pharmacotherapist believed that the patient's treatment had been undermined by an ideological conflict. In trying to help the patient gain greater awareness of his feelings, the well-intentioned ward staff had unwittingly interfered with his medication compliance. The significance of lithium's pharmacologic effects had been discounted by too exclusive a focus on its dynamic meanings.

In each of these interactions, ideologic disagreement between caregivers harmed the patient's treatment. In each case a clinician viewed the patient in terms suggested by one theoretical model and rejected input from the alternative model, leaving the patient confused, unsure which viewpoint was correct, and potentially fearful of being mistreated. Perhaps of greatest importance to the patient, the possibility of combining treatment approaches and obtaining the differential benefits of each treatment approach was made very difficult.

Dogmatic adherence to either the biological or the psychodynamic model oversimplifies the rich complexity of human behavior and constricts the range of treatment alternatives. Patients should never be led to believe that their behavioral symptoms are purely chemical. A solely biological formulation of a patient's problems may foreclose consideration of potentially valuable psychotherapy or may leave a patient who is already in psychotherapy feeling mistreated by the psychotherapist's insistence on self-exploration. Conversely, a patient who is told that medications are a form of resistance to self-exploration and growth, or that they gratify unhealthy needs, may lose an opportunity to facilitate psychotherapy by relieving a component of suffering that arises from a biochemical vulnerability. Clinicians who share an awareness of these issues are able to collaborate flexibly, emphasizing one or the other modality of treatment at different stages, as in the following case.

Case 3. A 35-year-old woman was referred by her psychotherapist to a pharmacotherapist because of her increasing depression and her decision to stop psychotherapy. The patient had found it more and more difficult to attend psychotherapy sessions because of the pain involved in exploring angry and hopeless feelings about her family and upbringing. As the psychotherapy stirred up feelings of deprivation, she had responded with an increase in bingeing on highly caloric food. Her sleep and concentration were impaired and at times she suffered from an intense physical sense of fatigue.

The pharmacotherapist formulated her symptoms as evidence of a major depressive episode complicated by bulimia and suggested that the disturbance of sleep, energy, and concentration as well as the bingeing might respond to antidepressant treatment. With agreement among caregivers and patient, an antidepressant trial was begun. Improvement in sleep, energy, and bingeing occurred within several weeks. After several months the patient reported to the pharmacotherapist that she now wished to resume psychotherapy, to better understand life issues she had been unable to address until medication allowed her to feel less acutely out of control.

Incompatible assumptions about caregivers' roles provide another important source of mixed messages and conflict in many disputes during combined treatment. Again, differing conceptual frameworks may underlie these disputes. Psychotherapists, emphasizing the importance of the psychotherapeutic relationship, may consider themselves to be the primary therapist, using a pharmacotherapist as a consultant to treatment. This belief may not be shared by the pharmacotherapist, whose medical training emphasizes the physician's authority and medicolegal responsibility. Covert interdisciplinary and/or sexual issues also complicate the matter of roles, since many combined-treatment agreements pair a male psychiatrist with a female social worker, psychologist, or nurse. Undiscussed assumptions of hierarchy may be present, for example, when the pharmacotherapist makes a major change in medication without involving the psychotherapist, or the psychotherapist supports the patient's decision to discontinue medication without involving the pharmacotherapist. Referral patterns can reinforce hierarchical role definitions, as when one clinician attempts to ensure greater control over a consultant by referring downward to a more junior colleague or to a discipline perceived as subordinate in a given setting.

Treatment priorities in the face of multiple, competing goals can represent a further manifestation of underlying conceptual discord between pharmacotherapist and psychotherapist. It is astounding how easily an argument about "what to do first" can arise between providers of care. The psychotherapist, for example, may prize adaptation, growth, and the development of intimacy, even at the cost of increased emotional turmoil, insomnia, and interpersonal strife. The pharmacotherapist may value symptom relief to a much greater degree, believing that mere survival is a more practical initial goal than emotional growth. In the following case, a conflict over priorities is made explicit by communication between psychotherapist and pharmacotherapist.

> Case 4. Mr. A, a 40-year-old man with a 12-year history of bipolar affective disorder, had for eight years been in the care of Dr. X, who monitored his medication. Mrs. Y had been the patient's psychotherapist for four years. Mr. A had a history of multiple hospitalizations, but none since beginning treatment with Mrs. Y. After many years of unemployment, Mr. A considered returning to a more active life, and signed up for a six-week training program which would increase his employability. Soon after, he reported to Mrs. Y that he planned to drop out of the course. He explained that Dr. X "said he was worried that my nerves are worse. The doc thinks the course is bad for me." Mrs. Y was startled both by Mr. A's report and by Dr. X's involvement.
>
> Mrs. Y wondered what was occurring dynamically for the patient as well as in the combined treatment team. Had there been a simple misunderstanding? Was the patient playing psychotherapist and pharmacotherapist against each other? Was the pharmacotherapist intruding inappropriately into the treatment, or did he understand the patient in a way that led him to offer appropriate support to the patient?
>
> Mrs. Y asked the patient how he noticed that his nerves were worse. Mr. A replied that he was sleeping poorly, pacing more, making more phone calls, and experiencing more anxiety. He was very worried. He could not concentrate. He thought his course was definitely making his nerves worse. Exploring the way in which the course was problematic, Mrs. Y learned that since high school Mr. A had not had to memorize anything. He feared his illness had ruined his mind and would cause him to flunk. Flunking would squelch his hopes of ever returning to a normal life and might lead to rehospitalization. Dr. X, therefore, had said he should stop the course if it bothered him so much. Mr. A added that he was "very confused about what is the best thing to do. You

know, Dr. X helped me last time I was in the hospital. He knows how sick I can get. You don't really know."

Mrs. Y tried to sort out her own feelings. She realized that she felt anxious because Dr. X had in fact known the patient longer and seen him at sicker moments, and because she and he usually saw eye-to-eye about treatment decisions. She realized as well that the patient was doubting her judgment and perhaps Dr. X was too. On the other hand, from what she knew of the patient's dynamics, the source of the patient's distress might have been his fears about getting better rather than just his fears of the course. Mrs. Y developed a dynamic formulation which understood Mr. A's current crisis as a conflict between his wish to progress and his fear of failure.

A conference of the caregivers allowed them to resolve their differences and agree on prioritization of the patient's goals. The pharmacotherapist, who knew the severity of the patient's former illness, felt reassured by the psychotherapist's assertion that Mr. A's anxiety was caused by a step forward rather than a regression. Mrs. Y, who had not witnessed Mr. A's previous regressions and hospitalizations, felt relieved by Dr. X's availability and experience with the patient.

An additional element of conflict in this episode with Mr. A, which emerged through further exploration, concerned his use of psychotherapist and pharmacotherapist as transference figures with whom he experienced a repetition of early relationship patterns. One of Mr. A's parents habitually had shown love by shielding him from anxiety. Dr. X assumed this role while Mrs. Y was cast in the role of Mr. A's less caring parent. Such transference reactions commonly occur, of course, whether one or two clinicians are involved with a patient. In the heat of a negative transference, a patient may present his psychotherapist to friends or relatives in such a pejorative and frightening way as to elicit alarmed and/or indignant inquiries. In a combined treatment relationship, such complaints are typically directed to the other caregiver, as in the following cases.

Case 5. A 40-year-old divorced woman was referred for antidepressant evaluation during the course of her psychotherapy with another clinician. She complained to the pharmacotherapist about her psychotherapist's unavailability, lack of caring, and tendency to give inane and useless advice. "I told him I feel so empty I could devour everything in my kitchen, and he asked if I could go on a diet!" The pharmacotherapist accepted the devaluation without exploration and neglected to call the psychotherapist. Instead, he offered several other psychotherapists' names to the patient, who interviewed one after another and found each more unacceptable than the last. A belated discussion with the initial psychotherapist clarified how this patient's early deprivation and nearly uncontainable rage led her to see any clinician as depriving and uncaring.

Case 6. A group psychotherapist phoned, in alarm, to speak with the pharmacotherapist prescribing antidepressants for one of the group patients. That day, the patient had occupied most of the group session with a litany of complaints about his pharmacotherapist, whose unavailability was allegedly exceeded only by his vindictiveness. This pharmacotherapist was reportedly continuing to prescribe a medication whose adverse effects had seriously injured the patient. Discussion with the pharmacotherapist led the psychotherapist to agree that appropriate treatment was being offered. The caregivers' discussion clarified that currently the patient was experiencing the pharmacotherapist as a sadistic and abandoning figure, reminiscent of the father of his early years.

As emphasized elsewhere in this book, the meaning of medication usually becomes a dynamic issue in combined treatment. When this is not appreciated by the pharmacotherapist or addressed when appropriate in psychotherapy, the pharmacotherapist may be alerted by an increasing sense of confusion about the treatment. Changes in medication or dosage begin to seem like moves in the game of "battleship," where each maneuver strikes an unseen target in an unknown way. When this predicament develops, it is time for a conference of caregivers, as in the following example.

Case 7. A 30-year-old man was referred to a pharmacotherapist by his psychotherapist when increasing insomnia and agitation threatened to interfere with his ability to remain employed. Noting symptoms of the type usually responsive to medication, the pharmacotherapist suggested an antidepressant trial. She was surprised when the patient vehemently resisted her suggestion and minimized the severity of his symptoms.

When the depressive symptoms increased, the patient agreed to take medication. He complained, though, of severe side effects and seemed to comply poorly with dosage instructions. The pharmacotherapist felt increasingly confused about her role in the patient's care. Her confusion prompted her to call for a discussion with the psychotherapist, who further explored with the patient his feelings about medications. It was in this way that both clinicians learned that the patient's father, a physician, had inappropriately supplied him during his adolescence with abusable drugs for his "nerves." This new piece of history helped to explain how any pharmacologic interventions would probably elicit doubt and fear from the patient.

In some cases, disruption of a combined treatment agreement arises from incompetence or unwillingness of either clinician or the patient to do what they're supposed to do in the arrangement. This can be for reasons of skill, dynamics, or personality. A pharmacotherapist, for example, may feel unsafe offering medication that could be lethal in overdose to a patient in psychotherapy with a clinician who seems to disagree about how to monitor suicidality. The psychotherapist may actually be incompetent; usually, however, there is a more specific disagreement about the needs of an individual patient or type of patient. Conversely, a psychotherapist justifiably fears involvement with a pharmacotherapist who prescribes in a potentially dangerous manner. Concern is appropriate, for example, when a pharmacotherapist allows a suicidal patient access to large amounts of toxic medication or seems too casual about monitoring drug levels or adverse reactions. For either clinician, unwillingness to communicate with the other therapist can be considered a sign of noncompliance with the demands of combined treatment. Sometimes conflicts of this type amount primarily to differences in the personality styles of the clinicians, which may prove an insurmountable obstacle in the busy pace of the real world.

When noncommunication of caregivers is requested by the patient, a complex situation arises. While it is the patient's right to restrict communication, it is often more productive to explore the reasons for this request than to merely acquiesce. While many psychotherapeutic details simply need not be shared between caregivers, a patient's request for restricted communication often leaves one clinician in the dark about important issues and constitutes a type of noncompliance with the needs of combined treatment.

PREVENTING CONFLICT

An ounce of prevention is better than a late-night phone call, so attention to potential conflicts in combined treatment best begins the moment consultation is considered.

An assessment of the pharmacotherapist's competence as a psychopharmacologist must be one of the psychotherapist's first considerations in finding a collaborator. It is tempting to seek medication evaluation and backup from the first psychiatrist available, and sometimes, as in an agency, it may be necessary to do so. This, however, may be a prescription for disaster. While one wishes all psychiatrists to be thorough, careful, well informed, and up-to-date, these qualities become especially necessary in pharmacotherapy, a subspecialty that deals with an individual's subjective experience of reality and with therapeutic agents that alter that experience. The drugs involved are potent and can have life-threatening side effects. Many require careful and consistent monitoring. The difference between a subtherapeutic dose, a therapeutic dose, and an overdose may be small and may differ from patient to patient, requiring individualized dosage determination. To provide effective pharmacotherapy, a psychiatrist must be invested in keeping up-to-date with a specialized and rapidly expanding field.

Second, the psychotherapist is well advised to assess the pharmacotherapist's ideological stance. Does he believe in psychotherapy? In combined treatment? Does he believe that a psychotherapist without medical training is capable of helping a patient? If so, what kinds of psychotherapy does he think are efficacious? Perhaps he favors cognitive therapy over insight-oriented psychodynamic treatment. If that is the case, how does he feel about working with a psychotherapist who uses a different modality? What does he think about the way pharmacotherapy and psychotherapy fit together?

Third, one needs to pick a psychopharmacology consultant with whom one senses a good personal fit. This does not mean that the pharmacotherapist and psychotherapist must see eye-to-eye on everything, but mutual respect, appropriate trust, the capacity to talk things through, and a genuine willingness to work together are essential. It is inevitable that patients in crisis will at times evoke radically different responses from the two providers. The psychotherapist, for example, may have just concluded that a depressed alcoholic patient needs a detoxification center, Alcoholics Anonymous, and six months of sobriety without medication, when the pharmacotherapist expresses a strong opinion that in this case an antidepressant medication should be started without delay. Without a solid relationship between caregivers to facilitate negotiation of differences, the patient will be the biggest loser.

While medical competence and ideologic issues can be initially assessed through having conversations and checking with references (do not be afraid to ask a pharmacotherapist for references you can telephone), the eventual comfort of the fit may not be easily apparent from the outset. But answers to the following questions will emerge over time: Does the relationship feel collegial or hierarchical? What are the sexual politics? How do patients describe their experiences with the pharmacotherapist? Do they feel that they are respected and taken seriously? Do you? If the answers are not positive, it is time to reassess the combined treatment relationship.

RESOLVING COMBINED TREATMENT CONFLICTS

Even carefully formulated treatment plans are prone to unexpected twists and turns over the course of time. Sometimes an intertherapist conflict that appeared resolved will reemerge at a later stage of treatment. In other cases, a new difficulty arises in a previously successful collaboration. Most such conflicts can be resolved; it is exceptional when the only recourse is disengagement from the combined treatment agreement.

The key to working through combined treatment conflicts is communication. A willingness to discuss conflicting ideologies is generally facilitated when the colleagues are familiar with one another's clinical work and share a history of successful combined treatments. It is within the context of this type of relationship, which is based on mutual trust and respect, that differences of opinion may be discussed, resolved, or tolerated without adversely affecting the therapeutic process.

Many conflicts can be directly discussed or can be explored with the help of outside consultants. When ideologic conflicts have led to conflicting ideas about case formulation, treatment planning, or caregiver's roles, discussion is crucial to the process of coordinating treatment. When medication or the pharmacotherapist who prescribes it has taken on a special transferential significance to the patient, discussion will help the pharmacotherapist to be aware of the dynamic significance of the medication or person, and help the psychotherapist to provide appropriate psychological interventions. When the matter appears to be one of competence or professional conduct, communication is again crucial, in this case either to verify that the combined treatment is not sustainable or to understand the problem as a transferential reenactment or distortion by the patient.

Combined treatment begins with the introduction of a second modality of treatment and second clinician into an ongoing treatment, whether the initial treatment was pharmacotherapy or psychotherapy. The patient's initial meeting with the new clinician should be preceded, whenever possible, by a discussion between therapists. During this discussion the initial caregiver can communicate the patient's history, the reasons for referral, and the expectations of the consultation. Following the patient's initial meeting with the new caregiver, a second conversation should take place, this time followed up by a note to the referrer detailing any additional relevant history, findings of the consultant's examination or results of additional laboratory or psychological testing, and treatment recommendations. This second discussion facilitates consensus in treatment planning.

A disagreement between caregivers may become clear during one of these initial conversations. The pharmacotherapist, for example, may evoke concern by expressing doubt that psychotherapy has a role in the treatment of severe depression. The psychotherapist may reveal the basis for a potential ideologic conflict by requesting that a patient's panic attacks be treated with something mild that can be taken when needed rather than taken on an ongoing basis. Major disagreements may occur during the second conversation with respect to the patient's diagnosis or formulation. One clinician, for example, may see the patient as far more ill than does the other, or at far more acute risk of acting in a self-destructive or homicidal manner. The caregivers may find at this stage that they have concerns about each others' competence or personality styles. When communication between caregivers is direct, the opportunity exists to unravel distortions or misconceptions, reach a consensus about the patient's treatment, and address any other concerns.

Beyond the initial discussions, it is the responsibility of each clinician to inform the other of such important matters as prolonged absences, coverage, changes in treatment approach, crises relevant to the other clinician's work, or major clinical changes in the patient's status of which the other caregiver may not be aware. In addition, it is wise to be in touch periodically (perhaps monthly or bimonthly) to allow an opportunity for discussion of changes in the patient's status or treatment. The patient, of course, must be aware that communication is occurring periodically or during acute crises, as in the following example.

Case 8. A pharmacotherapist was surprised when a young schizophrenic woman called to cancel all future appointments. "My therapist says I don't need medications anymore ... He and I are going to talk about what's bothering me." The pharmacotherapist, upon contacting the psychotherapist, found that the patient had been told her improved clinical condition suggested considering a lowering of medication. The patient ardently wished to be rid of the medication's side effects and to increase her independence by stopping the medication.
The psychotherapist and pharmacotherapist explored further with their patient her feelings about her symptoms and treatment. They reviewed with her the risks and benefits of stopping or lowering antipsychotic medication and together supported her attempt to decrease her dosage on a trial basis. Through prompt communication and discussion, the caregivers clarified the meaning of the patient's communication to the pharmacotherapist, shared information and ideas about the treatment, and returned to the patient with a unified approach. The result was a greater likelihood of success and compliance in the lowering of medication.

When ideologic conflicts between clinicians surface after a combined treatment is already under way, the potential disruption of treatment can often be resolved through discussion of the interplay between biological and psychodynamic factors in the patient's behavior. Clarification of the underlying assumptions about diagnosis, treatment goals, and caregivers' roles will often resolve the conflict.

In a smoothly functioning combined treatment, in fact, the roles of caregivers overlap to some extent. The psychotherapist, for example, often is aware of medication issues and may wish to play a role in educating the patient about the positive and adverse effects of the medication. The pharmacotherapist generally has some awareness of psychotherapy, too, and may be the first to sense that a patient is developing a conflictual transference toward the medication or the person who prescribes it. On occasion, the pharmacotherapist may be the first to note a patient's negative transference to the psychotherapist, as the patient may feel freer to air concerns in the less intense setting of a medication visit. When the pharmacotherapist thinks it necessary to offer psychotherapeutic interventions which go beyond basic support, however, the psychotherapist should be informed. Interpretation of transference issues, for example, is handled more effectively if it is discussed with the psychotherapist. This is illustrated in the following case.

Case 9. A 20-year-old graduate student became moderately depressed after an understandably stressful experience. As his insomnia increased, he agreed to see a pharmacotherapist regarding the possibility of antidepressant treatment. The pharmacotherapist, noting the patient's mild depression and reluctance to accept medication, asked how psychotherapy was going. This elicited the report of a dream that had occurred the night following his psychotherapist's suggestion of a consultation.

In his dream, the patient had been hit by a car. As he lay in terror on the ground, a group of onlookers rushed toward him. His psychotherapist, among them, insisted he be lifted and moved. The patient knew this was wrong for him and could be dangerous, since his back might be broken, but he felt helpless to resist. As he associated to this dream (which he had neglected to tell his psychotherapist) he said he liked his psychotherapist but felt less hopeful about psychotherapy since reading a magazine article that claimed that psychologists, when they socialize together, spend most of their time commiserating about how rarely psychotherapy helps anyone.

The pharmacotherapist discussed with the patient how his reluctance to share his hopelessness had distanced him from his psychotherapist. With the patient's knowledge and consent, the caregivers discussed the dream and associations. With input from both clinicians, the patient decided to postpone pharmacotherapy and continue with psychotherapy.

Case 10. A year after her most recent manic episode, a young woman who was taking lithium on a maintenance basis appeared for her monthly medication visit. The pharmacotherapist was impressed by the patient's cheerful mood, apparently stable functioning at work and home, and enthusiasm about attending night school classes. A routine discussion with the individual psychotherapist added important information that had not been revealed during the medication visit. Even though there was no evidence of a hypomanic mood or a shift in sleep or eating, the patient was quarreling more frequently with her husband. She was also beginning to mention a belief that an important administrative job at the night school was secretly being held for her, to be offered on graduation. Graduation, in fact, was an impending and significant stress for this woman. Alerted to the importance of this stress, the pharmacotherapist assessed the patient's mental status on her next visit and thought it appropriate to suggest a temporary increase in lithium. The open communication between caregivers had facilitated the pharmacotherapist's assessment of the patient's medication needs.

When the conflict between caregivers appears to hinge upon matters of competence or professional conduct, communication is absolutely essential. A patient's allegation that improper treatment is being provided may be correct but professional courtesy dictates that any conclusions remain tentative until the allegation is further investigated. When improper professional conduct is claimed, the first step in investigation is an open discussion with the accused caregiver.

Certain types of personality conflicts between clinicians (for example, lack of respect, unwillingness to return phone calls, apparent or real devaluation of the patient, or sadistic treatment) are fortunately rare occurrences, but they may become so intolerable in a combined treatment that they lead to the dissolution of a treatment contract and referral to another clinician. There may be reasons, however, for trying to work out the relationship even with a colleague one finds disagreeable. The patient's regard for the individual or success with his or her treatment plan, the clinician's special competence or skills, or the difficulty of obtaining needed services elsewhere (for example, when the only pharmacotherapist in a mental health center is difficult to work with) might provide a reason for tolerating involvement with a disliked clinician. The bottom line in such a decision is whether the combination of two caregivers is providing more help to the patient than would be available if the association with one were to be terminated. It is also worth emphasizing that abandonment during a crisis may endanger a patient and entangle the clinician(s) in a sticky web of medicolegal issues. Dissolution of a combined treatment, when it occurs, needs to be handled in an orderly manner and in a time of lesser or no crisis. For both ethical and medicolegal reasons, a patient who is to be refused treatment must be offered suggestions for feasible alternatives.

Obviously, some combined treatment contracts should be dissolved when they are working to a patient's detriment. Interpersonal or interagency conflicts may make it virtually impossible for a combined treatment to be sustained. Unwillingness to communicate or actual incompetence of one clinician may lead to the other's unwillingness to remain involved. Even at the stage when an impasse between caregivers seems unresolvable, however, the treatment may be salvaged on occasion through the use of an objective consultant. The consultant may recognize factors of which one or both caregivers were unaware, or may be able to educate one or both caregivers or the patient about treatment, as in the following example.

>Case 11. A psychology intern sought help from his supervisor in dealing with the psychiatric resident assigned to medicate his patient. "This patient's completely off the wall," complained the intern, who knew he had heard delusional material and loose associations when the patient confided long-standing, profound impairment and distress.
>
>The resident, a thoughtful and very independent young man, asked, "How can I medicate a man in whom I see no sign whatever of psychosis?" In his brief and structured evaluation of the medication, he had observed a coherent, organized individual. He did not wish to expose such a person to the side effects of an antipsychotic drug.
>
>In a case conference that included both trainees' supervisors, the patient's two sides were integrated and the trainees came to understand how differently some patients will appear under different clinical (and life) circumstances. The validity of the intern's observations was supported while he also was shown that his patient functioned much more effectively in other settings. The psychiatric resident helped to give greater weight to the intern's observations and to recognize the diagnostic limitations of a structured interviewing approach. Recommendations for limiting the depth of psychotherapy and strengthening the patient's reality testing with a low dose of antipsychotic medication facilitated the continuation of this combined treatment.

CONCLUSION

Intertherapist conflicts are often inevitable during the course of combined treatment. The most productive tools for resolving combined treatment conflicts are those (usually shared to some degree) of the psychotherapist. With respectful professional discussion and attention to communication from the outset of treatment, many intertherapist disagreements can be prevented or resolved.

REFERENCES

1. Chiles JA, Carlin AS, Beitman BD: A physician, a nonmedical psychotherapist, and a patient: The pharmacotherapy-psychotherapy triangle, in Beitman BD, Klerman GL (eds): *Combining Psychotherapy and Drug Therapy in Clinical Practice*. New York, Spectrum Publications, 1984, pp 89–101.
2. Weissman MM, Klerman GL: Depression: Interpersonal psychotherapy and tricyclics, in Beitman BD, Klerman GL (eds): *Combining Psychotherapy and Drug Therapy in Clinical Practice*. New York, Spectrum Publications, 1984, pp 149–165.
3. Goldstein MJL: Schizophrenia: The interaction of family and neuroleptic therapy, in Beitman BD, Klerman GL (eds): *Combining Psychotherapy and Drug Therapy in Clinical Practice*. New York, Spectrum Publications, 1984, pp 167–185.
4. Mavissakalian MR: Agoraphobia: Behavioral therapy and pharmacotherapy, in Beitman BD, Klerman GL (eds): *Combining Psychotherapy and Drug Therapy in Clinical Practice*. New York, Spectrum Publications, 1984, pp 187–211.
5. Lipper S, Davidson JRT, Grady TA, et al: Preliminary study of carbamazepine in post-traumatic stress disorder. *Psychosomatics* 1986;27:849–854.
6. Garfinkel PE, Garner DM (eds): *The Role of Drug Treatments for Eating Disorders*. New York, Brunner/Mazel, 1987.
7. Ellison JM, Adler DA: Psychopharmacologic approaches to borderline syndromes. *Compr Psychiatry* 1984;25:255–262.
8. Samuelly I: Dual treatment by psychiatrists — beware. *Psychiatric Times*, September 1986, pp 8–9.
9. Lazare A: Hidden conceptual models in psychiatry. *N Engl J Med* 1973;288:345–351.
10. Klerman GL: Ideologic conflicts in combined treatment, in Beitman BD, Klerman GL (eds): *Combining Psychotherapy and Drug Therapy in Clinical Practice*. New York, Spectrum Publications, 1984, pp 17–34.

# Section II
A Psychopharmacology Knowledge Base for Psychotherapists

# 6

Medications for Mental Disorders:
A Brief History and an Overview
of Current Uses

James M. Ellison

Psychotropic medications are a fact of modern life. More than 1% of American adults take antipsychotic drugs and at least twice as many take antidepressants.[1] Data from household surveys show that more than 10% of adults have taken an antianxiety drug once or more frequently within the preceding year.[2] These numbers reflect psychotropic drug use among the general population. Among individuals with mental disorders, of course, the rates are far higher.

For mental health clinicians, it is virtually impossible to practice without encountering patients whose treatment includes medication. As medications become increasingly ubiquitous, it is essential that psychotherapists acquire a basic knowledge of their benefits and risks. This chapter discusses the evolution of pharmacotherapy (treatment with medications) and provides an overview of current indications for its use.

THE EVOLUTION OF PHARMACOTHERAPY

Many clinicians know that the modern era of pharmacotherapy in psychiatry dates from the late 1940s and early 1950s, a period of explosive progress that gave us many of the drugs still in clinical use. It is less widely appreciated, though, that the pharmacologic treatment of behavioral disorders is a discipline with ancient roots and a colorful history. The use of somatic therapies such as trephining (boring holes in the skull, presumably to allow the escape of demons) dates back to prehistoric times.[3] The ingestion of mind-altering substances is thought to date back at least as far, and is documented to have been important in several ancient civilizations. In the ancient civilizations of Babylonia and Egypt, where hysterical symptoms and mood disorders were described as early as 2600 BC, psychoactive medications were administered by priests as part of a healing ritual. Since their theory of mental illness was one of possession, drugs were used to help free the patient from demons responsible for the production of insanity. In Greece, when medical care was offered in the Temples of Aesculapius (1000 BC), possessed individuals received treatment in a ritualized setting where priests are believed to have employed opiates to promote healing visions.[3]

The Greek physician Hippocrates (460–377 BC) localized disturbances of mentation to the brain and classified their manifestations into four categories: epilepsy, mania, melancholia, and paranoia. The son of an Aesculapian priest, Hippocrates nonetheless espoused a nonreligious theory of mental illness. Of epilepsy, for example, he wrote that "... one disease is neither more divine nor more human than another."[4] Proposing a model prophetic of the modern notion of chemical imbalance, he attributed insanity to an excess or deficiency of certain vital bodily fluids or humors: blood, phlegm, black bile, and yellow bile. His followers prescribed medications, primarily plant extracts, for their emetic or laxative effects. Through purging, an attempt was made to restore humoral balance. The removal of excessive blood, through phlebotomy, was also a valued form of therapy.

Hippocrates' work was later systematized by Galen (131–200 AD), who extended the theory of the humors and emphasized the four qualities of heat, cold, dryness, and moisture. Each humor combined two of these qualities, and each was also affected by food, climate, location, age, occupation, sexual activity, and other factors.[5] Galen classified diseases and prescribed medications based on their complementary qualities. Mint (a hot and dry medication), for example, was given to soothe phlegmatic nausea, a cold and moist disorder. The phrase "cool as a cucumber" points back to Galen's system of classification of medications and foods.[6]

Galen's theories were passed along in Europe through the Middle Ages and were essentially unquestioned in academic circles. His humoral conception of mental illness was taught and his therapeutic strategies were codified. At the same time, a revival of the demonic view of mental disorders grew increasingly influential as the Church acquired the power which culminated in the Inquisition. By 1487, two Dominican monks, Sprenger and Kraemer, published their textbook of the Inquisition, *Malleus Maleficarum* (The Witches' Hammer), a compendium of lore about witchcraft and its eradication. Among its advice to physicians was the dictum, "If the patient can be relieved by no drugs, but rather, seems to be aggravated by them, then the disease is caused by the devil."[3] The notion that refractory symptoms were the devil's work and not the physician's failure was undoubtedly face-saving for frustrated clinicians of the time, but also assisted the persecution of many mentally ill individuals as witches.

During Europe's Middle Ages, Greek and Roman medical knowledge was preserved and extended in the academic institutions of the Arabian Empire. Formerly, physicians had compounded medications for their own use, but Arabian expansion of the pharmacopeia with such drugs as arsenic, camphor, senna, and cassia increased the complexity of pharmacotherapy so much that a new type of professional, the apothecary, became necessary. Then, as now, interdisciplinary skirmishes flashed along the shifting professional borders between the medical profession and these new drug specialists. As in modern times, pharmaceuticals were a costly item and the spice trade (which actually provided spices more for pharmaceutical than culinary use) was a powerful economic force. The fierce competition between apothecaries reportedly included duels between experts in which poisons were exchanged. Each had to find an antidote to the other's potion or suffer the consequences.

As the Renaissance approached, the supremacy of Galen's theories was increasingly coming under rational scrutiny. A more empirical approach was beginning to affect therapeutic practices.

Pare, a French surgeon who lived from 1510 to 1590, is credited with performing an early controlled trial. Having burned himself, he applied a remedy to one area and compared its healing with that of the untreated area. He also experimented with some of the most revered therapeutic agents of his time: mummy powder (purportedly derived from mummies), unicorn horn, and bezoar stone (the solidified tear of a unicorn). Unicorn horn, believed to neutralize any poison, was especially valued in royal households. Experimenting on a condemned prisoner who chose a potential death by poisoning over a more certain demise by public strangulation, Pare demonstrated a royal horn cup's powers to be less than satisfactory, especially to the prisoner.[6]

With the growth of medical empiricism during the Renaissance, physicians also began to approach mental illness with less mysticism. Johannes Weyer, for example, argued that witches were actually mentally ill and therefore should not be persecuted. Alongside these more rational observations, however, a staunch popular belief in the supernatural basis of insanity persisted. One source of Renaissance theory about mental illness, Robert Burton's learned compendium entitled *The Anatomy of Melancholy*, gives a cross section of popular and academic beliefs from the early 1600s.[7] Listing the causes of melancholy (a generic term for depression, psychosis, and several other categories of mental illness), Burton mixed together sorrow and loss alongside sorcery, witchcraft, and possession. His lengthy catalogue of physic (therapeutics) for melancholy included an array of mineral, animal, or plant preparations used as emetics, laxatives, or enemas. Blood-letting, leeches, cauteries (burning), and blisters (use of an irritant substance to raise blisters) were also advocated. The persistence of magical beliefs is apparent in his description of one medication:

> Take a ram's head that never meddled with an ewe, cut off at a blow, and the horns only taken away, boil it well, skin and wool together; after it is well sod, take out the brains, and put these spices to it, cinnamon, ginger, nutmeg, mace, cloves ... mingle the powder of these spices with it, and heat them in a platter upon a chafing-dish of coals together ... and for three days give it the patient fasting, so that he fast two hours after it. It may be eaten with bread in an egg or broth, or any way, so it be taken.[7]

Though the sheer care and attention required to administer a treatment of this complexity may have alleviated the isolation and alienation of melancholia, the pharmacologic effects of such a concoction may have been quite toxic. Burton both expressed his distrust of Renaissance polypharmacy and covered himself in case he should someday require treatment when he wrote:

> ... common experience tells us that they live freest from all manner of infirmities that make least use of apothecaries' physic. Many are overthrown by preposterous use of it, and thereby get their bane [a pun on henbane, a common medicine of the time], that might otherwise have escaped; some think physicians kill as many as they save ... How many murders they make in a year ... that may freely kill folks, and have a reward for it? ... But I will urge these cavilling and contumelious arguments no farther, lest some physician should mistake me, and deny me physic when I am sick: for my part, I am well persuaded of physic.[7]

The best and worst traditions of European pharmacotherapy crossed the Atlantic to Colonial America. Early on, somatic therapies were a component of a management approach that relied heavily on confinement. Some mentally ill individuals were imprisoned, while others were auctioned off to private bidders who were allowed to use them as laborers.

Established in 1752, the Pennsylvania Hospital is the site of this country's first psychiatric inpatient ward. Though progressive for its time, it consisted of tiny basement cells where treatment relied on the time-honored approaches of confinement, restraint, bleeding, purging, and blistering. Benjamin Rush (1745–1813), who came to work there in 1783, brought with him the ideas of his teacher William Cullen (1710–1790), a major advocate of the organic conception of mental illness. Rush, regarded as the father of American psychiatry, adhered to Cullen's theory that mental disorders originated in a disturbed functioning of the nervous system. He advocated more rational use of the unfortunately toxic somatic therapies of his time. His respect for patients led him to invent a restraint system, the tranquilizer, which, while more humane than previous means of confinement, would still be considered barbaric by today's standards.[8]

Around the turn of the 19th century, following on the model of England's York Retreat, humane asylums were developed in

America as an alternative to the state hospital system. While these catered to those who were able to afford their fees, they also accepted some subsidized patients. Moral treatment, based on respect, minimal restraints, and involvement of patients in productive activities, was espoused in these asylums. The asylums also served as an important site for experimentation with the effects of somatic therapies. By 1844 their directors formed the Association of Medical Superintendents of American Institutions for the Insane (later the American Psychiatric Association) for the purpose of sharing their therapeutic experiences and knowledge at meetings and through their publication, the *American Journal of Insanity*.

In a review of the medical treatment of insanity for this journal in 1850, Dr Samuel Woodward (a former superintendent of the Massachusetts State Lunatic Hospital at Worcester) summarized pharmacotherapeutic approaches of his time. He is most enthusiastic about the somatic treatment of what he calls mania, melancholia, and dementia. The available drugs are reminiscent of the days of Hippocrates: in common use were such anticholinergic plant-extracts as stramonium, belladonna, and hyoscyamus; emetics such as nux vomica, sanguinaria, and hellebore; and sedatives including cannabis indica and morphia. Woodward chronicled the humane discarding of some previously common but cruel and ineffective treatments:

> The abandonment of depletion, external irritants, drastic purges and starvation, and the substitution of baths, narcotics, tonics, and generous diet, is not less to be appreciated in the improved conditions of the insane, than the change from manacles, chains, by-locks and confining chairs, to the present system of kindness, confidence, social intercourse, labor, religious teaching, and freedom from restraint.[9]

With the synthesis of truly safer and more effective sedatives (bromide in 1865, chloral hydrate in 1870), the ancient drugs departed from psychiatry. Not every one of them, however, was retired from medicine. Veratrine (an extract of the hellebore plant), for example, was used until recently in treating hypertension. Sanguinaria extract, from the bloodroot plant, is an effective treatment for dental plaque. Morphine, of course, continues to be a valuable analgesic, and cannabis remains in use both medicinally and recreationally.

At the beginning of the 20th century, much of the interest in treating mental illness focused on effects of syphilis, the victims of which comprised a substantial proportion of institutionalized patients. The demonstration of a microorganism, the spirochete, in syphilitic brain tissue provided suggestive evidence that physical factors could produce the psychotic symptoms seen in the later stages of that disease. Von Jauregg, in Austria, introduced malarial fever therapy in 1917 as an effective treatment for this condition. Using the fever induced by a malarial infection to kill the delicate syphilis organism without, hopefully, harming the patient, he stimulated optimism and interest in developing new organic treatments in psychiatry.

Progress in chemical synthesis of pharmaceuticals in the early 20th century provided a variety of new drugs for clinical application. Barbiturates, synthesized first in 1903, gave physicians a superior sedative, which was applied to the treatment of a variety of mental disorders. Klaesi's "Dauernarkose" or sleep treatment of schizophrenia was one use of barbiturates popular in the early 1920s. This treatment used long periods (10 days) of barbiturate-induced sleep to interrupt a psychosis. (It probably offered a risky but welcome respite to families and hospitals as well.) Amphetamine, synthesized in Germany in 1930, was widely used to treat depression but ultimately lost favor because of its rapid production of tolerance and because of the rebound depression which followed its withdrawal.[10]

The mid-1930s witnessed the development of the shock therapies and psychosurgery. Beginning in 1934 with von Meduna's use of camphor injections to induce therapeutic seizures in schizophrenic patients, convulsive therapy evolved rapidly and spread quickly. By 1938, Cerletti and Bini had found electrical induction of convulsions safer and more easily controllable. Subsequent investigators refined this technique and clarified electroshock's greatest areas of effectiveness. Insulin shock, which involved production of coma rather than seizure, remained in use into the 1950s, though like the crude psychosurgery of the 1930s it was ultimately discredited as a therapeutic tool.

The modern era of pharmacotherapy (see Fig 6-1) is appro-

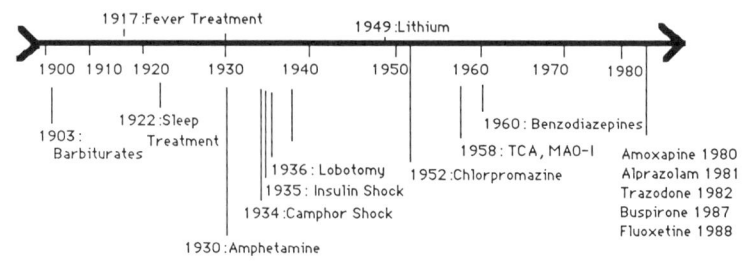

```
      1917:Fever Treatment        1949:Lithium
  |------|------|------|------|------|------|------|------|------>
  1900  1910   1920   1930   1940   1950   1960   1970   1980

         1922:Sleep                        1960: Benzodiazepines
 1903:     Treatment                       1958: TCA, MAO-I
 Barbiturates                                                    Amoxapine 1980
                        1936: Lobotomy    1952:Chlorpromazine    Alprazolam 1981
                        1935: Insulin Shock                      Trazodone 1982
                        1934:Camphor Shock                       Buspirone 1987
                                                                 Fluoxetine 1988
                     1930:Amphetamine
```

Figure 6-1 Progress in Somatic Therapies since 1900.

priately dated to 1949, the year lithium salts were first tested on severely ill psychiatric patients. Lithium was rapidly followed by the introduction of the antipsychotic drugs chlorpromazine and haloperidol, the tricyclic and monoamine oxidase (MAO) inhibiting antidepressants, and the first benzodiazepine (chlordiazepoxide), all of which came into use before 1960. Over the subsequent two decades a series of drugs with similar therapeutic mechanisms but varied side effects were developed, tested, and marketed.

During the early years of the 1980s, advances in the understanding of synaptic physiology and receptor function have led to greater understanding of old drugs and the development of several new ones. New classes of antidepressant and antianxiety agents have recently been marketed and new antipsychotic agents may soon be available as well. A wide range of new antidepressants, antianxiety agents, and antipsychotic agents now being investigated offers the hope that future pharmacotherapy will be more specific and effective. In addition, modern pharmacotherapists have found psychiatric uses for drugs adopted from other branches of medicine. Some anticonvulsants or antiarrhythmics, for example, have been found helpful in the treatment of mood disorders. These medications are described in detail in chapter 7.

A role for medications can be found today in the treatment of many DSM-III-R disorders, though emphasis remains on treating "Axis I" conditions.[11] In schizophrenia, the major and minor mood disorders, and several of the anxiety disorders it is routine to include pharmacotherapeutic interventions in a treatment plan. Newer approaches to the use of medications emphasize the use of minimal doses, briefer durations of treatment, the combination of synergistic actions in refractory cases, and attention to the prevention or minimization of adverse effects. Some of the disorders more recently found responsive to pharmacotherapy include obsessive-compulsive disorder, bulimic bingeing, some symptoms seen in severe personality disorders (especially schizotypal, borderline, and paranoid disorders), and attention-deficit disorder in adults. The remainder of this chapter will review some of the advances in each of these areas. Generic drug names will be used in this section, so the reader is referred to chapter 7 for brand names.

ANXIETY DISORDERS

The most ubiquitous of anxiety states, *adjustment disorder with anxious mood*, has traditionally been treated, if at all, by crisis intervention or other forms of focused psychotherapy. Drugs have played a role primarily in assuring that patients would be able to obtain an adequate amount of sleep and to control the most severe of daytime anxiety symptoms. In the 1980s, the range of drugs available to treat insomnia and acute anxiety allows for safe and effective short-term treatment. No less than 11 benzodiazepines are marketed in the United States. Their spectrum of side effects, half-lives, and rapidity of onset of action allows treatment choices to be tailored to the needs of a specific patient.

Panic disorder, among the anxiety disorders, has increasingly come to be understood as involving biological factors which are responsive to pharmacotherapy. Recent research exploring the biochemistry of panic disorder has demonstrated that panic attacks can be provoked in vulnerable patients by pharmacologic means (lactate, yohimbine, CO_2) and that these provoked attacks can be blocked by drugs including clonidine, tricyclic antidepressants, MAO inhibitors, and at least two benzodiazepines (alprazolam and clonazepam).[12] In clinical trials, some of these same medications have been shown to decrease the frequency and severity of panic attacks in patients with panic disorder.[13]

Research has shown both medications and behavioral therapy to be effective treatments for panic disorder. The behavioral approaches studied have included educative/cognitive treatment, relaxation, and therapist-assisted or self-paced exposure with systematic desensitization.[13] Behavior therapy is often enhanced by the addition of medications, which can provide quick relief of attacks and reduction of anticipatory anxiety while the patient is in the process of learning behavioral skills. Treatment with medications alone is most appropriate for patients unable or unwilling to practice behavioral techniques.

When medications are used, they are most often chosen from one of three classes: the tricyclic antidepressants, the MAO inhibitors, and the high-potency benzodiazepines (alprazolam and clonazepam). While these drugs are considered to be equally effective, the MAO inhibitor phenelzine has been suggested to have an advantage in refractory patients and alprazolam has been suggested to be more rapidly effective while more difficult to discontinue than the other drugs. Clonazepam, which has a longer duration of action than alprazolam, is finding increasing use among patients who find alprazolam to produce interdose anxiety.

In the treatment of *agoraphobia*, the traditional approach has been behavioral therapy, which repeatedly has been shown to be effective. The recent hypothesis, based on learning theory, that understands agoraphobia primarily as a secondary complication of panic disorder has led to the treatment of this condition with imipramine and other antidepressants. Mavissakalian and colleagues demonstrated imipramine's ability to enhance behavioral treatment of agoraphobia.[14] Again, for patients unwilling or unable to pursue behavioral approaches, antidepressants alone provide an effective treatment alternative.[13]

Performance anxiety, a state known to all but as yet unclassified in the DSM-III-R, has recently been treated on a systematic basis with beta-adrenergic receptor blockers in performers of many varieties.[15,16] The results have been surprisingly good, though popular controversy has been aroused as to whether or not this use of medication is legitimate. Behavioral therapy, which has a longer tradition in this complaint, has also been shown to be helpful. A promising area for further study is the nature of interaction between pharmacologic and behavioral therapies in performance anxiety.

Generalized anxiety, a heterogeneous syndrome often present in combination with other anxiety syndromes, has been treated with a variety of medications but with only modest success. The most popular drug class remains benzodiazepines, which during the 1970s superseded classes of drugs now considered abusable and dangerous (methaqualone, glutethimide, and meprobamate). The benzodiazepines have received criticism for the frequency with which they are prescribed, their potential for dependence or abuse, their potentiation of other sedating drugs or alcohol, and the potentially dangerous withdrawal symptoms that follow overly rapid discontinuation. Until recently, there were few pharmacologic alternatives to benzodiazepines in the treatment of prolonged anxiety states, though tricyclic antidepressants have provided a relatively effective and less abusable alternative for some patients. The recent introduction of buspirone, the first of a new class of nonbenzodiazepine anxiolytic drugs, may significantly affect the treatment of generalized anxiety.[17] Buspirone is still new, so there may be as-yet-unanticipated adverse effects, but results of preliminary testing in a large number of anxious patients have suggested that this drug may be superior to benzodiazepines in the treatment of some patients, perhaps especially those who have not previously been treated with benzodiazepines. Buspirone is thought not to induce sedation, tolerance, addiction, or withdrawal symptoms. It is also believed to be an unlikely drug for recreational abuse, since known drug abusers in one study refused buspirone in favor of taking a placebo. Patients perceive as buspirone's major drawbacks its lack of a high and the two-week lag time often required before its effects are experienced.

Obsessive-compulsive disorder, a relatively rare but extremely disabling anxiety disorder, has increasingly been treated pharmacologically. Studies demonstrate a modest effectiveness of clomipramine, a tricyclic antidepressant not yet available in the United States except for investigational purposes.[18,19] For patients unable to obtain clomipramine, other antidepressants have been tried and some success has been documented, especially with the recently released drug fluoxetine.[20] Phenelzine has been anecdotally effective, even in a particularly refractory group, those patients who suffer from obsessions without compulsions. Behavioral therapy, alone or in combination with medications, has also been advocated and shown to be of value for some patients.[13,21]

Post-traumatic stress disorder seems an unlikely diagnosis for which to prescribe medication, but recent investigators into the nature of this disorder suggested that drugs may indeed play a useful role.[22-24] This disorder includes a heightened activation of the sympathetic nervous system, so drugs that reduce sympathetic activity have been used adjunctively to reduce symptoms that otherwise might prevent participation in psychotherapy or effective social and occupational functioning. Clonidine has investigationally been used to reduce sympathetic hyperactivity; imipramine and other antidepressants have been advocated for depressive and/or anxiety symptoms; propranolol has been suggested to diminish autonomic hyperarousal; carbamazepine has been tried for episodic symptoms such as flashbacks. Each of these drugs has been used only in small numbers of patients but preliminary results suggest that drugs may provide an often helpful support to ongoing psychotherapy.

MOOD DISORDERS

The development of new drugs and the creative application of synergistic agents in the treatment of mood disorders during the 1980s have been major areas of progress. Second only to the anxiety disorders in prevalence, the mood disorders are estimated to affect 5% of the population at any time and to account for a substantial number of mortalities through suicide. The refinement of diagnostic criteria for mood disorders, their extension to include a "soft spectrum" of chronic minor mood disorders, the development of several classes of new antidepressants, and the creative application of synergistic anti-depressant "potentiators" have been the most significant recent advances in the treatment of mood disorders.

In terms of diagnosis, the development of the DSM-III-R and the delineation of *melancholic depression* have facilitated recognition of drug-responsive symptoms. The discovery of biological markers of mood disorders such as reduced rapid eye movement (REM) latency (an alteration of sleep EEG architecture) or nonsuppressing responses to the dexamethasone suppression test (which reflects disordered endocrine functioning) has stimulated further searches for increasingly sensitive and specific objective measures of physiological disturbances in depressed patients. Some of these biological markers have also been found in individuals with chronic minor mood disorders, which has encouraged clinicians to use medications in their treatment. The result has been an increasing interest in refining predictive criteria for which patients are likely to obtain relief from medication and which are likely to respond poorly.

Tricyclic and MAO-inhibiting antidepressants are thought to be effective in at least 70% of appropriately chosen patients. Of those remaining, a substantial number have been helped by the introduction of plasma tricyclic-level measurements, the use of potentiating synergistic drugs such as lithium, and the introduction of new drugs. Because they can be given without dietary restriction, the tricyclic antidepressants are often chosen initially in a course of treatment. Recent experimental evidence suggests that MAO inhibitors may have a small advantage in the treatment of atypical depressives (patients whose depression is characterized by hypersomnia, hyperphagia, leaden feeling, and sensitivity to rejection), especially when panic attacks are also present.[25]

An important technical advance in the treatment of mood disorders has been the standardization of measurements of tricyclic levels in blood. Appropriate use of these tests can help to ensure that an apparently refractory patient is achieving sufficient drug levels in the blood (and presumably the brain).[26] Until an adequate blood level of an antidepressant has been achieved for several weeks, a true treatment trial cannot be said to have occurred. In the face of an adequate but ineffective trial of one tricyclic agent, there is a limited likelihood of improving response by simply giving more medication. Instead, potentiators such as lithium, thyroid hormone, tryptophan, or stimulants are increasingly being used. These additional drugs are hypothesized to enhance the effectiveness of antidepressants by activating a different population of neurotransmitter receptors. The best effects have been demonstrated with lithium, which when added to tricyclic or MAO-inhibiting antidepressants has been reported to convert about half of refractory patients to responders within periods ranging from a few days to a few weeks.[27-30] Thyroid hormone, usually triiodothyronine, has also been claimed effective in this role.[31-34] Tryptophan has received some attention as an enhancer of MAO inhibitors, but has also been reported to be capable of inducing a toxic "central serotonergic" toxic syndrome when combined with an MAO inhibitor. Stimulants such as methylphenidate or amphetamine have been claimed to enhance antidepressant responsiveness but their potentially dangerous interaction with antidepressants (especially of the MAO-inhibitor class) requires caution when they are used adjunctively.[35]

Among the new antidepressants introduced as second generation drugs, maprotiline and trazodone have remained useful alternatives to tricyclic or MAO-inhibitor antidepressants. Maprotiline, structurally similar to the tricyclics, is an antidepressant of comparable efficacy and shares the same adverse effects, including an unfortunately high rate of seizures when dosage is too rapidly increased. Trazodone, whose structure differs from other available antidepressants, is a drug with comparable efficacy and a clearly different spectrum of side effects. Its lack of anticholinergic effects is welcome to patients who are able to withstand its sedative effects. Reports of priapism (sustained penile erection), rare though they have been, have raised anxiety of clinicians about prescribing this drug for men. It remains, nonetheless, an acceptable alternative when tricyclics or MAO inhibitors are not tolerated.

Recently, a new class of antidepressants entered the clinical arena: the selective serotonin reuptake blockers. Fluoxetine, the first of these to be marketed in the United States, is a bicyclic chemical that has been demonstrated to be an effective antidepressant.[36] One quality that will make it welcome is its purported lack of causing appetite increase and weight gain. Besides depression, preliminary findings suggest it will be useful in the treatment of patients with obsessive-compulsive disorder. It will be followed by another selective serotonin reuptake blocker, fluvoxamine.

Concern that the use of an antidepressant drug will undermine a psychotherapeutic treatment is often raised, but research has so far failed to validate that viewpoint. In fact, a study has shown that patients receiving antidepressants are more likely than unmedicated patients to remain in psychotherapy.[37] A recent review of research on psychotherapy and pharmacotherapy in depression stated that combined therapy resulted in "greater overall improvement in symptoms, lower attrition and lower chance of symptomatic failure, lower risk of relapse and greater improvement in social functioning."[38]

An estimated 10% of patients with mood disorders have *bipolar affective disorders*. The importance of distinguishing these mood disturbances from unipolar mood disorders has been emphasized by Akiskal, who asserts that in their more and less overt forms the bipolar disorders are more common than previously believed.[39] Lithium has been the major therapeutic agent in the treatment of patients with these disorders, but as many as 20% to 30% of patients have been refractory to lithium's effects or unable to tolerate its toxic side effects. A major treatment advance in the 1980s has been the discovery that a variety of drugs share lithium's mood-regulating effects but present a different spectrum of adverse effects which may be more acceptable to individual patients. The most popular current alternatives to lithium include carbamazepine and valproate (used also as anticonvulsants) and verapamil (an anti-angina drug).

A number of studies support the use of carbamazepine in bipolar patients, whether they have been responsive or refractory to lithium.[40-42] Each drug seems to offer relief to 70% of patients but each treats some patients who were refractory to the other. As with lithium, carbamazepine appears helpful for prophylaxis as well as in the treatment of acute manic or depressive episodes. Because of its capacity to induce agranulocytosis (failure of blood-forming bone marrow cells) its use is closely supervised during the initial months of treatment and carefully monitored thereafter with checks of blood, liver functions, and blood levels of carbamazepine. Its use with antipsychotic drugs has generally been regarded as safe and it is regarded as safe to combine with lithium, a combination anecdotally reported to induce better mood control in some refractory patients. Unlike lithium, its use in combination with MAO inhibitors is not recommended, because of concern over additive side effects.

Another anticonvulsant drug used as a mood regulator,

valproate sodium (also called valproic acid), has received particular attention though its psychiatric efficacy remains insufficiently documented.[43] Valproate, like carbamazepine, can have toxic effects on the liver or bone marrow, which necessitate careful monitoring of these organs and valproate's blood level. A small number of patients have responded to valproate with severe platelet dysfunction, hepatitis, or pancreatitis. The drug should not be prescribed during early pregnancy, as it is considered teratogenic (capable of causing birth defects).

An intriguing and different drug that has recently received attention as a mood regulator is verapamil.[44] While it will still require further study, this drug seems to be effective in treating or preventing bipolar disorder episodes in some patients. If proven effective in larger studies it will be of particular value as a lithium alternative because of its minimal side effects and apparent lack of necessity for monitoring blood levels. Its cardiac and liver effects, however, require at least a baseline ECG and testing of liver function as well as periodic checks during therapy.

SCHIZOPHRENIA

The major modern breakthroughs in the pharmacotherapy of *schizophrenia* date from the early 1950s, when the French surgeon Laborit experimented with chlorpromazine for preoperative use. Observing that the drug produced a state of "artificial hibernation," he suggested that it be used in psychiatric patients.[45] The initial trials, in manic patients, were not more encouraging than those for electroshock therapy. Experiments with schizophrenic patients, however, yielded such extraordinary results that within several years the previously popular treatment approaches (electroconvulsive therapy [ECT], insulin shock, lobotomy, reserpine) began to fall into disuse.

Studies have repeatedly demonstrated the efficacy of antipsychotic drugs in the acute, continuation, and maintenance phases of the treatment of schizophrenia. Most acute psychotic episodes respond to these medications and attempts to find superior psychosocial approaches have been unsuccessful. Studies of treatment using a combination of modalities have confirmed the central role of medications, and have shown medications' effectiveness to be enhanced by concurrent supportive psychotherapy, family therapy, or psychoeducational treatment.[46-48]

In the treatment of acute psychosis, advances have consisted of increasingly sophisticated balancing of therapeutic and adverse effects. Since it is now known that a very large number of patients experience disturbing side effects with these medications even in the short run, clinicians are paying increasing attention to selection of drugs with a tolerable spectrum of side effects. Attention is also being paid to minimization of dosage, given evidence that an acute phase daily dosage range of 400 to 600 mg of chlorpromazine equivalents should suffice for the treatment of the average patient.[49]

Following an acute episode, the maintenance or prophylactic phase of treatment begins. Studies in which schizophrenic patients were randomly switched, in a double-blind manner, from active medication to placebo have shown a consistently high rate of relapse.[49] Even when patients have been in remission while taking medication for two to three years, the relapse rate during the first 12 months after medication discontinuation approaches 65%. For patients emerging from an initial episode of schizophrenia, a similarly high rate of relapse has been noted when pharmacotherapy is not sustained.[49]

Unfortunately, the ubiquitous presence of acute and long-term adverse effects has hampered the effective treatment of schizophrenia. Sedation, orthostatic hypotension, acute extrapyramidal effects including tardive dyskinesia, and anticholinergic effects are problematic concomitants of treatment. The presence of unpleasant side effects of these drugs has led, during the 1980s, to advances in their use, which focus on maximizing their therapeutic effectiveness and minimizing their adverse effects. Two strategies in particular have been advocated for this purpose: low-dose treatment and intermittent treatment.

The low-dose approach dates back at least to the observations in 1964 of Caffey and associates, who found that when patients taking 350 to 400 mg/d of chlorpromazine were reduced to 3/7 of their starting dose, they developed a relapse rate (15% over four months) between that observed with the original dose (5%) and that observed with placebo (45%).[50] Using injectable fluphenazine enanthate (which, like fluphenazine decanoate, is a long-acting intramuscular antipsychotic medication) Goldstein and colleagues compared recently discharged schizophrenic patients treated with high (25 mg every two weeks) or low (6.25 mg every two weeks) doses and concurrent crisis-oriented family therapy or no psychotherapy.[48] During the first six weeks after discharge, 24% of the low-dose/no therapy patients relapsed. None of the high-dose/therapy patients relapsed. The other two groups showed intermediate and equivalent relapse rates, suggesting that a psychosocial treatment approach might allow use of a lower dosage of medication. In a longer term study, Kane followed stable schizophrenic outpatients during a year and assigned them randomly to treatment with either fluphenazine decanoate, 12.5 to 50 mg, 2.5 to 10 mg, or 1.25 to 5 mg intramuscularly (IM) every two weeks.[49] On the lowest dose regimen, 56% of patients relapsed, while only 24% of those who received the intermediate range and 14% of those who received the standard dosage relapsed. Evidence favored the lower doses despite a higher rate of relapse in several ways: firstly, the restabilization of relapsed patients was easily accomplished by a temporary dosage increase; secondly, there were significantly fewer early signs of tardive dyskinesia among the low-dose patients; and finally, the low-dose patients achieved better ratings on some psychosocial measures, for example showing less emotional withdrawal. Taken together, these studies suggest that a lower dose of antipsychotic medication is appropriate for some patients in a maintenance phase of treatment. A higher rate of exacerbation or relapse is to be anticipated, but may be worth accepting in exchange for livelier psychosocial functioning and a potentially diminished risk of tardive dyskinesia.[49]

The approach called intermittent or targeted medication has been advocated by clinicians who maintain that some schizophrenic patients may remain in remission for significant lengths of time with no medication at all. Fundamental assumptions underlying this approach include the notion that patients can recognize their impending relapse and that long-term adverse antipsychotic effects can be diminished by reduced total exposure to the drugs. The observations of Herz and Melville showed that many patients exhibit characteristic signs or symptoms during early stages of relapse.[51] Patients or family members were found capable of observing these signs and predicting a relapse with considerable accuracy. Carpenter and Heinrichs incorporated these observations into a treatment protocol, which allowed patients to remain unmedicated until relapse symptoms occurred.[52] While this treatment approach proved effective for patients, no controlled comparison of low-dose to targeted treatment has yet been completed. It is therefore premature to espouse one or the other approach as superior at this time.[49]

While antipsychotic medications have greatly improved the treatment of schizophrenic patients, clinicians are familiar with the persistent impairment seen in partial responders or nonresponders. Although advances in the treatment of refractory schizophrenia have been limited, some patients have been found to benefit from the addition to antipsychotic medication of lithium carbonate, benzodiazepines, propranolol, or carbamazepine. ECT, initially developed to treat schizophrenics, remains an alternative for some drug nonresponders. There are currently no guidelines for choosing among these alternatives for a specific refractory patient.[53]

Hope for the near future rests on two new pharmacologic approaches emerging in the atypical neuroleptics now being explored.[54] One class of drugs, exemplified by haloperidol, pimozide, or sulpiride, binds very specifically to the class of dopamine receptors termed D2 receptors. This subpopulation of receptors is thought to be most relevant to the therapeutic effects of the medications. Sulpiride has appeared less likely to induce tardive dyskinesia, perhaps because it does not induce dopamine-receptor supersensitivity. Another class of neuroleptics, exemplified by clozapine, binds to a broad spectrum of receptors and may exert some of its effects through nondopaminergic neurotransmitter effects. In high doses, clozapine actually suppresses tardive dyskinesia without leading to a rebound exacerbation. Lower doses have sometimes been observed to induce improvement in dyskinetic symptoms. The availability of clozapine in this country has been delayed by a serious side effect, agranulocytosis (destruction of blood-producing bone marrow cells), which may affect between 0.06% and 0.38% of treated patients. Because there is a 19% to 42% mortality of patients with this condition, clozapine is currently restricted to experimental use. It is of note that agranulocytosis is not unheard of with use of conventional phenothiazines, where the rate is 0.1%.[54]

FRONTIERS OF PHARMACOTHERAPY

Among the diverse and frustrating group of eating disorders, *bulimic bingeing* has been most responsive to pharmacotherapy. Studies have supported the use of tricyclic antidepressants, atypical antidepressants (such as trazodone), and MAO inhibitors, reporting improvement in as many as 90% of patients. While rates of improvement with use of placebo have also been high in some studies, clear therapeutic effects have been demonstrated and proven to be more than mere relief of concurrent depressive symptoms.[55] Further work is needed to define the optimal choice of drug, dosage, or duration of treatment. In the only published observations extending beyond two years, Pope and his colleagues at McLean noted that many patients relapsed once medications were discontinued. They claimed extended remission of bingeing, however, in a sizeable group of medicated patients and even in a few patients who were successfully off of medications.[56]

Another class of disorders in which systematic investigations of pharmacotherapy have recently begun is that of the *personality disorders*. Given the lack of persistent psychotic or mood disturbances in these disorders, the use of drugs even in conjunction with psychotherapy has prompted controversial discussions about the nature of these disorders and the proper bounds of pharmacotherapy. For the treatment of symptoms of borderline, schizotypal, or paranoid personality disorders, the final assessment of pharmacotherapy is far from being made. Recent studies, however, offer some suggestions as to when drugs are most useful in these conditions.

When carefully assessed, the target borderline symptoms which have shown greatest medication responsiveness are mood lability, depressive symptoms, severe and especially phobic anxiety, brief psychotic regressions, ideas of reference, obsessive-compulsive symptoms, and some types of impulsivity or self-injurious behavior.[57] Low-dose neuroleptic regimens (such as 4 to 6 mg of haloperidol or 5 to 10 mg of thiothixene per day) are currently popular and seem to have modest but significant beneficial effects in treating these target symptoms.[58,59] Antipsychotic drugs, of course, bring with their use the risk (over a longer time course) of tardive dyskinesia. It is essential, therefore, to note that studies of antipsychotic drugs in the treatment of borderline patients are all short term, and none have suggested the continuous use of these drugs for more than several months' duration. Some other interesting approaches, especially for the treatment of self-injurious behavior, have been suggested by Cowdry and Gardner's careful study of 16 borderline patients. In their group, carbamazepine showed a general ability to reduce out-of-control harmful behavior,[60] but also induced depression in a few patients. Tranylcypromine, an MAO inhibitor-antidepressant, produced some beneficial effects, though the use of an MAO inhibitor carries with it the risk of severe self-destruction if taken inappropriately (for example, if dietary restrictions are not observed). Of great interest in this era of alprazolam's popularity, this drug was beneficial to a small number of borderline patients. In the majority, however, it exacerbated severe self-injurious behavior. This result suggests that clinicians should exert caution in prescribing alprazolam to any patient with a history of self-harm.

Attention deficit hyperactivity disorder, now known to affect adults as well as children, has been recognized to produce a syndrome of motor hyperactivity, attentional difficulty, affective lability, inability to complete tasks, volatile temper, impulsivity, impaired interpersonal relationships, and stress intolerance. This cluster of symptoms is often associated with or mistaken for conduct disorder in children or personality disorder in young adults (see chapter 11). Pharmacologic approaches have helped both affected children and adults. In adults, the use of stimulants such as methylphenidate or pemoline has been shown particularly to alleviate the symptoms of attentional impairment, impulsivity, motor hyperactivity, and stress intolerance.[61] This in turn can improve psychosocial functioning or perhaps allow an individual to make better use of psychosocial therapies.

CONCLUSION

Looking over the long course of pharmacotherapy's history and the wide range of current indications for psychotropic medications, it is apparent that astounding progress has been made. Recent years have seen advances in the scientific evaluation of drug effects, the development of new drugs with lesser toxicity or alternative mechanisms of action, the expansion of pharmacotherapeutic approaches beyond the most severe disorders, and the integration of pharmacotherapeutic with psychotherapeutic techniques. While much remains to be accomplished, the use of drugs to treat behavioral disorders and to ease human emotional suffering has evolved substantially and offers even greater hope for the future.

REFERENCES

1. Escobar JI, Anthony JC, Canino G, et al: Use of neuroleptics, antidepressants, and lithium by U.S. community populations. *Psychopharmacol Bull* 1987;23:196–200.
2. Griffiths RR, Sannerud CA: Abuse of and dependence on benzodiazepines and other anxiolytic/sedative drugs, in Meltzer HY (ed): *Psychopharmacology: The Third Generation of Progress*. New York, Raven Press, 1987, pp 1535–1541.
3. Alexander FG, Selesnick ST: *The History of Psychiatry*. New York, Harper and Row, 1966.
4. Gordon BL: *Medieval and Renaissance Medicine*. New York, Philosophical Library, Inc., 1959.
5. Kroll J: Reappraisal of psychiatry in the middle ages. *Arch Gen Psychiatry* 1973;29:276–283.
6. Haggard HH: *Devils, Drugs, and Doctors*. New York, Harper & Brothers, 1929.
7. Burton R: *The Anatomy of Melancholy*. New York, Random House, 1977.
8. Deutsch A: *The Mentally Ill in America, ed 2*. New York, Columbia University Press, 1949.
9. Woodward SB: Observations on the medical treatment of insanity. *Am J Insanity* 1850;7:1–34.
10. Moriarty KM, Alagna SW, Lake RC: Psychopharmacology: An historical approach. *Psychiatric Clin N Am* 1984;7:411–433.
11. Baldessarini RJ: *Chemotherapy in Psychiatry, ed 2*. Cambridge, Harvard University Press, 1985.
12. Shear MK, Fyer MR: Biological and psychopathologic findings in panic disorder, in Frances AJ, Hales RE (eds): *American Psychiatric Press Review of Psychiatry* vol 7. Washington, DC, American Psychiatric Press, 1988, pp 29–53.
13. Roy-Byrne PP, Katon W: An update on treatment of the anxiety disorders. *Hosp Comm Psychiatry* 1987;38:835–843.
14. Mavissakalian M, Michelson L, Dealy RS: Pharmacological treat-

ment of agoraphobia: imipramine versus imipramine with programmed practice. *Br J Psychiatry* 1983;143:348–355.
15. Brantigan CO, Brantigan TA, Joseph N: Effect of beta blockade and beta stimulation on stage fright. *Am J Med* 1982;72:88–94.
16. James I, Savage I: Beneficial effect of nadolol on anxiety-induced disturbances of performance in musicians: A comparison with diazepam and placebo. *Am Heart J* 1984;108:1150–1155.
17. Goa KL, Ward A: Buspirone: A preliminary review of its pharmacological properties and therapeutic efficacy as an anxiolytic. *Drugs* 1986;32:114–129.
18. Zohar J, Insel TR: Obsessive-compulsive disorder: Psychobiological approaches to diagnosis, treatment, and pathophysiology. *Biol Psychiatry* 1987;22:667–687.
19. Volavka J, Neziroglu F, Yaryura-Tobias JA: Clomipramine and imipramine in obsessive-compulsive disorder. *Psychiatry Res* 1985; 14:83–91.
20. Fontaine R, Chouinard G: An open clinical trial of fluoxetine in the treatment of obsessive-compulsive disorder. *J Clin Psychopharmacol* 1986;6:98–101.
21. Baer L, Minichiello WE: Behavior therapy for obsessive-compulsive disorder, in Jenike MA, Baer L, Minichiello WE (eds): *Obsessive-Compulsive Disorders: Theory and Management*. Littleton, MA, PSG Publishing Co., 1986.
22. Burstein A: Treatment of post-traumatic stress disorder with imipramine. *Psychosomatics* 1984;25:681–687.
23. Vander Kolk BA: Psychopharmacologic issues in posttraumatic stress disorder. *Hosp Comm Psychiatry* 1983;34:683–691.
24. Lipper S, Davidson JRT, Grady TA, et al: Preliminary study of carbamazepine in post-traumatic stress disorder. *Psychosomatics* 1986;27:849–854.
25. Quitkin FM, Stewart JW, McGrath PJ, et al: Phenelzine versus imipramine in the treatment of probable atypical depression: Defining syndrome boundaries of selective MAOI responders. *Am J Psychiatry* 1988;145:306–311.
26. Task Force on the Use of Laboratory Tests in Psychiatry: Tricyclic antidepressants — Blood level measurements and clinical outcome: An APA task force report. *Am J Psychiatry* 1985;142:155–162.
27. Heninger GR, Charney DS, Sternberg DE: Lithium carbonate augmentation of antidepressant treatment: An effective prescription for treatment-refractory depression. *Arch Gen Psychiatry* 1983;40:1335–1342.
28. Price LH, Conwell Y, Nelson JC: Lithium augmentation of combined neuroleptic-tricyclic treatment in delusional depression. *Am J Psychiatry* 1983;140:318–322.
29. Louie AK, Meltzer HY: Lithium potentiation of antidepressant treatment. *J Clin Psychopharmacol* 1984;4:316–321.
30. Price LH, Charney DS, Heninger GR: Efficacy of lithium-

tranylcypromine treatment in depression. *Am J Psychiatry* 1985; 142:619-623.
31. Prange AJ, Wilson IC, Rabon AM, et al: Enhancement of imipramine antidepressant activity by thyroid hormone. *Am J Psychiatry* 1969;126:457-469.
32. Earle BV: Thyroid hormone and tricyclic antidepressants in resistant depressions. *Am J Psychiatry* 1970;126:1667-1669.
33. Goodwin FK, Prange AJ, Post RM, et al: Potentiation of antidepressant effects by L-triiodothyronine in tricyclic nonresponders. *Am J Psychiatry* 1982;139:34-38.
34. Schwarcz G, Halaris A, Baxter L, et al: Normal thyroid function in desipramine nonresponders converted to responders by the addition of L-triiodothyronine. *Am J Psychiatry* 1984;141:1614-1616.
35. Wharton RN, Perel JM, Dayton PG, et al: A potential clinical use for methylphenidate with tricyclic antidepressants. *Am J Psychiatry* 1971;127:1619-1625.
36. Sommi RW, Crismon ML, Bowden CL: Fluoxetine: A serotonin-specific, second-generation antidepressant. *Pharmacotherapy* 1987; 7:1-15.
37. Rounsaville BJ, Klerman GL, Weissman MW: Do psychotherapy and pharmacotherapy for depression conflict? *Arch Gen Psychiatry* 1981;38:24-29.
38. Weissman MM, Jarrett RB, Rush JA: Psychotherapy and its relevance to the pharmacotherapy of major depression: A decade later (1976-1985), in Meltzer HY (ed): *Psychopharmacology: The Third Generation of Progress*. New York, Raven Press, 1987, pp 1059-1069.
39. Akiskal HS: The milder spectrum of bipolar disorders: Diagnostic, characterologic and pharmacologic aspects. *Psychiatric Ann* 1987; 17:32-37.
40. Okuma T, Inanaga K, Otsuki S, et al: Comparison of the antimanic efficacy of carbamazepine and chlorpromazine: a double-blind controlled study. *Psychopharmacology* 1979;66:211-217.
41. Ballenger JC, Post RM: Carbamazepine (Tegretol) in manic-depressive illness: A new treatment. *Am J Psychiatry* 1980;137:782-790.
42. Post RM, Uhde TW: Clinical approaches to treatment-resistant bipolar illness, in Hales RE, Francis AJ: *American Psychiatric Association Annual Review*, vol 6, Washington, DC, American Psychiatric Press, 1988, pp 125-150.
43. Emrich, Okuma, Muller: *Anticonvulsants in affective disorders*. Amsterdam, Excerpta Medica, 1984.
44. Pollack MH, Rosenbaum JF, Hyman SE: Calcium channel blockers in psychiatry. *Psychosomatics* 1987;28:356-360.
45. Deniker P: Introduction of neuroleptic chemotherapy into psychiatry, in Ayd FJ, Blackwell B (eds): *Discoveries in Biological Psychiatry*. Baltimore, Ayd Medical Communications, 1984, pp

155–164.
46. Schooler NR, Hogarty GE: Medication and psychosocial strategies in the treatment of schizophrenia, in Meltzer HY (ed): *Psychopharmacology: The Third Generation of Progress*. New York, Raven Press, 1987, pp 1111–1119.
47. Carpenter WT, Keith SM: Integrating treatments in schizophrenia. *Psychiatric Clin N Am* 1986;9:153–164.
48. Goldstein MJ, Rodnick EH, Evans JR, et al: Drug and family therapy in the aftercare of acute schizophrenics. *Arch Gen Psychiatry* 1978;35:1169–1177.
49. Kane JM: Treatment of schizophrenia. *Schizophrenia Bull* 1987;13:133–156.
50. Caffey EM, Diamond LS, Frank TV, et al: Discontinuation or reduction of chemotherapy in chronic schizophrenics. *J Chronic Dis* 1964;17:347–358.
51. Herz MI, Melville C: Relapse in schizophrenia. *Am J Psychiatry* 1980;137:801–805.
52. Carpenter WT, Heinrichs DW: Intermittent pharmacotherapy of schizophrenia, in Kane JM (ed): *Drug Maintenance Strategies in Schizophrenia*. Washington, DC, American Psychiatric Press, 1984, pp 70–82.
53. Donaldson S, Gelenberg A, Baldessarini R: Pharmacologic treatment of schizophrenia: A progress report. *Schizophrenia Bull* 1983;9:504–527.
54. Tamminga CA, Gerlach J: New neuroleptics and experimental antipsychotics in schizophrenia, in Meltzer HY (ed): *Psychopharmacology: The Third Generation of Progress*. New York, Raven Press, 1987, pp 1129–1140.
55. Garfinkel PE, Garner DM (eds): *The Role of Drug Treatments for Eating Disorders*. New York, Brunner/Mazel, 1987.
56. Pope HG, Hudson JI, Jonas JM, Yurgelun-Todd D: Antidepressant treatment of bulimia: A two-year follow-up study. *J Clin Psychopharmacol* 1985;5:320–327.
57. Ellison JM, Adler DA: Psychopharmacologic approaches to borderline syndromes. *Compr Psychiatry* 1984;25:255–262.
58. Goldberg SC, Schulz C, Schulz PM, et al: Borderline and schizotypal personality disorders treated with low-dose thiothixene vs placebo. *Arch Gen Psychiatry* 1986;43:680–686.
59. Soloff PH, George A, Nathan RS, et al: Progress in pharmacotherapy of borderline disorders. *Arch Gen Psychiatry* 1986;43:691–697.
60. Gardner DL, Cowdry RW: Positive effects of carbamazepine on behavioral dyscontrol in borderline personality disorder. *Am J Psychiatry* 1986;143:519–522.
61. Wender PH, Reimherr FW, Wood DR: Attention deficit disorder ("Minimal brain dysfunction") in adults. *Arch Gen Psychiatry* 1981;38:449–456.

7

An Introduction to Psychiatric Medications

James M. Ellison

Virtually every psychiatric medication in current use began its clinical life within the past four decades. During this brief time, nonetheless, psychiatric drugs have flourished and diversified. Currently they account for 20% of all prescriptions filled in the United States. Ten percent of the general population uses psychiatric medications, and the percentage of psychotherapy patients taking such medications is much higher. Because these medications profoundly affect the way people feel, think, and act, a familiarity with their effects is essential knowledge for a psychotherapist. This chapter explains how these drugs work and how the body handles them. The major classes of medications are discussed, with attention to specific drugs, dose ranges, and side effects.

HOW DRUGS WORK TO AFFECT BEHAVIOR

The brain is composed of groups of specialized cells (neurons), which communicate with each other in order to achieve the incredible synchronization of activity necessary to perform even the most simple of functions. Currently the classic model of synaptic transmission is being revised on the basis of new discoveries. For heuristic purposes, however, this model still provides a useful framework for understanding many of the synaptic effects of psychotropic drugs.

In the classic model, intercellular communication (neurotransmission) occurs when one neuron releases a membrane-bound packet containing many molecules of a chemical messenger (neurotransmitter) into the specialized interface separating it from neighboring neurons. The interface is called a synapse, so the contiguous cells are called presynaptic and postsynaptic neurons. The molecules of neurotransmitter released from the postsynaptic neuron have a strong affinity for receptor molecules (complex molecules within the postsynaptic neuron's membrane) and tend to cling or bind to specialized sites on those molecules. This binding of receptors and neurotransmitters activates chemical processes that excite or inhibit cellular activity. The release of an inhibitory neurotransmitter onto a postsynaptic cell, for example, may make that cell less likely to discharge and pass on its received impulse to a subsequent cell. Released neurotransmitter does not accumulate endlessly in the synapse because its presence is regulated in several ways. Some is taken up through a special transport system into the presynaptic cell, to be destroyed chemically or reused. Some is destroyed within the synapse or nearby, through the chemical action of specialized molecules called enzymes. Over a longer time course, some neurotransmitters are also regulated through inhibitory presynaptic receptor sites. When large amounts of neurotransmitter have been released into the synapse, binding of these inhibitory sites is increased and the result is a reduction of presynaptic neurotransmitter release (see Fig 7-1).

The summing up of many excitatory and inhibitory neurotransmitter-induced communications among individual cells leads to coordinated activity among large groups of brain cells, which form systems. The output from these systems forms the brain's instructions to the body. Output from the brain channelled to the muscles, for example, is what initiates and controls physical movement. Perceptions, thoughts, and emotions also depend on the coordination of neuronal activity, so an excess or shortage of neurotransmitters (or a problem in neurotransmitter regulation) can affect cognition and mood.

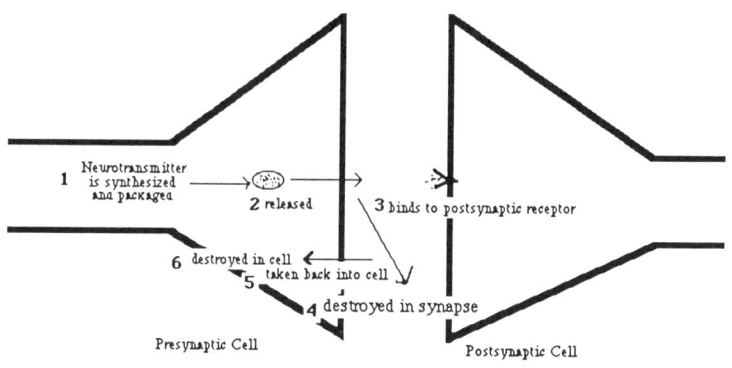

Figure 7-1 Neurotransmitter Synthesis, Release, and Destruction at the Synapse.

Many psychopharmacologic drugs exert their desired effects by modulating the availability or regulation of neurotransmitters. They may enhance neurotransmitter effects, for example, by interfering with the presynaptic reuptake process, which removes excess neurotransmitter from the synapse. Or they may reduce neurotransmitter effects through a kind of molecular "musical chairs" process in which they competitively occupy available presynaptic or postsynaptic binding sites but do not produce the further chemical actions of neurotransmitters. Still other drugs go within the postsynaptic cell and produce direct chemical effects. And, finally, some drugs modulate synaptic regulatory activity over a longer time period through mechanisms only partially understood, accounting for the clinically observed time lag necessary for the effects of these drugs. Well over 100 neurotransmitters have been identified, yet the following five have been of particular interest to psychopharmacologists because their activities are affected by so many of the drugs currently prescribed:

Acetylcholine is the neurotransmitter in the cholinergic pathways of the brain and also in the parasympathetic part of the autonomic peripheral nervous system. (Neuronal pathways, after they exit the skull or spine, are called the peripheral nervous system. They connect the brain to muscles or other target organs, and can be involved in unwanted side effects of drugs. For example, the accelerated heart rate sometimes accompanying antidepressant treatment is related to peripheral blocking of acetylcholine receptors on the heart, which otherwise would receive "slowing" messages from the brain via the parasympathetic part of the autonomic nervous system.) Psychotropic drugs which block the cholinergic receptors on neurons are called anticholinergic. A special class of anticholinergic drugs is described later in this chapter. Antidepressants and antipsychotic drugs also block cholinergic receptors, though this seems unrelated to their therapeutic activities. Any drug that blocks cholinergic receptors can produce annoying anticholinergic side effects (see Table 7-1).

Dopamine is the neurotransmitter in the dopaminergic pathways and systems of the brain, which include regulators of emotional activity and muscular tone and coordination. The seemingly effortless movements of facial expressions or the smooth maintenance of balance while standing or walking are modulated by dopamine's activity or drugs that block its effects. Dopamine is believed to be functionally overactive (either too much is available or the receptors are too sensitive) in schizophrenia and some acute psychotic states. Antipsychotic medications probably exert their therapeutic effects by blocking postsynaptic dopamine receptor sites, thereby reducing the excess activity of dopamine. The familiar syndrome of Parkinson's disease (which includes rigid posture, slow trembling of the hands, shuffling gait, drooling, and a masklike facial expression, often accompanied by depression) is caused by a functional underactivity

Table 7-1
Anticholinergic Side Effects

Dry mouth
Blurred vision
Constipation
Dilated pupils
Increased heart rate
Dry skin
Difficulty urinating
Confusion, disorientation
Irritability
Hallucinations, delusions
Exacerbation of glaucoma

of dopamine — the opposite of what happens in schizophrenia. Dopamine-blocking antipsychotic medications currently used to treat schizophrenia are not specific enough to reduce the neurotransmitter's effects solely in the mesolimbic pathway, where psychotic symptoms seem to originate. They also block dopamine's important functions in the nigrostriatal pathway, the area of the brain affected in Parkinson's disease. This is how the dopamine-blocking antipsychotic drugs can cause parkinsonian side effects in patients treated for psychosis.

Norepinephrine (sometimes called noradrenaline) is the transmitter in noradrenergic pathways of the brain, which include regulators of pleasure and alertness. Norepinephrine is also an active neurotransmitter in the sympathetic part of the autonomic nervous system, where it helps to maintain blood pressure. When a person rises suddenly after sitting or lying, the body's ability to maintain blood pressure depends on the normal functioning of the noradrenergic pathways. Drugs that block the receptor sites for norepinephrine tend to lower the blood pressure and cause dizziness when a person suddenly stands up (orthostatic or postural hypotension). This is generally undesirable but is especially dangerous with a patient whose stability is already impaired (for example, an elderly person with difficulty walking). It is also particularly dangerous for a person with cardiac ischemia (reduced oxygen availability to the muscles of the heart, usually because of coronary artery disease) who requires a steady blood pressure to fill diseased coronary arteries in order to maintain the heart's functioning. Too low a blood pressure, caused by drugs, can lead to a disturbance of the heart's rhythm in such an individual, and this can be fatal, which is one reason so much careful attention is given to a patient's cardiac functioning when psychoactive drugs are prescribed.

Alpha receptors and beta receptors are two molecularly distinct populations of noradrenergic receptors. Norepinephrine's effects on a neuron depend in part on whether the receptors to which it binds are of the alpha or the beta type. Alpha and beta receptors, when bound, have different physiologic effects, often opposite to each other. Alpha-receptor stimulation, for example, will increase the constriction of blood vessels (vasoconstriction) and raise blood pressure, while beta-receptor stimulation expands (vasodilates) the vessels. To exploit the broad range of the noradrenergic system's physiological properties, drugs that bind especially well to a specific receptor type have been developed. This helps to fine-tune the drug's effects. Such specialized drugs are called alpha agonists, alpha blockers (or antagonists), beta agonists, or beta blockers (or antagonists) depending on which receptor type is more tightly bound and whether the effect is to enhance or oppose the receptor's effect.

Serotonin is the neurotransmitter in the serotonergic pathways and systems of the brain. It seems to be involved in the normal processes of sleep and mood regulation, and may be important in causing disturbances of appetite and in the development of obsessions and compulsions. Many psychiatric medications affect the amount of serotonin available at synapses. Serotonin is manufactured, in the body, from an amino acid constituent of protein in food) called tryptophan. Tryptophan is an important component of the glass of warm milk that many people find helpful to promote sleep on occasion, an effect thought to result from an increase in the brain's level of serotonin.

Gamma amino butyric acid (GABA) is the neurotransmitter in the gaba-ergic pathways of the brain and spinal cord. GABA is an important inhibitory neurotransmitter (that is, it reduces the excitability of neurons). It appears to be involved in modulating anxiety; when anxiety-reducing drugs such as benzodiazepines are used, they work through an enhancement of the GABA system's inhibitory activities.

In addition to the neurotransmitters just mentioned, a plethora of chemical messengers in the body may affect behavior. Of particular research interest at present are the endorphins, endogenous opioid substances that among other functions, may affect mood and pain sensitivity, and the neuropeptides, molecules that are more complicated than the simpler neurotransmitters and that possess many complex regulatory functions.

HOW THE BODY ABSORBS, METABOLIZES, AND ELIMINATES DRUGS

A drug's effects on neurotransmitters depend on its concentration in the brain and other parts of the body. This in turn depends on the drug's absorption, elimination, and brain concentration (usually estimated on the basis of its concentration in the blood or in the plasma, which is blood from which blood cells have been removed). Absorption, elimination, and concentration have practical implications with respect to dosage amounts, schedules, and drug interactions. A detailed explanation of pharmacokinetics, the branch of pharmacology concerned with the body's handling of drugs, is beyond the scope of this chapter. Here, though, is a whirlwind overview of the important issues.

Drug absorption is characterized by *rate* and *completeness*. These depend on the *route of administration*, the *physical properties of the drug,* and the *presence of food or other drugs* which interfere with absorption. The usual routes for administration of psychiatric drugs are *oral* (pills and liquids) or *parenteral* (intramuscular or intravenous injections). Drugs that are administered intravenously are completely and rapidly absorbed, while intramuscular administration produces rapid but sometimes less complete absorption because some drugs get trapped within the muscle tissue (diazepam, for example, is known to do this). The oral route is slower but much more convenient. An oral drug is absorbed more rapidly if the body does not have to wait for a pill to dissolve, so elixir or concentrate liquid forms of drugs tend to exert their effects more quickly. Though some drugs are irritating to the stomach and so should be taken with food, absorption is usually decreased by the presence of food in the stomach. Some drugs that reduce stomach emptying and intestinal movements (for example, anticholinergic drugs) reduce the rate of drug absorption by this mechanism.

Obviously, the body cannot afford to accumulate drugs unendingly! The processes of elimination inactivate drugs and discharge them from the body. There are not many routes of elimination, and the most significant routes are fecal (for unabsorbed drugs) and urinary (for drugs which pass from the blood, through the kidney, and into the urine). Some drugs are easily absorbed but unable to leave the body very quickly through the urine. These drugs are chemically altered by the liver to facilitate their ability to dissolve in urine and thus be eliminated. Oxidation, reduction, dealkylation, and the attachment of water-soluble chemical components (conjugation) are the main chemical mechanisms used for this purpose. The activity level of the liver enzymes responsible for this housecleaning activity (microsomal enzymes) is very responsive to the presence of certain other drugs. The presence of one drug that alters liver activity, therefore, can have unexpected effects on the blood concentration of another drug metabolized by the liver. A dangerous example of this is the decrease in the blood level and effectiveness of a liver-metabolized anticoagulant (blood thinner) once an anticonvulsant such as carbamazepine (which induces increases in liver enzymes) is added to the patient's medications. If the same patient were a schizophrenic taking chlorpromazine, the blood level of the antipsychotic drug would also decrease following the addition of carbamazepine, potentially leading to the recurrence of hallucinations and delusions.

Drug elimination rates are compared by a standardized measurement, the elimination half-life, defined as the length of time it takes for half of the drug to leave the body. The half-life is taken into account when planning dosing schedules in order to avoid large *peaks* (maximal blood levels) or *troughs* (minimal levels) in drug concentration. Drugs with a long half-life such as nortriptyline ($t1/2 = 24$ hr) need be given only once a day, while a drug like alprazolam ($t1/2$ closer to 6 hr) would be given on a twice (bid), three (tid), or four (qid) times a day basis to avoid high peaks and low troughs that might manifest themselves in a patient becoming intoxicated and unsteady an hour after each dose but jumpy and restless before the next dose.

Ultimately, for most psychoactive medications, the intensity of effect is greater when more drug reaches the brain. For more drug to reach the brain, greater absorption and less elimination are desirable. Two other important factors affecting plasma drug concentration are lipid solubility and plasma protein-binding. Lipids are fats. A drug that dissolves not only in water but also in lipids has more places to go in the body — the *volume of distribution* is larger — so the concentration of the drug in blood reaching the brain will be lower and less drug will get to important sites in the brain. Most of the antipsychotic and antianxiety drugs are very lipid soluble, while lithium has just the opposite quality of being very water soluble.

In addition to cells and plasma, blood contains a variety of plasma proteins that can tie up drugs by attaching to them electrostatically. When a drug is tied up in this way, it is not able to exert its effects, so the amount of drug in the blood is deceptively larger than the amount available for interaction with the brain.

A rough estimate of the amount of drug reaching the brain is obtained by measuring the concentration in the fluid surrounding blood cells, the plasma. With antidepressants, the recent availability and standardization of plasma tricyclic-level measurements has helped to guide the treatment of patients who are nonresponsive to standard treatment. Plasma levels are indispensable to the monitoring of lithium therapy. Whether blood level measurements will become equally useful with antipsychotic or antianxiety drugs remains to be seen.

NONPHARMACOLOGIC DRUG EFFECTS

Though evidence continues to accumulate in the search to understand psychoactive drugs' mechanisms of action, a number of mysteries remain. One of the most intriguing is the observation that drugs can act in ways that seem totally unrelated to their chemistry. With remarkable consistency, for example, it has been observed that many people have unpleasant side effects when they are given an inert pill if they are led to believe it is an active drug. Similarly, some patients experience beneficial effects so immediately after taking an active medication ("as soon as I took the first pill") that it seems impossible to believe that they are related to the drug's chemistry. These effects, which may be mediated through endorphins or other bodily chemical messengers, are termed placebo effects.

THE MAJOR CLASSES OF PSYCHOPHARMACOLOGIC DRUGS

Having laid a basis for understanding the actions of drugs and their handling by the body, I will now discuss the major classes of psychopharmacologic drugs in clinical use, beginning with antianxiety drugs, then antipsychotic drugs, stimulants, antidepressants, mood regulators, anticholinergic agents, and beta-adrenergic blockers. For each class of drugs, I will discuss the mechanism of action, uses or indications, abuse potential, side effects, specific agents, and dosages.

Antianxiety Drugs

Anxiety, in its more and less severe forms, accounts for the largest number of patients with symptoms severe enough to warrant a psychiatric diagnosis. The search for safer and more efficacious drugs has provided modern clinicians with an array of agents from which to choose. Some of the earlier antianxiety drugs, because of their addictiveness or danger in overdose, have been largely replaced by the safer drugs available today. Methaqualone (Quaalude), ethchorvinyl (Placidyl), glutethimide (Doriden and others), and meprobamate (Miltown and others), for example, were common in the 1950s and 1960s both for treatment and for recreational abuse but are now only rarely prescribed in the treatment of anxiety.

The barbiturates, once exceedingly common in the treatment of anxiety, have also fallen largely into psychiatric disuse because of their adverse effects and potential toxicity. Taken in overdose or in combination with other CNS depressants such as alcohol, their respiratory and CNS depressant effects can be lethal. They remain, nonetheless, very useful anesthetic agents and anticonvulsants for certain varieties of seizure disorders. Methohexital (Brevital) is used as a brief anesthetic agent during electroconvulsive therapy (ECT), and pentobarbital (Nembutal and others) remains of use in helping addicted patients withdraw from a variety of sedative/hypnotic drugs. Short-acting barbiturates, in the technique known as the Amytal interview, are also useful in obtaining diagnostic information from dissociative or catatonic patients.

The antihistamines remain a useful alternative for the treatment of anxiety in patients for whom other drugs are contraindicated. Diphenhydramine (Benadryl and others) and hydroxyzine (Atarax and others) are the most frequently used antihistamines in the treatment of anxiety symptoms and insomnia. They are not physically addictive and are relatively safe in overdose. The amounts of these drugs required to relieve anxiety, however, often produce unwanted sedation or anticholinergic effects, limiting their usefulness. When a patient is considered inappropriate for benzodiazepine treatment, however, antihistamines may provide a relatively safe alternative with less potential for abuse.

By far the most popular antianxiety drugs at present are the benzodiazepines, accounting currently for over 60 million prescriptions per year. Introduced in 1960 with the marketing of chlordiazepoxide (Librium and others), the class of benzodiazepines now comprises more than 13 drugs. Some are approved in the United States as hypnotics (sleeping pills), others as anxiolytics (antianxiety agents), but all share the same mechanism of action and differ primarily in their rate of onset of action, duration of action, and degree of hepatic metabolism (important when the drug is prescribed for someone with a damaged or diseased liver). A more rapid rate of onset of action produces the sense that the drug is starting to work. In street terminology this is called a buzz. A longer duration of action is associated with desirable longer-term anxiety relief or undesirable prolonged sedation. Table 7-2 compares the currently marketed benzodiazepine drugs in terms of these characteristics.

Investigations into the mechanism of action of the benzodiazepines have pushed forward with enthusiasm, because the discoveries which lie ahead promise to yield profound insights into the biochemical nature of anxiety. In 1977 a benzodiazepine receptor molecule was identified, and the presence of this molecule suggested the existence of a naturally occurring benzodiazepine receptor ligand, a chemical manufactured by the body which could serve as a regulator of anxiety, sleep, and seizure threshold. The search for this endogenous ligand continues, but has already identified several interesting chemicals which have stimulated further investigations. Benzodiazepines are believed to act in concert with the GABA system to regulate the intracellular concentration of chloride, an ion whose presence reduces the electrical activity of a neuron. The binding of a benzodiazepine to its receptor facilitates the binding of GABA and the influx of chloride into the cell. On a larger scale, the use of benzodiazepines reduces activity in a part of the brain that regulates alertness called the brainstem reticular formation. Additionally, activity is diminished in areas of the brain involved in

Table 7-2
Benzodiazepines Currently Available in the United States

Generic Name	Brand Name	Dose Equivalent, mg	Duration of Action, hr[*]	Rapidity of Onset[+]	Oral Dosages, mg
Chlordiazepoxide[‡]	Librium	10	24–48	++	5,10,25
Diazepam[‡]	Valium	5	20–70	+++	2,5,10
Alprazolam	Xanax	0.5	8–15	++	0.25,0.5,1
Oxazepam	Serax	15	5–15	+	10,15,30
Chlorazepate	Tranxene	7.5	36–96	+++	3.75,7.5,15
Lorazepam[‡]	Ativan	1	10–20	++	0.5,1,2
Prazepam	Centrax	10	36–96	+	5,10,20
Halazepam	Paxipam	20	36–96	++	20,40
Temazepam[‡][§]	Restoril	?	8–20	++	15,30
Flurazepam[‡][§]	Dalmane	?	36–120	+++	15,30
Triazolam	Halcion	?	1.5–5	+++	0.125, 0.25

[*] These numbers reflect duration of action following a single dose. For some of these drugs, the range of numbers refers to actions of an active metabolite. Data are from Greenblatt DJ, Shader RI: Pharmacokinetics of antianxiety agents, in Meltzer HY (ed): *Psychopharmacology: The Third Generation of Progress.* Raven Press, NY, 1987, p 1381.

[+] Relative speed of onset is reflected by the presence of more + signs. The benzodiazepines, which are more slowly absorbed, reach peak serum levels after several hours. The most quickly absorbed benzodiazepines reach peak serum levels within less than an hour.

[‡] Available generically.

[§] Marketed for use as sleeping pills (hypnotic use).

emotion: the locus ceruleus, septal region, amygdala, hippocampus, and hypothalamus. Benzodiazepines have other effects as well, including anticonvulsant effects and muscle-relaxant effects.

Benzodiazepines have proven useful and received governmental approval for the treatment of anxiety disorders, but they are not equally useful for each of the DSM-IIIR anxiety disorders. In adjustment disorder with anxious mood and in some cases of generalized anxiety disorder they have been used effectively. They are not considered to be as effective in the treatment of agitation associated with depression, prepsychotic anxiety, obsessive-compulsive disorder, or post-traumatic stress disorder. In panic disorder, two high-potency benzodiazepines, alprazolam (Xanax) and clonazepam (Klonopin) have been carefully studied. Rigorous trials have shown them to produce relief on a par with standard antidepressant treatment. Other benzodiazepines may also have a beneficial effect on panic disorder. Benzodiazepines are also used in the treatment of insomnia, alcohol withdrawal, and seizures. When benzodiazepines are used to treat situational anxiety, the best results have been obtained in nonpsychotic, nondepressed individuals with good premorbid adjustment and recent onset of symptoms.

Because benzodiazepines exhibit cross-tolerance with alcohol, there has been considerable debate as to the appropriateness of their use with patients who have a history of substance abuse. People prone to develop addictions (often having personality disorders with anxiety intolerance and impulse or affect dysregulation) may tend to increase their benzodiazepine dosage independent of medical advice, leading to psychological and physiological dependence. Addiction is considered to have occurred when increased drug amounts are required to achieve the same effect (tolerance) and discontinuation of the drug results in uncomfortable and even dangerous physical responses (withdrawal). While the benzodiazepines are far less addictive than some earlier antianxiety drugs, several of them have developed a reputation for being difficult to discontinue. Alprazolam in particular often requires a very slow tapering of dosage to minimize withdrawal symptoms and support the patient's cooperation.

The side effects of the benzodiazepines in general resemble the effects of alcohol (see Table 7-3). Of particular annoyance to

Table 7-3
Benzodiazepine Side Effects

Common side effects
  Sedation
  Clumsiness (ataxia)
  Increased appetite/weight gain
  Nausea
  Headache

Uncommon but potentially serious side effects
  Skin rash
  Depression
  Uncharacteristic irritability
  Physical dependence
  Withdrawal reactions (agitation, insomnia,
    irritability, tremulousness, seizures)

many patients are sedation and impairment of fine-motor coordination, which may interfere with driving; slurred speech, which may give an appearance of drunkenness; and the danger of fetal malformations, of concern to any woman of childbearing age. Controversy remains as to whether fetal malformations can be ascribed to the use of these drugs during the first trimester of pregnancy. Some studies support this notion, while others offer evidence that the malformations are uncommon or due to other factors. Until more definitive evidence comes along, however, these drugs carry a warning against their use during the early months of pregnancy and this should be heeded.

Several of the benzodiazepines have been marketed primarily as hypnotics, that is, as sleep-inducing drugs. Most differ insignificantly from the other benzodiazepines in rate of onset of action and duration of action. Three frequently prescribed benzodiazepine hypnotics are temazepam (Restoril), triazolam (Halcion), and flurazepam (Dalmane and others). Temazepam and triazolam have the advantage of a shorter elimination half-life, which theoretically means less of a drug hangover the next morning. Dalmane has a longer half-life and its metabolic elimination generates active metabolites as well, so it carries a greater risk of next-day drowsiness — a quality which may be desirable for a patient during a period of acute stress and anxiety but undesirable for one who must remain alert. All hypnotics have the unfortunate property of rapidly including tolerance. The problem of insomnia, especially when it is chronic, should never be simply medicated. A complete workup is necessary to rule out medical illness or serious psychiatric illness that might manifest as chronic insomnia.

A recent addition to the antianxiety drugs is buspirone (BuSpar), a novel drug that acts by a mechanism different from that of other antianxiety agents. Though the precise mechanism of its action remains unclear, buspirone's affinity for serotonergic receptors may mediate its antianxiety effects. Because of its different mechanism of action, buspirone lacks some valuable therapeutic properties possessed by benzodiazepines: it is not an effective sleeping pill, anticonvulsant, or muscle relaxant. On the other hand, it has been shown to be as effective as diazepam, lorazepam, or clorazepate in the treatment of persistent, generalized anxiety symptoms (generalized anxiety disorder) in large study populations. Whether it will have any role in the treatment of panic disorder remains unclear.

Assessing buspirone's abuse potential by offering it to known drug abusers, investigators have predicted a low likelihood of abuse. It causes less drowsiness than benzodiazepines and appears not to enhance the CNS depressant effects of alcohol. Side effects have so far been mild and uncommon, affecting less than 10% of users. The most common complaints have been headache, dysphoria, dizziness, nervousness, nausea, or paresthesias. Evidence suggests that buspirone is discontinued more easily than are benzodiazepines. Its danger in overdose is small. Among its drawbacks are its expense, which is higher than that of generically available benzodiazepines; its slow onset of action (taking as long as two weeks to reach a degree of anxiety relief equivalent to that of benzodiazepines); and its short half-life, which will require two to three doses per day to maintain a steady blood level of the drug.

Antipsychotic Drugs

The antipsychotic drugs have elicited fully as much controversy and fascination as the antianxiety drugs. Revered by some as the liberating factor that made possible deinstitutionalized and community-based care of chronic patients, they are nonetheless condemned by others as dulling the mind and rigidifying the body. Used judiciously, these medications have offered freedom to many patients who in former times would have been permanently institutionalized; yet these drugs certainly can produce disturbing adverse effects, especially when they are used inappropriately.

Current treatment approaches emphasize the minimization of dosage and duration of treatment with antipsychotics, preferring the risk of more frequent but more easily controllable relapses to that of greater sedation and endocrine or neurologic side effects. The terms *major tranquilizers* or *ataractics* are old-fashioned names for this class of drugs. The terms *neuroleptics* (which literally means drugs which seize the nervous system as in dystonic reactions) and *antipsychotic drugs* are currently favored.

Antipsychotics are postulated to act clinically by blocking the effect of the neurotransmitter dopamine, a substance crucial to the functioning of the brain's emotional centers. Every effective antipsychotic drug has been shown to block postsynaptic dopamne receptors, thereby reducing dopaminergic transmission. Unfortunately, many antipsychotic side effects are produced in this way, since dopamine pathways also facilitate endocrine function and modulate muscle activity. The search for ways to affect dopamine receptors involved in psychosis while sparing the others has discovered distinct receptor subpopulations. In time, specialized drugs now in a testing phase of development may allow more effective control of psychotic symptoms. In addition, evidence, which includes the success of drugs with prominent effects on other neurotransmitter systems, suggests that psychosis must involve more than just the dopamine system. Clozapine (Clozeril), an atypical antipsychotic drug now under special surveillance because of its unfortunate propensity for suppressing the blood-forming cells of bone marrow, may eventually provide an alternative treatment for patients who have failed to respond to conventional antipsychotics.

Though known primarily for their dopamine-blocking effects, the antipsychotics each affect a spectrum of other neurotransmitter systems. Their blockade of cholinergic transmission produces anticholinergic symptoms (see Table 7-1). Their blockade of alpha-adrenergic receptors produces orthostatic hypotension.

Their blockade of histaminic neurotransmission is partly responsible for their sedative effects.

Three distinct therapeutic effects of the antipsychotic drugs have been identified. A sedative effect, which begins within an hour after oral administration or about half an hour after intramuscular administration, is the most noticeable initial effect. It increases with higher dosage, and generally diminishes after days to weeks of taking the medication regularly. In excess, this therapeutic effect is the unwanted side effect of oversedation. An antianxiety effect, usually beginning within several hours after starting the medication, continues even after prolonged administration, although for many patients this property of the drug is weak. The antipsychotic effect, not usually evident until several days of adequate dosage, becomes increasingly apparent over time. In treating patients with chronic psychotic symptoms, the full effect may not be achieved for weeks. Hallucinations, ideas of reference, delusions, hostility, agitation, and self-neglect are among the symptoms which often are responsive to antipsychotic treatment. The diagnostic categories of patients in whom these symptoms are most prominent and antipsychotic drugs have been most helpful include acute or chronic schizophrenia, hypomania or mania, brief reactive psychoses, organic psychoses, aggressive or impulsive states related to organic dysfunction, paranoid states, Huntington's disease, Gilles de la Tourette syndrome (multiple motor and vocal tics), and psychotic depression, where they are usually given in combination with an antidepressant drug. Some clinicians have advocated using these drugs to treat anxiety in nonpsychotic patients with a thought disorder manifested by vagueness or distractibility, a use which is controversial because the usually limited efficacy of the drugs for this purpose may not justify the risk of tardive dyskinesia in a chronic nonpsychotic patient. When clear psychotic or psychotic-like symptoms (eg, hallucinations, delusions, ideas of reference, depersonalization, derealization) are present in a personality-disordered patient, the trial use of an antipsychotic drug is justified at least for temporary relief of symptoms, though this is not yet approved by the Food and Drug Administration. One nonpsychiatric use of these medications has developed as a result of their effects on brain systems that control nausea and vomiting.

Patients afflicted with severe vomiting, for example because of cancer chemotherapy, can obtain relief through the use of antipsychotic drugs.

Because of their often unpleasantly dulling effects in high doses, antipsychotic medications are rarely abused. Persons with more anxiety than they can tolerate, however, may attempt to relieve their dysphoric state by increasing these medications to large amounts. Such an approach is rarely effective and can even lead to the opposite outcome, because with increasing dosage there is a greater likelihood of producing an anxiety-like state of restlessness called akathisia (to be discussed).

The significant side effects of antipsychotic drugs are listed in Table 7-4. Among the most common are anticholinergic effects, unwanted sedation, and orthostatic hypotension. These tend to be worst early in treatment and may diminish over time. Antipsychotic drugs potentiate the effects of alcohol or other CNS depressants, such as sedative-hypnotic drugs, and the combination can therefore cause impairment of driving or other attention-requiring activities. They can also lower the threshold for seizure activity, increasing the likelihood of seizure in a vulnerable individual, such as an epileptic who is not taking anticonvulsant

Table 7-4
Antipsychotic Drug Side Effects

Common side effects
   Sedation/spaciness
   Anticholinergic effects (see Table 7-1)
   Postural hypotension
   Extrapyramidal effects (see text)
   Menstrual and sexual function changes

Uncommon but potentially serious side effects
   Tardive dyskinesia (see text)
   Skin rash
   Sensitization to sunlight
   Impaired cardiac conduction
   Impaired liver function
   Seizures
   Neuroleptic malignant syndrome
   Retinal damage (very uncommon)

medication. Antipsychotics impair the body's ability to react to temperature changes with appropriate regulatory responses, which can be hazardous in very hot or cold conditions. They also can sensitize the skin to the effects of sunlight, leading to easy sunburning. In rare cases, liver function has been impaired by the antipsychotic drugs. Changes in alertness can accompany the use of these drugs, especially in the early phase of treatment. The dysphoria and spaciness that may occur with these drugs are unpleasant for many patients, and can lead to refusal of medication or poor compliance. Regarding use during pregnancy, there is no conclusive evidence of increased fetal danger but in light of the paucity of available information treatment should be continued during pregnancy only when there are very clear and necessary indications.

Given dopamine's widespread roles in normal brain functioning, it is not unexpected that some of the adverse effects of antipsychotics represent unwanted interruption of dopaminergic functions. Some hormone-related antidopaminergic side effects include disturbance of menstrual functioning, breast enlargement, induction of lactation (galactorrhea), and weight gain. A particularly important site of adverse antidopaminergic effects is in the part of the brain called the extrapyramidal tract. That tract, so named for its location outside the pyramidal nerve pathway involved in voluntary muscular activity, is essential to the smooth coordination of movements that usually pass unnoticed except when they are malfunctioning. Balance, relaxed muscle tone, and flexible facial expressiveness can all be affected by the antipsychotic drugs' effects on extrapyramidal functions. The significant extrapyramidal side effects include acute dystonic reactions, drug-induced Parkinson's syndrome, akathisia, and tardive dyskinesia. These will be discussed in order of time of onset during treatment.

Acute dystonic reactions are painful acute muscle spasms which tend to occur very early (hours to days) in treatment. Commonly the spasms affect the neck (torticollis), eyes (oculogyric crisis), or back (opisthotonos). They often appear dramatic or even histrionic, and they are exacerbated with increased anxiety. They tend to disappear over time but are very alarming and uncomfortable, and are easily treated with anticholinergic medications. Though very rare, an acute laryngeal dystonic reaction can produce labored breathing. The resulting respiratory impairment can be life-threatening.

Drug-induced parkinsonism tends to occur during the first few weeks of treatment and resembles naturally occurring Parkinson's disease. The symptoms include shuffling gait, stooped posture, pill-rolling tremor (a slow hand tremor which looks like the person is rolling a pill between thumb and forefinger), and cogwheeling of the limbs (the combination of rigidity and tremor leads to jerky movements when the limb is passively flexed or extended). Treatment with anticholinergic drugs is often helpful.

Akathisia, the most frequent extrapyramidal side effect of antipsychotic therapy, affects up to 30% of patients treated with antipsychotic drugs but too often goes undetected or is mistaken for functional anxiety. It often begins several days to weeks after the initiation of treatment. Akathisia is the subjective sense of having to keep in motion, and leads to pacing or agitation so uncomfortable that it has precipitated suicide attempts. The symptom disappears with drowsiness and sleep. This syndrome is relatively resistant to pharmacologic treatment, though some patients' akathisia diminishes with the lowering of their antipsychotic dosage, the switch to a lower-potency antipsychotic, or the addition of an antianxiety or beta-blocking drug.

Tardive dyskinesia, the most dreaded extrapyramidal adverse effect, is a syndrome characterized by involuntary movements of the tongue, face, hands, fingers, or other parts of the body. It is no more frequent with any particular antipsychotic drug, but seems to claim an additional several percent of patients on antipsychotics with each successive year of treatment, up to a plateau somewhere near 30%. It is very rarely seen in patients who are treated for a few months or less. In half of acutely affected patients, the involuntary movements subside after antipsychotic medications are tapered or discontinued. With increasing duration, however, the symptoms become less likely to disappear. Since there is currently no very effective treatment for tardive dyskinesia, emphasis is increasingly placed on primary prevention: reducing the risk of this problem by using antipsychotics only when it is necessary and at the lowest effective dosage.

A final rare but important side effect of antipsychotic drugs

Table 7-5
Antipsychotic Drugs Currently Available in the United States

Drug Name	Brand Name	Available Dosage Forms	Dose Equivalent to 100 mg Chlorpromazine
Phenothiazines			
Chlorpromazine[*]	Thorazine and others	10-,25-,50-,100-,200-mg tablets, sustained release tablets, elixir, injectable	100 mg
Thioridazine[*]	Mellaril and others	10-,15-,25-,50-,100-,150-,200-mg tablets, concentrate, suspension	100 mg
Mesoridazine	Serentil	10-,25-,50-,100-mg tablets, concentrate, injectable	50 mg
Perphenazine	Trilafon	2-,4-,8-,16-mg tablets, concentrate, injectable	10 mg
Acetophenazine	Tindal	20-mg tablets	16 mg
Trifluoperazine[*]	Stelazine and others	1-,2-,5-,10-mg tablets, elixir, injectable	5 mg
Fluphenazine HCL[*]	Prolixin, Permitil	1-,2.5-,5-,10-mg tablets, elixir, injectable	2 mg
Fluphenazine decanoate	Prolixin-D	10-mL vial, 25mg/mL for IM use	[‡]

Butyrophenones			
Haloperidol*	Haldol and others	0.5-,1-,2-,5-,10-,20-mg tablets, elixir, injectable	2 mg
Haloperidol decanoate	Haldol	50 mg/ml in 1 ml (capsule) for IM use	§
Dephenylbutylpiperidines			
Pimozide	Orap	2-mg tablets	4 mg
Thioxanthenes			
Thiothixene	Navane	1-,2-,5-,10-mg capsules, elixir, injectable	4 mg
Chlorprothixene	Taractan	10-,25-,50-,100-mg tablets	100 mg
Oxoindolones			
Molindone	Moban	5-,10-,25-,50-,100-mg tablets, concentrate	10 mg
Dibenzoxazepines			
Loxapine	Loxitane, Daxolin	5-,10-,25-,50-mg tablets, concentrate, injectable	10 mg

* Available generically.
‡ No exact formula for conversion of IM dose to equivalent oral dose is available. One study suggests that 0.5 mL of Prolixin IM every 3 weeks is roughly equal to 10 mg of oral Prolixin HCl daily, though clinical experience suggests the depot Prolixin to be less potent than what those numbers suggest.
§ One conversion formula suggests multiplying a daily oral dose of haloperidol by 15 to achieve the number of mg suitable for monthly IM injection. For individual patients this must be adjusted on the basis of clinical factors.

is the neuroleptic malignant syndrome, thought to be more common with the high-potency agents. Occurring in between 0.4% to 1.4% of patients receiving antipsychotics, this potentially lethal syndrome is characterized by high fever, muscular rigidity, and mental status changes which often include disorientation. A patient with these symptoms requires emergency care and any neuroleptic medication should be discontinued while physiologic supportive care is given, usually in an intensive care setting. Dantrolene (Dantrium) and bromocriptine (Parlodel) are two medications that have proved useful in the treatment of this condition. Attempts to predict in just whom neuroleptic malignant syndrome is likely to develop have not yet arrived at definitive answers, but it does appear that patients who are exhausted or dehydrated are at increased risk. Patients taking high-potency antipsychotics are also at greater risk for this very dangerous reaction.

The currently available antipsychotic medications are listed in Table 7-5. At present there are six different chemical groups of these drugs, the most popular being the phenothiazines, butyrophenones, and thioxanthenes. Another way of classifying these drugs is to consider them in terms of potency, since they fall broadly into two classes: the high potency (low dose) and the low potency (high dose). For sake of comparison, potency is usually expressed in terms of chlorpromazine equivalents, the number of milligrams of a drug which would produce an effect equivalent to 100 mg of chlorpromazine. While no specific drug has been shown more effective against psychosis than the others, the range of side effects varies, allowing a clinician to pick a medication appropriate to the needs of an individual patient. As a general rule, the low-potency drugs produce more intense sedation, orthostatic hypotension, and anticholinergic effects than do the high-potency ones. This generalization does not hold true for the extrapyramidal syndrome of tardive dyskinesia, which is apparently no less common with any of the available drugs.

Stimulants

Since the synthesis of amphetamine in the 1930s, stimulants have been enlisted in the fight against depression, fatigue, appetite,

Table 7-6
Stimulants Currently Available in the United States

Generic Name	Brand Name	Available Dosage Forms, mg tablets
Amphetamine sulfate	Obetrol	10,20
Dextroamphetamine*	Dexedrine	5,10
(Sustained release)	Dexedrine Spansules	5,10,15
Methamphetamine*	Desoxyn	5
(Sustained release)	Desoxyn Gradumet	5,10,15
Methylphenidate	Ritalin	5,10,20
(Sustained release)	Ritalin SR	20
Pemoline	Cylert	18.75,37.5,75

* Available generically.

and excess weight (see Table 7-6). Though effective in lifting mood, energizing the body, and squelching appetite for brief lengths of time, these drugs are usually ineffective over the long haul. They have found, nonetheless, a few niches in modern medicine: they are useful in appetite suppression for as long as two weeks; they promote wakefulness in narcoleptics, individuals with a disorder of alertness; they enhance concentration and attention in children and adults with attention deficit disorder or hyperactivity; and they may be helpful even over a longer time course in elderly patients with a fatigued, depressed condition, especially when concurrent illnesses or medications prevent the use of conventional antidepressants.

This class of drugs exerts its effects by provoking release of dopamine and norepinephrine from neurons in the brain. These effects are short-lived, with most stimulants lasting only a few hours. During prolonged use, stimulants' effects diminish as neurons become depleted of their neurotransmitters. This development of tolerance undermines the effectiveness of long-term use, which is why for indications other than narcolepsy or attention deficit disorder stimulants are prescribed for short-term use. The rapid development of tolerance becomes a particular problem when chronically dysphoric, addiction-prone personalities take or abuse these drugs as mood elevators. Experiencing diminishing drug effects, these individuals may unilaterally raise their own dosages, leading to dangerously high levels of use.

As uppers, energizers, and diet pills, stimulants have been

Table 7-7
Stimulant Side Effects

Excessive arousal
Anxiety or jitteriness
Restlessness
Tremors
Sweating
Diarrhea
Tachycardia
Headache
Insomnia
Physical dependence
Depression and fatigue following discontinuation

abused extensively. Taken alone, orally or intravenously, or in combination with other drugs, they are highly addicting substances. At high doses for prolonged periods, they are capable of inducing a psychotic state clinically indistinguishable from mania or paranoid schizophrenia. With discontinuation, especially when abrupt, a rebound state of depression (the crash) occurs, and this can be severe enough to require psychiatric hospitalization. Whether the drug is prescribed or taken illicitly, adverse effects can be seen with stimulant use and primarily result from the drugs' sympathomimetic effects (see Table 7-7).

Antidepressant Drugs

Several years after the introduction of chlorpromazine in 1952, the first tricyclic antidepressant came into use. This was no coincidence, since imipramine and the other tricyclics that soon followed bear a striking chemical resemblance to the antipsychotic class of phenothiazines and reflect the flurry of pharmaceutical industry interest in related drugs that followed chlorpromazine's success. A small structural difference seems to amount for the antidepressants' immensely different clinical effects: unlike the antipsychotics, the tricyclic antidepressants are not helpful in treating uncomplicated schizophrenia but effect improvement in the majority of appropriately diagnosed depressed patients. The tricyclics are the most commonly prescribed class of antidepressants but not the only one. Several monoamine oxidase (MAO) inhibiting drugs are effective antidepressants, and a group of chemically dissimilar drugs introduced during the 1980s share a classification as second-generation antidepressants.

Antidepressants' mechanism of action remains a subject of controversy more than 30 years after their introduction. One important theory stresses tricyclics' capacity to block presynaptic cell reuptake of previously released neurotransmitters. By blocking this reuptake, an excess of neurotransmitter remains present in the synapse. This presumably compensates for a transmitter deficiency related to the basic nature of the biochemical disturbance in depression. This catecholamine theory of depression was an early attempt to understand depression in terms of catecholamine deficiency. It has since been modified to include other neurotransmitters (especially serotonin) and longer term synaptic changes that occur over a longer time period more pertinent to the two-week lag seen clinically before antidepressant effects establish themselves.

Tricyclic antidepressants are most effective at treating depression in patients in whom vegetative signs and symptoms (such as loss of the capacity for pleasure, early morning awakening, loss of appetite, decreased concentration, and decreased energy) have been present for at least two weeks. In at least 70% of patients with such depressions tricyclics provide a substantial degree of relief. When ineffective in treating an appropriately diagnosed depression, an increasingly aggressive program of pharmacologic treatments may be used, beginning with trials of other antidepressants or the combined use of an antidepressant with another drug that potentiates its effects. ECT, a highly effective but socially stigmatized treatment for severe depression, generally is tried after pharmacotherapy, except when medical disorders or severe urgency make pharmacotherapy unacceptable.

An adequate trial of a tricyclic antidepressant requires four weeks at a dosage that produces a plasma level within the therapeutic range (ie, the range within which most depressed patients have been observed to benefit from treatment). Meaningful standards have been established particularly for the levels of nortriptyline, imipramine, and desipramine. Plasma level measurements are now readily available to help guide therapy when a patient does not respond to treatment, as nonresponse may be due to inadequate absorption or rapid metabolic destruction of the medication.

Though called antidepressants, the tricyclics' chemical properties make them suitable for the treatment of several other disorders. Their use in these conditions has been studied but not all of these applications are FDA-approved. Of particular importance to psychotherapists are the tricyclics' effectiveness in treating panic disorder, agoraphobia, obsessive-compulsive disorder, bulimic bingeing, narcolepsy, childhood enuresis, and attention deficit disorder or hyperactivity of childhood.

The tricyclic antidepressants make poor drugs of abuse because of their anticholinergic and sedative effects. As a drug of overdose, however, they produce some of the most serious effects seen in an emergency room or intensive care unit. An overdose equivalent to a one-week therapeutic supply can induce lethal cardiac arrhythmias.

At therapeutic dosages their side effects can be severe enough to discourage compliance with treatment (see Table 7-8). The most common adverse effects are anticholinergic symptoms, sedation, and orthostatic hypotension. As with the antipsychotics, usage during pregnancy is discouraged though it has not been definitively proven harmful during the early stages of fetal development. Some days prior to delivery, a mother receiving treatment should taper or discontinue her tricyclic antidepressant. This will prevent delivering an infant whose blood drug level is high enough to impair activity and responsiveness, since the infant's immature liver will only slowly metabolize and inactivate the drug. A clinical problem often of importance is whether to treat depression in a patient who may be bipolar. Antidepressants, when they are given in the absence of a mood regulator such as lithium, may be capable of actually inducing a manic state and therefore are given only with caution to potentially bipolar patients.

Of the available tricyclics, none has been demonstrated clinically superior. They are listed for comparison in Table 7-9. As with the antipsychotics, they fall into two broad classes characterized by a different spectrum of side effects. The tertiary amines (amitriptyline, imipramine, trimipramine, doxepin) tend to

Table 7-8
Tricyclic Antidepressant Side Effects

Common side effects
    Sedation/spaciness
    Anticholinergic effects (see Table 7-1)
    Appetite increase/weight gain
    Sexual dysfunction
    Postural hypotension

Uncommon but potentially serious side effects
    Impaired cardiac function
    Induction of mania
    Withdrawal reactions

Table 7-9
Tricyclic Antidepressants Currently Available in the United States

Drug Name	Brand Name	Available Dosage Forms	Typical Daily Dose Range for Adult, mg/d
Amitriptyline*	Elavil and others	10-,25-,50-,75-,100-,150-mg tablets, injectable solution	100-300
Imipramine*	Tofranil and others	10-,25-,50-mg tablets, injectable solution	100-300
Desipramine	Norpramin, Pertofrane	10-,25-,50-,75-,100-,150-mg tablets	100-250
Nortriptyline	Aventyl, Pamelor	10-,25-,50-,75-mg tablets	50-150
Protriptyline	Vivactil	5-,10-mg tablets	10-60
Doxepin*	Sinequan and others	10-,25-,50-,75-,100-,150-mg tablets, oral concentrate	100-300
Trimipramine	Surmontil	25-,50-,100-mg tablets	50-200
Perphenazine/amitriptyline	Etrafon, Triavil	2/20-,2/25-,4/10-,4/25-mg tablets	
Chlordiazepoxide/amitriptyline	Limbitrol	5/12.5-,10/25-mg tablets	

* Available generically.

produce more sedation, anticholinergic symptoms, and orthostatic hypotension. The secondary amines (desipramine, nortriptyline, protriptyline) produce less of those side effects but may be too activating, producing unwanted restlessness or insomnia. Table 7-9 also includes two combination preparations, perphenazine/ amitriptyline and chlordiazepoxide/amitriptyline. More popular in the past, these combinations are less frequently prescribed now because they make it difficult to adjust the component drugs individually. Table 7-9 does not include clomipramine (Anafranil), a tricyclic available in the United States only for experimental use at present. This drug is an effective antidepressant but is of greater interest for its apparently superior effects in treating obsessive-compulsive disorder.

Monoamine oxidase (MAO) inhibitors comprise the other main class of antidepressants. They are as effective as tricyclics in treating unipolar depression, and may be even more effective in treating atypical depression, especially with concomitant panic attacks. MAO inhibitors are regarded as the most effective drug in the treatment of panic disorder and have also been effective in treating agoraphobia and social phobia. Bulimic bingeing has responded to MAO inhibitors. As an alternative to stimulants, MAO inhibitors also play a role in the treatment of narcolepsy.

This class of antidepressants works by competitively binding the enzyme MAO, a protein responsible for destroying certain neurotransmitters in presynaptic neurons. With less presynaptic intracellular destruction of neurotransmitters, the synaptic presence of these chemicals is enhanced, consistent with the catecholamine theory's prediction that drugs which increase norepinephrine's availability will also relieve depression. MAO, however, also plays an important role at another location. In the lining of the intestines, it detoxifies the peptide tyramine and other substances which would otherwise be absorbed into the body from food or medications and be misinterpreted by the brain as chemical messengers. When MAO is inhibited the body loses its defenses against these potential toxins and serious damage can ensue in the form of a hypertensive crisis when they are absorbed into a defenseless body. Researchers have now delineated fairly clearly which foods or medications must be avoided by a patient taking an MAO inhibitor, so this adverse effect is preventable (see Table 7-10). It is worth emphasizing that these substances should be avoided several days before starting an MAO inhibitor and seven to ten days after stopping an MAO inhibitor. Recent case reports have also emphasized the danger of switching too rapidly from one MAO inhibitor to a tricyclic antidepressant or to a different MAO inhibitor, between which 14 days should elapse.

Three MAO-inhibitor antidepressants are in current use

Table 7-10
Foods and Medications Incompatible with
MAO-Inhibitor Treatment

Foods to avoid:
- Aged cheeses (including cheddar, American cheese, and mozzarella as in pizza; cream cheese, farmer cheese, and cottage cheese are considered safe)
- Yeast extract (may be a component of certain canned soups; baked products raised with yeast are acceptable)
- Red wine (especially Chianti; white wine in moderation will rarely cause a hypertensive reaction)
- Beer or ale (tyramine content varies from lot to lot)
- Pickled herring, canned sardines, anchovies, caviar
- Any meat or fish which is not fresh, freshly canned, or freshly frozen (including lox, salami, sausage, corned beef, liver pate)
- Broad beans or fava beans
- Canned figs, stewed or overripe banana, overripe avocado
- Caffeine[*]
- Soy sauce[*]
- Raisins[*]
- Liver (dangerous when not fresh)

Medications to avoid (ask your physician about any other prescribed medications for safety)
- Decongestants
- Nasal drops or sprays
- Pain relievers[+] (NB: meperidine must be avoided)
- General and local anesthetics[+]
- Stimulants[+]
- L-dopa[+]
- Propranolol[+]
- Other antidepressants[+]

[*] Considered safe in limited amounts.
[+] May be usable with precautions and careful monitoring.

(see Table 7-11). None has been proven clinically superior, though phenelzine and isocarboxazid are regarded as less stimulating than tranylcypromine, an important difference when drug-induced insomnia complicates treatment. Dosage adjustment with MAO inhibitors requires even more clinical art than is needed with tricyclics, since blood levels of MAO inhibitors are not obtainable as a routine test. Platelet levels of MAO inhibition are available from specialized laboratories, but provide only a rough guideline for treatment decisions. As with the tricyclics, the required dosages of these drugs vary widely from patient to patient. The duration required for a full therapeutic trial is at least one month at adequate dosage, and full effects may not be seen for up to two months or more.

There are no euphoriant or sedative effects with MAO inhibitors, so abuse is unlikely. They do potentiate alcohol and other drugs but often in an unpleasant way. Tolerance to the drugs does not develop. They are not considered to be addictive.

The "cheese reaction" or hypertensive crisis is the most dangerous of MAO-inhibitor side effects but fortunately is preventable when dietary precautions are observed. Other potential side effects seen with MAO-inhibitor treatment include increased appetite and weight gain, induction of mania or hypomania, orthostatic hypotension, sexual dysfunction including inhibition of orgasm, swelling of the ankles or feet, increased sweating, skin rash, constipation, drowsiness, dry mouth, insomnia, nightmares, or fatigue. Because MAO inhibitors can cause damage to the liver, periodic measurements of liver function are useful and require only a simple blood test. In overdose or in combination with forbidden foods or medications, these drugs can be lethal by causing very severe elevation of blood pressure, leading to catastrophic events such as cerebral hemorrhage. Any patient taking an MAO inhibitor who has a severe headache should immediately get his or her blood pressure checked and in general should also promptly visit a physician or emergency room. Since the crisis is due to an excess of norepinephrine's effects, an alpha-adrenergic agonist, the severe reaction can be treated in an emergency setting with an alpha-adrenergic antagonist such as phentolamine (Regitine), 5 mg given intravenously slowly over five minutes. More recently, the antihypertensive calcium-

Table 7-11
MAO-Inhibitor Antidepressants Currently Available in the United States

Drug Name	Brand Name	Available Dosage Forms	Typical Daily Dose Range for Adult
Phenelzine	Nardil	15-mg tablets	15–90 mg/day
Isocarboxazid	Marplan	10-mg tablets	10–30 mg/day
Tranylcypromine	Parnate	10-mg tablets	10–60 mg/day

channel blocker nifedipine (Procardia, Adalat) has been effectively used with some patients in whom hypertensive reactions developed. A 10-mg capsule is chewed, then held under the tongue, where it is rapidly absorbed into the bloodstream.

The group of drugs known as novel or second-generation antidepressants includes a variety of agents unrelated by structure or mechanism of action but all introduced during the 1980s. New drugs' reputations tend to follow a predictable course: first, there is unbridled enthusiasm as patients and clinicians anticipate liberation from previous drugs' limitations; next, the occurrence of side effects or incomplete therapeutic efficacy elicits a period of condemnation and rejection; and finally, the drug takes an appropriate place in the pharmacological armamentarium after several years of open clinical experience. The second-generation antidepressants have not been around long enough yet to objectively assess what their contribution to treatment will be. It is clear, however, that they broaden the scope of treatment and theory in several ways: at least one works by a mechanism which challenges the formerly popular catecholamine theory of depression, several may offer a different (and for some patients a more tolerable) spectrum of side effects, and some patients refractory to treatment with the standard (first-generation) antidepressants may respond to one of these. The newer antidepressants currently available are amoxapine, alprazolam, trazodone, maprotiline, and fluoxetine (see Table 7-12). Each will be discussed individually with respect to its special characteristics.

Amoxapine (Asendin), essentially a tricyclic antidepressant, is unique among antidepressants for possessing postsynaptic dopamine-blocking activity, resulting from its chemical relationship to the antipsychotic drug loxapine. For this reason it was initially expected to excel in the treatment of psychotic depressions. Many clinicians, however, dislike exposing depressed patients unnecessarily to the side effects of a dopamine blocker that cannot be independently discontinued after the psychotic symptoms remit. Instead, a conventional antidepressant can be combined with an antipsychotic drug for greater ease in individualized dose adjustment of the two agents. An additional concern with amoxapine is its propensity to induce seizures when it is taken in overdose. At therapeutic dosages, its side effects

Table 7-12
Second-Generation Antidepressants Currently Available in the United States

Drug Name	Brand Name	Available Dosage Forms	Typical Daily Dose Range for Adult
Amoxapine	Asendin	25-, 50-, 100-, 150-mg tablets	100–300 mg/day
Alprazolam	Xanax	0.25-, 0.5-, 1-mg tablets	0.75–4 mg/day
Trazodone*	Desyrel and others	50-, 100-, 150-mg tablets	150–400 mg/day
Maprotiline	Ludiomil	25-, 50-, 75-mg tablets	75–225 mg/day
Fluoxetine	Prozac	20-mg tablets	20–80 mg/day

* Available generically.

include those associated with antipsychotic drugs as well as those associated with tricyclic antidepressants. Amoxapine, nonetheless, is clinically effective in treating depression and has achieved response in some patients refractory to other single drugs.

Alprazolam (Xanax), controversial because of its potential for abuse and addiction, is a triazolobenzodiazepine, which means it bears a chemical relationship to diazepam (Valium and others) and other benzodiazepine antianxiety drugs. While it appears to be an effective drug for treating anxiety and panic disorder, its efficacy as an antidepressant is not secure (some studies support this and others do not). When used as an antidepressant, alprazolam's role should probably be restricted for now to the treatment of milder depressive states, especially when panic attacks are present and there is little potential for drug abuse. Alprazolam also provides an alternative for antidepressant treatment of medically ill patients in whom the use of other antidepressants might be specifically contraindicated. Its side effects are similar to those of other benzodiazepines. Tapering and discontinuation have proven particularly difficult for some patients and must be handled with tact and patience.

Trazodone (Desyrel), a triazolopyridine, has been considered a valuable addition to the pharmacopeia because it is relatively safe in overdose and because it lacks anticholinergic side effects. Given in adequate dosages, it may be as effective an antidepressant as any of the tricyclics. Unfortunately, it has some disadvantages: it is very sedating; it has occasionally caused priapism in men; and several reports implicate trazodone in causing arrhythmias, though these have been controversial. Of the antidepressants, it is probably significantly less effective in treating panic disorder, though equally effective for several other purposes.

Maprotiline (Ludiomil) is a tetracyclic antidepressant, a chemical relative of the tricyclics created by the addition of an ethylene bridge across the tricyclic's middle ring. It is considered as effective as any tricyclic but shares a similar range of side effects. Maprotiline's major disadvantages are its long half-life (which means a slow development of a steady-state serum level and longer illness following overdose) and its tendency to produce seizures, even in patients with no history of seizures, when the dosage is raised too quickly. Additionally, it occasionally causes a skin rash which clears after discontinuation of the drug.

Fluoxetine (Prozac), recently released for clinical use, is an antidepressant with distinctly different properties than those of the tricyclics or MAO inhibitors. Its structure, being bicyclic, differs from that of other antidepressants. Fluoxetine's efficacy in the treatment of depression is comparable to that of tricyclics or MAO inhibitors, and it may have special effectiveness in reducing the symptoms of obsessive-compulsive disorder. It is a highly selective inhibitor of serotonin reuptake, with little effect on other neurotransmitters. This means that it lacks the anticholinergic effects, the anti-adrenergic orthostatic hypotension, and the sedation that are so often a problem with less specific antidepressants. It also seems not to potentiate the CNS depressant effects of alcohol. Cardiac toxicity is not seen at therapeutic dosages, and fluoxetine is less dangerous than most other antidepressants in overdose. It has no known deleterious effects during pregnancy or breast-feeding, but like the other antidepressants it cannot conclusively be considered safe. This antidepressant's adverse effects include the production in some patients of skin rash, nausea, anxiety, anorexia, diarrhea, dizziness, nervousness, headache, or insomnia. Fluoxetine has been reported capable of inducing mania in susceptible patients.

Mood Regulators (Drugs for Treating Bipolar Affective Disorder)

Lithium, recognized as a useful agent for the treatment of mania by John Cade in Australia in 1949, was for many years the only available non-antipsychotic drug effective in controlling the symptoms of mania. In contrast to the antidepressants, it is a mood regulator, because it treats either mania or depression. It also diminishes the frequency and intensity of both manic and depressive episodes in bipolar patients. For years, it has stood in a class by itself, which was a misfortune to the 30% of patients with bipolar disorder who were either unable to tolerate its side effects or unable to benefit from its therapeutic effects. In recent years, the lack of other mood regulators has been remedied by the adoption from medicine of several drugs still used medically as anticonvulsants or antiarrhythmic agents. Specifically, clinical research has demonstrated that carbamazepine, valproic acid, or verapamil provide effective alternatives to lithium, though they are not FDA-approved yet for this usage (see Table 7-13).

Lithium is available as either a salt, lithium carbonate, or a liquid, lithium citrate. Because it has a relatively short elimination half-life, standard lithium carbonate is often prescribed on a thrice daily schedule in order to maintain a steady blood level of the drug. A slow-release form of lithium, which allows twice daily dosing with less interdose level fluctuation, is marketed. Lithium's mechanism of therapeutic action remains difficult to extricate from among its many physiologic effects, but current theories focus on lithium's enhancement of serotonergic neurotransmission and its metabolic effects on intracellular actions of calcium.

The sole FDA-approved uses of lithium are acute treatment of bipolar affective disorder, manic type, and maintenance therapy (prophylaxis) for reducing the frequency of bipolar episodes. It is effective in preventing manic breaks in about 70% of patients, and may ameliorate the course of those episodes that it does not prevent. Because lithium usually takes 10 to 14 days to establish its effect, it is less useful as an acute treatment for mania than are antipsychotic drugs. In acute mania, if behavioral control must be established more rapidly, antipsychotics are generally used in conjunction with lithium or alone for the first week or so of an episode.

Though it is FDA-approved only in the treatment of mania and prophylaxis of bipolar episodes, lithium has clinically established its usefulness in several other areas, including the treatment of schizoaffective disorder, manic type; cyclothymic disorder, probably a mild form of bipolar disorder; depression, especially in bipolar individuals; aggressive states; and alcoholism which is associated with mood swings or affective disorder. It may also be useful in the treatment of some chronic schizophrenic patients who are unresponsive to antipsychotic medications alone, even when there are no clear affective symptoms.

Lithium's side effects, unfortunately, are common and varied (see Table 7-14). Many patients are annoyed by lithium's tendency to induce weight gain (often 10 to 15 lb) by increasing

Table 7-13
Mood Regulators Currently Available in the United States

Drug Name	Brand Name	Available Dosage Forms	Typical Daily Dose Range for Adult
Lithium carbonate[*]	Eskalith and others	300-mg capsules or tablets, syrup (1 tsp = 300 mg)	900–1800 mg/day[+]
Lithium citrate[*]			900–1800 mg/day[+]
Lithium sustained release	Lithobid, Eskalith CR	300-,450-mg capsules	900–1800 mg/day[+]
Carbamazepine[*]	Tegretol and others	200-mg tablets	400–1200 mg/day[+]
Valproic acid[*]	Depakene and others	250-mg capsules	250–1250 mg/day[+]
Verapamil[*]	Isoptin, Calan, and others	80-,120-mg tablets; 240 mg slow release	160–320 mg/day

[*] Available generically.
[+] Dosage adjusted according to measurements of serum drug level.

Table 7-14
Lithium Side Effects

Common side effects
  Diarrhea
  Dizziness
  Dry mouth
  Increased thirst and urination
  Nausea
  Sedation
  Appetite increase/weight gain
  Swelling of feet
  Worsening of acne

Uncommon but potentially serious side effects
  Confusion, slurred speech
  Muscle aches or weakness
  Clumsiness (ataxia)
  Impaired function of thyroid gland
  Impaired function of kidney

both appetite and metabolic efficiency. Careful dietary management is usually required in battling this side effect. Lithium can also produce a rapid tremor of the hands, which makes a patient appear highly anxious and can interfere with precise manual tasks. This side effect can usually be controlled by the adjustment of dosage or the addition of a beta-blocking medication. Many patients express concern about another side effect of lithium, its capacity to interfere with memory and cognitive function. This is dependent upon dosage and can sometimes be diminished by finding the lowest effective lithium level for a specific patient.

Among the most important side effects of lithium is its potential for affecting thyroid function. After even one year of treatment, a reversible decrease of thyroid function, which may produce symptoms of hypothyroidism including fatigue, cold intolerance, weight gain, hair loss, puffy skin, and a hoarse voice, develops in a few percent of patients. Since some of these symptoms overlap with those of depression, the true cause might be missed, which is why periodic assessment of thyroid function is part of the monitoring of lithium treatment. Kidney function is also affected in some patients taking lithium, though current opinion stresses the rarity of truly dangerous kidney damage from lithium when it is maintained below toxic levels. To ensure the greatest possible safety, two indicators of kidney function, BUN and creatinine, are monitored periodically. More intensive monitoring is pursued should any evidence of decreased function be noted. In women of childbearing age, lithium must be prescribed with caution because it has been shown to be capable of producing fetal malformations when it is taken during the first trimester of pregnancy. Toward parturition, a pregnant woman taking lithium should be advised to decrease the dosage or discontinue it, because of toxicity to mother and child which may occur as a result of rapid changes in fluid balance and kidney function following delivery.

Because lithium causes little or no subjective pleasant effect, it is rarely abused. At higher than effective dosages, it causes toxic effects including nausea and vomiting. In overdose, it can be lethal, by causing neurological deterioration leading to seizures, coma, and death. Because toxic levels are so close to therapeutic levels, serum lithium measurements are periodically taken to ensure that dosage remains within the effective yet safe range. Current practice favors a therapeutic range of 0.8 to 1.2 mEq/L in acute treatment and 0.6 to 0.8 mEq/L in maintenance treatment.

Carbamazepine (Tegretol and others) was used as an anticonvulsant in the treatment of temporal lobe epilepsy before it also proved helpful in the treatment of bipolar disorder. One explanation of its mechanism of action conceptualizes bipolar disorder as a kind of electrical abnormality of limbic system functioning, responsive to carbamazepine's electrically stabilizing effects. Clinical studies have shown it to be as effective as lithium, though not necessarily in the same patients, in acute treatment of mania in bipolar patients, for prophylaxis of manic or depressive episodes, and possibly in the treatment of depressive episodes in bipolar patients. In patients with aggressive outbursts or rage attacks, carbamazepine also provides an alternative to lithium. As with lithium, the toxic range of carbamazepine is only slightly above the range of clinical effectiveness, so periodic measurements of its blood level are necessary. Its short half-life suggests that it be given on a twice to thrice daily dosing schedule. Carbamazepine is usually used as a second-line drug (that is, only when lithium is ineffective or not tolerated) because it is newer and has some potentially dangerous side effects.

The most serious of these side effects, though it is an uncommon one, is suppression of the blood-forming cells of the bone marrow. Though rarely lethal (1:20,000 to 1:40,000), this potential danger of this adverse effect requires that any patient taking carbamazepine obtain frequent blood counts (weekly for the first three months, every one to three months subsequently). The occurrence of a rash in a patient taking carbamazepine may require discontinuation of the medication, since this may be an indication of a reaction which could adversely affect the marrow.

Liver damage may also rarely occur, so liver functions (SGOT, SGPT, alkaline phosphatase, and bilirubin) are also checked every three months. Hyponatremia (low sodium) can occur with carbamazepine treatment, requiring periodic checks of the serum sodium level.

Because it increases the liver's metabolic activity, levels of other concurrently administered drugs may be lowered by the addition of carbamazepine. Other side effects include ataxia (impaired coordination), drowsiness, or dizziness, which usually disappear after several weeks of treatment. Sexual dysfunction and potentiation of the sedating effect of alcohol or other depressants may occur. Disturbances of cardiac rhythm like those seen with tricyclic antidepressants are sometimes observed. Paradoxically, a depressive episode develops in an occasional patient treated with carbamazepine. Use during pregnancy is not advised. This drug appears to have little abuse potential.

Valproic acid or valproate (Depakene and others) appears to share many of the therapeutic and toxic effects of carbamazepine, though it presents less danger to marrow function and a greater hazard of liver toxicity. Another anticonvulsant, it is thought to work in a manner similar to that of carbamazepine, normalizing disturbed electrical activity in the limbic system. Its effectiveness has not, however, been as thoroughly demonstrated. Though not FDA-approved for psychiatric indications, it has shown promise in the treatment of bipolar disorder (manic or mixed) and schizoaffective disorder. The presence of EEG abnormalities may predict a greater likelihood of response to this drug. As with carbamazepine, periodic assessments of drug level, liver functions, and blood count are necessary for safe administration.

Verapamil (Isoptin, Calan, and others) is the first of a new class of mood regulators borrowed from the realm of cardiology, where it has for some time served as an antianginal drug. Verapamil has only begun to receive careful evaluation as a mood regulator and may be less effective than lithium or carbamazepine, but in selected patients who are unable to tolerate those other drugs it will provide a potential alternative. It is thought to be effective as an antimanic drug and a prophylactic treatment to avoid manic episodes. Whether it also alleviates or prevents depressive episodes or has other psychiatric indications is at present uncertain. The drug seems to work by affecting the metabolism of calcium, an ion deeply involved in the excitability of neuronal cells. Verapamil and its chemical relatives are called calcium channel blockers because they block calcium's entry through special passages into nerve cells. They also block several calcium-related chemical actions within the neurons.

Verapamil's more common side effects include fatigue, headache, dizziness, skin rash, and swelling of the feet and ankles. It can also produce slowing of cardiac conduction and heart rate, constipation, heartburn, nausea, and flushing. It should be given with caution in patients with impaired cardiac function, especially conduction abnormalities. Such patients would require careful ECG monitoring while taking verapamil or other calcium channel blockers. Usage during pregnancy has not been conclusively proven to be safe. Normal labor could conceivably be impaired or suppressed by the calcium channel blocking effects of these drugs.

Anticholinergic Agents

As implied by the name of this class of drugs, the anticholinergic agents act by blocking acetylcholine receptors. Additional effects may derive from lowering the absorption and serum levels of other drugs such as antipsychotics. The anticholinergic drugs may decrease the adverse effects of antipsychotic drugs, for example,

Table 7-15
Anticholinergic Medications Used in Psychiatry, Available in the United States

Drug Name	Brand Name	Available Dosage Forms	Typical Daily Dose Range for Adult
Benztropine[*]	Cogentin and others	0.5-, 1-, 2-mg tablets, injectable	0.5–6 mg/day
Trihexyphenidyl[*]	Artane and others	2-, 5-mg tablets, elixir	1–15 mg/day
Biperiden	Akineton	2-mg tablets, injectable	2–6 mg/day
Procyclidine	Kemadrin	5-mg tablets	7.5–20 mg/day

[*] Available generically.

partially by impairing their absorption. The main use of anticholinergic drugs is in the treatment of extrapyramidal side effects associated with antipsychotic treatment. These symptoms include acute dystonias, parkinsonism, and akathisia. Unfortunately they are of limited use in treating akathisia and of no use in treating tardive dyskinesia, which they may in fact exacerbate. The currently available anticholinergic agents are listed in Table 7-15.

Anticholinergic drugs' side effects are identical to the anticholinergic effects listed in Table 7-1. Some patients appear to enjoy a euphoriant, sedating, or hallucinogenic toxic effect and therefore abuse these medications. They are not proven to be safe during pregnancy.

Beta-Adrenergic Blockers

The beta blockers have been used for over 20 years for the treatment of heart disease, and have recently found roles (not yet FDA-approved) in psychiatry in the treatment of antipsychotic-induced akathisia, performance anxiety, and social phobia. In higher doses, they have also been used with some success to treat aggressive outbursts in psychotic or brain-damaged individuals. Some researchers advocate their use also in the treatment of schizophrenia. Eight different drugs of this class are available in the United States (see Table 7-16). Propranolol (Inderal and others), the most popular, has a half-life of four hours (which suits it especially for treating short-term conditions such as performance anxiety) but has the drawback of causing sedation for some. Atenolol (Tenormin) is beta-1-selective (acts preferentially on heart receptors), which means that it might be especially helpful for someone whose main problem in performance situations is rapid heartbeat, but it would theoretically provide less relief for shaking hands. Nadolol (Corgard) is nonselective and not very sedating but has a long half-life (24 hours), so its effects would persist for a period of hours. This has suited it for the treatment of akathisia, as it can be given on a once daily schedule.

The beta blockers are contraindicated in patients with concurrent asthma, diabetes, thyroid disease, or certain types of

Table 7-16
Beta Blockers Currently Available in the United States

Drug Name	Brand Name	Available Dosage Forms	Usual Adult Elimination Half-life (t1/2)
Propranolol[*]	Inderal and others	10-,20-,40-,60-,80-,90-mg tablets	3–6 hours
Propranolol slow-release	Inderal-LA	60-,80-mg capsule, solution for oral use	
Metoprolol	Lopressor	50-,100-mg tablets	3–6 hours
Nadolol	Corgard	20-,40-,80-,120-,160-mg tablets	20 hours
Atenolol	Tenormin	50-,100-mg tablets	6–9 hours
Timolol	Blocadren	5-,10-,20-mg tablets	4–5 hours
Pindolol	Visken	5-,10-mg tablets	3–5 hours
Labetalol	Trandate, Normodyne	100-,200-,300-mg tablets	4–6 hours
Acebutalol	Sectral	200-,400-mg capsules	3–4 hours

[*] Available generically.

heart disease (congestive failure, conduction delay) except under careful medical supervision because they can interfere with the body's protective mechanisms. Beta blockers may interact poorly with certain other drugs (such as MAO inhibitors or general anesthetics). They are possibly unsafe during pregnancy. In healthy individuals, they may cause sedation, fatigue, depression, light-headedness, insomnia, hallucinations, nightmares, dizziness, ringing in the ears, or other symptoms, though this would be unusual with the type of use and the low doses typical of their use in treatment of performance anxiety or akathisia.

SUGGESTED FURTHER READING

1. Hyman SE: Recent developments in neurobiology: Part I. Synaptic transmission. *Psychosomatics* 1988;29:157–165.
2. Appleton WS: Fourth psychoactive drug usage guide. *J Clin Psychiatry* 1982;43:12–27.
3. Barnhart ER (ed): *Physician's Desk Reference*, ed. 42. Oradell, N.J., Medical Economics Company, Inc., 1988.
4. Bassuk EL, Schoonover SC, Gelenberg AJ (eds): *The Practitioner's Guide to Psychoactive Drugs*, ed. 2. New York, Plenum Medical Book Company, 1983.
5. Baldessarini RJ: *Chemotherapy in Psychiatry*. Cambridge, Harvard University Press, 1985.
6. Goa KL, Ward A: Buspirone: A preliminary review of its pharmacological properties and therapeutic efficacy as an anxiolytic. *Drugs* 1986;32:114–129.
7. Greenblatt DJ, Shader RI: *Pharmacokinetics in Clinical Practice*. Philadelphia, WB Saunders Company, 1985.
8. Lake CR (ed): Clinical psychopharmacology I. *Psychiatric Clin N Am* 1984;7:409–654.
9. McElroy SL, Keck PE, Pope HG: Sodium valproate: Its use in primary psychiatric disorders. *J Clin Psychopharmacol* 1987;7:16–24.
10. Perry PJ, Alexander B, Liskow BI: *Psychotropic Drug Handbook*, ed. 3. Cincinnati, Harvey Whitney Books, 1981.
11. Pollack MH, Rosenbaum JF, Hyman SE: Calcium channel blockers in psychiatry. *Psychosomatics* 1987;28:356–360.
12. Sommi RW, Crismon ML, Bowden CL: Fluoxetine: A serotonin-specific, second-generation antidepressant. *Pharmacotherapy* 1987;7:1–15.

8
Child and Adolescent Pharmacotherapy Comes of Age

Kerim Munir

> Biology is like a Van Eyck painting; as you approach closer, clarity actually increases. The focus holds true down to the tiniest detail. Such perspective is not of the eye but of the mind; and I ask the reader to use an equal facility of focus as we traverse between broad and narrow views.
> James M. Tanner, MD, *Fetus into Man*[1]

Pharmacotherapy of children and adolescents has gained increasing recognition among clinicians, parents, and teachers during the past decade.[2-7] Once restricted to psychostimulant treatment of childhood hyperactivity, pediatric pharmacotherapy has recently expanded its horizons. Now a larger selection of medications are used and a broader range of childhood disorders are treated.[6]

Children suffer some of the same psychiatric disorders and respond to some of the same treatments as do adults. Depression, for example, can occur in children and may respond to antidepressant treatment. At the same time, clinicians have learned to respect the ways in which child and adult pharmacotherapy differ. This chapter summarizes developments in child psychiatry which have led to the present growth of child and adolescent pharmacotherapy. It will then emphasize some of the diagnostic and clinical issues that merit special attention when medications are used to treat children and adolescents.

THE EVOLUTION OF CHILD PHARMACOTHERAPY

The first American report of using psychotropic medications in children was in 1937, when Bradley discussed the effects of benzedrine (a CNS stimulant affecting mood and behavior) on the behavior of children in residential treatment.[2,8] Ironically, his findings appeared during a time when the previously dominant constitutional-mechanistic view of child psychiatry was increasingly being pushed aside by the psychoanalytic viewpoint. Psychoanalytic ideas, which emphasized the importance of developmental factors and early life experiences, ushered in a progressive and optimistic era of child psychiatry.[9] The psychoanalytic approach, however, was not supportive to the use of medications for child and adolescent disorders. During the psychoanalytic era, child psychiatrists focused on psychotherapeutic techniques, sometimes with little awareness of the empirical data being accumulated by the disciplines of developmental and social psychology, pediatrics, and the neurosciences.[9]

By the 1970s, biological and psychodynamic factions of the American mental health community began to integrate their findings and approaches. Beginning in 1976, the American Psychiatric Association exhorted psychiatrists to broaden their professional goals and deemphasize a more rigidly psychoanalytic approach. In 1978, President Carter's Commission on Mental Health highlighted the need for research by identifying methodological problems and gaps in our understanding of many psychiatric disorders.[10,11] The Commission emphasized that psychiatry, as it was then practiced, was based on speculations and formulations which lacked a basis in empirical data. To remedy this situation, increased federal funding was offered. This laid the foundation for major advances in psychiatric research and community-based epidemiologic studies. The Epidemiological Catchment Area (ECA) study, for example, was launched in 1978. The data gathered by this multicenter longitudinal study are providing important information on the prevalence, incidence, and risk factors of specific psychiatric disorders in the general adult population.[12] Since children and adolescents were not included in the ECA study, the paucity of empirical data on the epidemiology of child and adolescent psychiatric disorders persists.

In the early 1980s, the National Institutes of Mental Health (NIMH) recognized these gaps in child and adolescent psychiatry and defined priority areas for epidemiologic and psychopharmacologic investigations. In collaboration with the American Academy of Child and Adolescent Psychiatry, the NIMH sponsored workshops and symposia to stimulate research by child psychiatrists and trainees. At first, clinicians in child mental health were skeptical of these new developments. Their subsequent effect, however, has been the encouragement of high-quality research in numerous academic centers.

The area of pharmacotherapy, though it has attracted increasing research interest, remains an open frontier. Many questions persist regarding the efficacy, toxicity, long-term effects, and abuse potential of psychotropic medications. The coupling of pharmacotherapy research methods with observational and naturalistic studies of children and adolescents,[13,14] however, is a promising trend. Carefully designed epidemiologic and clinical studies are expected to lead to a better understanding of many disorders and to clarify the interactions of biological with environmental variables.

DSM-III-R: REFINEMENTS IN THE CLASSIFICATION OF CHILD AND ADOLESCENT DISORDERS

Prior to the 1980s one factor that made the collection and comparison of pharmacotherapy data nearly impossible was the absence of consensus about diagnostic criteria for child and adolescent disorders. Before the evolving series of the *Diagnostic and Statistical Manual of Mental Disorders* (DSM) provided such criteria,[13,14] assessments in psychiatry were subjective and reflected the views and idiosyncracies of influential teachers. Diagnostic labels were liable to be affected by therapeutic fashions, innovations, or changing etiological assumptions. Though there is no truth or gold standard in defining psychiatric disorders, precision and consensus have been facilitated by the DSM criteria. Standardized diagnostic labels have made possible meaningful comparisons between the work of researchers in different locations.

The current DSM version, the DSM-III-R, offers several improvements over previous editions in its classification of child and adolescent disorders. Of particular interest are changes in the definition of the newly named attention deficit–hyperactivity disorder (ADHD), which is now grouped with oppositional defiant disorder and the conduct disorders under the rubric of disruptive behavior disorders. Of great value to clinicians, the DSM-III-R also has partially operationalized the assessment of severity of these disorders as mild, moderate, or severe. For the first time, the DSM-III-R has linked symptom number with impairment of functioning at home, at school, and with peers.[14] This improvement makes diagnostic characterization more meaningful.

Though the DSM-III-R standardizes United States terminology, it is of interest that international diagnostic disparities persist.[15] The American concept of attention deficit–hyperactivity disorder (ADHD), for example, differs significantly from the United Kingdom's definition of childhood hyperactivity. This was emphasized by a recent US-UK diagnostic comparison study, which revealed that differences in the rates of DSM-III attention deficit disorder (ADD) between the two countries could be attributed to discrepancies in the diagnostic criteria used.[15] A child psychiatrist in London is likely to diagnose DSM-III ADD as conduct disorder, reserving the diagnosis of childhood hyperactivity for the pervasive cases of patients with neuropsychological dysfunction or soft neurological signs. Although it is meaningless to ask which view is correct, the achievement of greater accuracy and consensus is an important goal. Ongoing research in child psychiatry is addressing these issues.

Also of importance in the DSM-III-R is the emphasis on a broader assessment of functioning (Axis V). Prior to DSM-III-R, only social and occupational functioning were rated. These domains were generally difficult to define in children and adolescents in view of age-specific variations and subjective norms.

In addition, DSM-III-R has introduced a modification of the Children's Global Assessment Scale,[16] which assesses psychological functioning on a continuum of mental health. The value of DSM-III-R's Axis V is further enhanced by the inclusion of ratings of both current functioning and highest level of functioning during the year preceding the evaluation. Utilization of these diagnostic refinements allows clinicians to characterize adaptive functioning in a richer way.

By no means are all controversies about classification resolved by the DSM-III-R. The inclusion of three types of conduct disorder (group, solitary-aggressive, and undifferentiated), for example, has been justified by the implied clinical usefulness of the distinction,[14] but resolution of the question whether these conditions differ qualitatively or quantitatively must wait for future DSMs. A future DSM would also benefit from a section on adolescence, and from further delineation of the differences among disorders of childhood, adolescence, and adulthood. A classification scheme, of course, evolves and improves over time. "It cannot," as Kendell has eloquently stated, "as Athene did, spring fully armed from the head of Zeus."[17]

CRITICAL ISSUES IN THE PRACTICE OF CHILD AND ADOLESCENT PSYCHIATRY AND PHARMACOTHERAPY

Referrals for pharmacotherapy evaluation come from schools, psychologists, community mental health and social services, medical and nonmedical practitioners in individual and group practice, specialty clinics in medical centers, and parents. Characteristically, children referred for psychopharmacological evaluation have undergone prior psychological treatment. Most parents, apprehensive about exposing their child to medication, are reluctant to accept pharmacotherapy for their child except as a last resort. Often they need to hear from multiple resource persons (relatives, friends, teachers, pediatrician, or family practitioner) that their child may benefit from such treatment.

The younger the child is, the more reluctant a parent is likely to be in accepting the recommendation for a medication trial. When the child has failed to benefit from other therapeutic interventions, the psychotherapeutic treatment is at an impasse, or there is an outstanding crisis, consultation may be sought as a safety valve measure. Under these circumstances, expectations of pharmacotherapy's effects may be unrealistically high and attended by anxious hopes.

A comprehensive diagnostic, developmental, and psychosocial evaluation should always precede pharmacotherapy. The pharmacotherapist and other clinicians must make a concerted effort to obtain and include information from the child's family and school. The evaluation process also involves a medical examination including vital signs (blood pressure, heart rate, height, and weight) and baseline laboratory tests (blood count, urinalysis, and serum chemistry). Other diagnostic tests may be obtained as suggested by the clinical picture — for example, thyroid function tests when symptoms suggest disturbed endocrine function, ECG when cardiac symptoms are present, EEG when a seizure disorder must be ruled out, or tomographic brain scan (CAT or MRI) when an underlying structural neurological lesion is suspected. The child's pediatrician should participate in the evaluation and test results could be shared. Other specialty consultations can be requested as indicated. Further evaluation by a pediatric neurologist or by a neuropsychologist, for example, may be required to clarify diagnostic issues.

The disorders and behaviors considered most likely to respond to medication include attention deficit–hyperactivity disorder, separation anxiety disorder, major depression, functional enuresis, tic disorders (including Tourette's syndrome), obsessive-compulsive disorder, psychotic and various agitated/aggressive disorders including the bipolar variant disorder of childhood or adolescence, and various seizure disorders, as well as behavioral and psychiatric complications of mental retardation and pervasive developmental disorder (including autistic disorder).[4–7]

The choice of medication is based on the child's symptoms, age, weight, and general physical health. The symptoms to be targeted by medication should be assessed at baseline and reassessed throughout the course of treatment. Parents should understand that children may paradoxically need higher dosages of medication per unit weight than adults because of their ability to metabolize medications more quickly.

When pharmacotherapy is recommended, the potential risks and benefits of any suggested medication should be carefully explained to parents and school personnel in a clear and comprehensive manner. Consent for treatment ultimately rests upon the parent(s) or guardian, who must therefore understand these risks and benefits in order to represent the best interests of the child or adolescent. Ideally, the parent should be competent to supervise the child's use of medication and to help monitor beneficial and toxic effects. Pharmacotherapy may be too risky to recommend for a child or adolescent with an unreliable parent.[7]

When parents are separated or divorced and there is parental disagreement over the need for pharmacotherapy, the parent who has custody of the child is ultimately responsible for consent. This is usually an awkward situation for the older child or adolescent, who may be ambivalent about taking medication. If the child spends weekends with the parent who disapproves of pharmacotherapy, treatment is likely to suffer because of intermittent noncompliance. One such child often behaved poorly at the beginning of each week, following weekend visits with his father. His mother was unaware of the medication noncompliance on these weekends, but the child's withdrawal symptoms revealed the reason for his fluctuating behavior.

When the patient is an older child or adolescent, he or she can often be included in discussions of the risks and benefits of drug treatment. The adolescent's agreement to treatment should be sought. Older children and adolescents are particularly sensitive and may feel easily stigmatized about taking mood-altering drugs. Their feelings about medication should be elicited and discussed respectfully. In the context of current anti-drug education at schools and in the community, the patient may need help in understanding the distinction between substance abuse and the monitored use of prescribed medications.

It is often advisable to encourage adolescents to take responsibility for reminding their parent or school nurse about their medication schedule. In general, however, they should not be expected to store or carry their medications. Adolescents can be volatile, moody, and impulsive. When medications are available as a vehicle for acting out behaviors, the consequences can be disastrous.

In treating children and adolescents, the risk of suicide must always be considered. Recent years have seen a dramatic increase in the suicide rate for young men (both white and black) aged 15 to 24 years. The influence of media publicity and the role played by imitation have gained increased recognition.[18] There is firm psychiatric evidence that the presence of a mental disorder, especially depression, constitutes a strong risk factor. Recent follow-up studies suggest that the risk of suicide in a child with mental illness is increased by a factor of eight or more.[19] Children who have attempted suicide unsuccessfully have an increased risk of subsequently completing a suicide attempt. Although it is unlikely that psychiatric illness accounts for all suicides, suicide risk must be carefully assessed in any child or adolescent referred for pharmacotherapy.

Ongoing assesssment of medication response and side effects is essential in pharmacotherapy. Outcome of treatment should always be measured objectively and take into account several different domains: home, school, and social functioning. Any cognitive effects of medication, as well as any effects on growth in weight and height, should be monitored closely. Dosage levels may require adjustment in the attempt to optimize the balance between therapeutic and adverse drug effects.

Tapering or discontinuation of medication should be reconsidered periodically. Many clinicians prefer to attempt medication discontinuation during the academic year. This provides an opportunity to monitor the child's school performance before and after discontinuation and to obtain input from multiple resource persons interacting with the child.

CASE ILLUSTRATIONS

The following cases are presented as clinical vignettes to illustrate aspects of the practice of pharmacotherapy with children and adolescents. They are not intended to represent a cross section of patients.

> Case 1. An 8-year-old white boy was referred for pharmacotherapeutic evaluation because of his long-standing impulsivity, inattentiveness, and self-destructive behaviors. The latter included head-banging during temper outbursts, which had recently increased in frequency and intensity. The child was in the custody of

the Department of Social Services and had been living in foster care. His younger brother had been placed in a separate foster home. Their biological mother, who had a history of psychological problems and alcoholism, was contesting the state authorities for custody of her children. There was a substantiated history of emotional neglect and abuse associated with the mother's problems. On examination, both the patient and his younger brother showed traits of alcohol fetal syndrome consistent with mother having abused alcohol during both pregnancies. Both children were below the 3rd percentile for growth in height and in weight. The patient's DSM-III-R diagnostic profile was as follows:

Axis I: Attention deficit–hyperactivity disorder; oppositional defiant disorder; parent-child problem; adjustment disorder with mixed disturbance of emotions and conduct;

Axis II: No evidence for specific developmental (learning) disorder; average IQ;

Axis III: Fetal alcohol traits; below 3rd percentile for growth;

Axis IV: Level of psychosocial stressors: severe;

Axis V: Children's Global Assessment Score (CGAS): 50–41, moderate degree of interference in functioning in most social areas with severe impairment of functioning in one area.

The patient's outbursts were usually (but not always) precipitated by his mother's visits, during which she told her son she would fight the authorities in order to reclaim custody of him. An additional stressor was his fear that he would never again be reunited with his brother in a stable environment. The patient was in psychotherapy with an experienced psychologist, who substantiated the history that ADHD symptoms pre-dated the onset of self-destructive episodes and temper tantrums and most likely exacerbated his current difficulties. Therapeutic classroom, foster home, and psychotherapeutic interventions had in the past been satisfactory in addressing his problems, without a need for pharmacotherapy. Given his intense behavioral excitation and rage, the use of stimulant or antidepressant medications were thought to carry a risk of symptom exacerbation. Urgent containment of the aggressive and self-destructive behaviors took precedence over pharmacotherapy of ADHD. All caretakers concerned agreed on the need for therapeutic limitation of mother's visits.

Because of the potential danger of physical damage from the patient's head-banging, the pharmacotherapist suggested a trial of thioridazine, an antipsychotic drug potentially useful in controlling agitation, but this recommendation was contested by the boy's biological mother. Amazingly, and to everyone's relief, the boy began to calm down when a concerted effort was made to meet with him, his case worker, his therapist, his foster mother, and his brother. During this period, the court ruled that the patient could be given thioridazine as indicated for the treatment of his self-injurious behaviors. His self-destructive behaviors remitted without sustained pharmacotherapy, however, once he felt reassured that he would be able to visit his brother.

Case 2. A 10-year-old white boy was referred by his parents for evaluation and treatment of attention deficit–hyperactivity disorder. His parents, both of whom were grade-school teachers, were convinced that their son fitted the picture of ADHD described in a newspaper article. The boy was moody, restless, unable to sit still, and easily distractible at home and at school. In addition, he had difficulties getting along with his older sister. Always at the top of his class, the patient was unusually motivated in school but seemed uncomfortable with competition. Psychological testing showed him to be of superior intelligence with significant difficulties in attention span.

Diagnostic evaluation including a lifetime structured interview of parent and child revealed that he had experienced at least two episodes of major depression. One of these had been associated with suicidal ideation. There was also a family history of major depressive disorder in the patient's mother, who had been treated with antidepressant medications. Family assessment was otherwise unremarkable except for confirming the parents' high expectations of both children, at some cost to fun activities or time spent together as a family. The diagnostic picture was as follows:

Axis I: Major depressive disorder; attention deficit–hyperactivity disorder, mild;
Axis II: None;
Axis III: None;
Axis IV: Psychosocial stress: mild;
Axis V: Children's Global Assessment Score (CGAS): 70–61, some difficulty in a single area, but generally functioning well.

Of interest in this example was the uncovering of significant depressive episodes in association with mild to moderate ADHD.[20,21] In view of the boy's depression, stimulant medication was not the drug of first choice for the ADHD symptoms. A tricyclic antidepressant medication, desipramine, was chosen instead. In keeping with the parents' wishes, psychotherapy was deferred until completion of the medication trial. Within eight weeks a dramatic and sustained improvement was observed in the patient's depressed mood, distractibility, and inattentiveness. Initially, the parents expressed reservations about informing the school of his treatment because of concerns that he might be stigmatized. Their request for confidentiality was respected. At a later date, they felt comfortable sharing the facts of his treatment with school personnel.

Case 3. A 5-year-old boy living with his biological parents and younger sibling was referred by his pediatrician for a pharmacotherapy evaluation because of depression and stereotypical movements (habit disorder).[12] The boy had not been eating well. He looked depressed and seemed withdrawn. In addition, he had a series of somatic complaints which had been worked up by the pediatrician without any significant findings. Most noticeably, an excoriation of one cheek had resulted from his repetitive skin-picking over the preceding two months. During that time the child's sleep was reported to have been impaired, with initial and middle insomnia. Developmental history, family history, and physical examination were otherwise unremarkable. Psychological evaluation confirmed a depressive picture without cognitive deficits. After the initial evaluation parents were given further opportunity to consult their pediatrician and to discuss the recommendations. Pharmacotherapy was deferred until completion of psychological testing. These test results, the child's continuing symptoms, and the pediatrician's observations all confirmed the impression of major depression with stereotypy/habit disorder.

During a return visit to the pharmacotherapist, the parents expressed their willingness to begin the patient on medications. They also indicated that they were moving to a larger house since they felt "too cramped." Apparently the move had been planned for some time and they had been preparing for this move during the preceding month. Furniture and other objects had been put into storage, significantly disrupting the home environment. Based on this new information, pharmacotherapy was further deferred, until completion of the move. During the visit two weeks later, the boy appeared alert and less depressed. He engaged in meaningful play in the office for the first time. Over the course of the next few weeks he continued to improve, his face-touching gradually diminished, and the excoriation on his cheek began to heal.

The diagnostic picture was:
Axis I: Major depressive episode versus adjustment disorder

with depressed and anxious mood; Stereotypical movement-habit disorder;
Axis II: None;
Axis III: None;
Axis IV: Level of stress: moderate;
Axis V: Children's Global Assessment Score (CGAS): 60-50, variable functioning with sporadic difficulties or symptoms in several but not all areas.

This case illustrates the value of patience in pharmacotherapeutic assessment of young children. This is especially justified when confidence about the diagnosis is low or the nature of environmental stressors remains uncertain. If the patient had begun antidepressant treatment, the response to medication might have been illusory. A spontaneous remission based on psychological restabilization would not have been appreciated. When clear target symptoms are identified, however, pharmacotherapy should not be indefinitely deferred. Had the boy's symptoms persisted, a medication trial may have been indicated even in the presence of psychosocial stressors.

CONCLUSION

Despite exciting advances in child and adolescent pharmacotherapy, a caveat is necessary. Reliance on pharmacotherapy to the exclusion or deemphasis of other treatment modalities would be an undesirable trend. Current economic concerns have lessened face-to-face time spent with patients and family and have limited the accessibility of long-term treatment of children with a complex array of disorders and psychosocial problems. There is some risk of embracing pharmacotherapy, which appears to represent a more cost-effective approach, too enthusiastically. Eisenberg, recognizing the renewed emphasis on biological knowledge and technology, recently warned that we face the danger of "substituting a mindless psychiatry for the brainless psychiatry of the past."[22] Recent advances in pharmacotherapy give us an expanding armamentarium of useful medications for psychiatric disorders, but "hyperactive children or depressed adolescents need more than a drug prescription."[9]

Child and adolescent pharmacotherapy, nonetheless, can

become valuable components of a comprehensive treatment program. Over the past decade, the introduction of operational diagnostic criteria for classifying child and adolescent psychiatric disorders, the development of assessment instruments for their measurement, the application of improved research methods in observational studies, and the better selection of diagnostic groups in placebo-controlled clinical trials have begun to clarify how and where medications may be most usefully applied. When administered rationally and selectively for specific disorders with clear target symptoms, medications can help to alleviate suffering, but their use needs always to be part of a comprehensive treatment addressing complex psychological, educational, and social issues.

REFERENCES

1. Tanner JM: *Fetus into Man: Physical Growth from Conception to Maturity*. Cambridge, MA, Harvard University Press, 1978.
2. Weiner JM (ed): *Diagnosis and Psychopharmacology of Childhood and Adolescent Disorders*. New York, John Wiley and Sons, 1985.
3. Campbell M, Green WH, Deutsch SI: *Child and Adolescent Psychopharmacology*. Beverly Hills, CA, Sage Publications, 1985.
4. Biederman J, Jellinek MS: Psychopharmacology in children. *N Engl J Med* 1984;310:968–974.
5. Popper C (ed): *Psychiatric Pharmacosciences of Children and Adolescents*. Washington, DC, American Psychiatric Press, Inc., 1987.
6. Campbell M, Spencer EK: Psychopharmacology in child and adolescent psychiatry: A review of the past five years. *J Am Acad Child Adolescent Psychiatry* 1988;27:269–279.
7. Coffey BJ: Therapeutics III: Pharmacotherapy, in Robson KS (ed): *Manual of Clinical Child Psychiatry*. Washington, DC, American Psychiatric Association Press, 1986, pp 149–184.
8. Bradley C: The behavior of children receiving Benzedrine. *Am J Orthopsychiatry* 1937;94:577–585.
9. Chess S: Child and adolescent psychiatry comes of age: A fifty year perspective. *J Am Acad Child Adolesc Psychiatry* 1988;27:1–7.
10. President's Commission on Mental Health: *Report to the President from the President's Commission on Mental Health*, vol. 1. Washington, DC, US Government Printing Office, 1978.
11. Freedman DX: The President's Commission: realistic remedies for neglect (editorial). *Arch Gen Psychiatry* 1978;35:675–676.
12. Regier DA, Myers JK, Kramer M, et al: The NIMH Epidemiologic Catchment Area Program. *Arch Gen Psychiatry* 1984;41:934–941.

13. *Diagnostic and Statistical Manual of Mental Disorders*, ed. 3. Washington, DC, American Psychiatric Association, 1980.
14. *Diagnostic and Statistical Manual of Mental Disorders*, ed. 3, revised. Washington, DC, American Psychiatric Association, 1987.
15. Taylor EA: Childhood hyperactivity. *Br J Psychiatry* 1986;149:562–573.
16. Shaffer D, Gould GS, Brasic J, et al: A Children's Global Assessment Scale. *Arch Gen Psychiatry* 1983;40:1228–1231.
17. Kendell RE: What are mental disorders? in Freedman AM, Brotman R, Silverman I, Hutson D (eds): *Issues in Psychiatric Classification*. New York, Human Services Press, 1986, pp 23–45.
18. Philips DP, Carstensen LL: Clustering of teenage suicides after television news stories about suicide. *N Engl J Med* 1986;315:685–689.
19. Monk M: Epidemiology of suicide. *Epidemiol Rev* 1987;9:51–69.
20. Biederman J, Munir K, Knee D, et al: High rate of affective disorders in probands with attention deficit disorder and in their relatives: A controlled family study. *Am J Psychiatry* 1987;144:330–333.
21. Munir KM, Biederman J, Knee D: Psychiatric co-morbidity in patients with attention deficit disorder: A controlled study. *J Acad Child Adolesc Psychiatry* 1987;26:844–848.
22. Eisenberg L: Mindlessness and brainlessness in psychiatry. *Br J Psychiatry* 1986;148:497–508.

9

Organic Mental Disorder: When To Suspect Medical Illness as a Cause of Psychiatric Symptoms

Stephen J. Bartels

> It is the brain ... which is the seat of madness and delirium, of the fears and frights which assail us, often by night, but sometimes even by day; it is there where lies the cause of insomnia and sleep-walking, of thoughts that will not come, forgotten duties, and eccentricities. All such things result from an unhealthy condition of the brain.
>
> *Hippocrates*

Since the time of Hippocrates, the relationship of mind and body has fascinated and perplexed philosophers. For those who study psychiatric illness, the nature of this relationship becomes especially complex. For example, is psychosis to be understood as a disease of the brain or of the mind? In terms of psychopathology, what is meant by the distinction? Recent discoveries in neurobiology suggest clear links between altered brain structure and function in schizophrenia. But can all forms of schizophrenia be explained in this way? Studies of affective disorders have correlated depression with altered functioning of neurotransmitters and hormones. How does this fit with what we know about the psychodynamics of depression? And what of personality? We are beginning to appreciate that certain types of explosive or violent behaviors have a neurological basis. Yet clearly, we are far from understanding the biology of an individual's personality. Psychiatry is only just beginning to untangle the biological underpinnings of major mental illness. Another aspect of the mind-body question confronts us every day in our clinical work. Faced with behavioral symptoms, we must always consider whether they may be a manifestation of medical illness requiring special attention. Organic diseases of the body are known to dramatically affect and alter mental functions.[1] *In fact, no psychiatric symptom exists that cannot be caused or exacerbated by various physical illnesses.*[1-3] Depression, anxiety, panic, elation, hallucinations, delusions, confusion, sexual dysfunction, and changes in personality can occur under the influence of organic disturbances. For this reason, organic mental disorders have been called the great imposters of psychiatric illness.[2] In assessing the emotionally or behaviorally disturbed patient, the possibility of organic illness must be considered as part of the initial evaluation or at a later stage if treatment has not proved as effective as expected. To aid the psychotherapist in this process, this chapter reviews information about medical illness in psychiatric patients and offers guidelines for suspecting the presence of an undiagnosed organic mental disorder.

MEDICAL ILLNESS IN PSYCHIATRIC PATIENTS

An alarming body of research reveals how common medical illness occurs in psychiatric patients. From 24% to 80% of psychiatric outpatients have a major medical illness.[4-8] These illnesses are often unknown to the patient's psychotherapist or physicians, though many are easily found when sought. In a study of over 2,000 psychiatric outpatients, approximately one-half had major medical illnesses undiagnosed by the referring clinicians. Clinicians from *all* disciplines demonstrated deficiencies in medical diagnosis. Referring medical physicians were unaware of major medical illness one-third of the time. Psychiatrists missed medical diagnoses approximately one-half of the time. Social worker and social agencies had no knowledge of existing major medical illness in 83% of patient referrals. Self-referred patients were unaware of their own medical illness 84% of the time.[9]

These undiagnosed medical illnesses frequently have a direct impact on psychological health and functioning.[9-12] Physical illness exacerbates psychiatric symptoms in as many as two-thirds of psychiatric outpatients.[12] Physical illness is the sole cause of the presenting psychiatric disorder in as many as one-fifth of patients.[9,11,12] In most cases these medical problems are previously unrecognized.[7-9]

Undiagnosed medical illness is also a significant cause of the higher than average death rate of psychiatric patients. Many psychiatric patients die needlessly as a result of undetected physical illnesses that could have been discovered by a routine medical evaluation consisting of a psychiatric and physical examination, full blood chemistries, urinalysis, ECG, and sleep-deprived EEG.[5,13] In one study, these procedures detected more than 90% of the medical illnesses that were identified in patients subjected to extensive research examinations.[5]

GENERAL GUIDELINES FOR IDENTIFYING THE MEDICALLY ILL PSYCHIATRIC PATIENT

To ask the fundamental question *"Could this be organic?"* is the most important step in detecting medical illness. In answering this question the clinician should follow three basic principles: (1) perform a thorough history and mental status examination on all patients, (2) request that patients obtain a routine physical examination, and (3) continue to consider the possibility of organicity throughout the course of treatment.

The first of these principles is the most important. Findings that should alert the psychotherapist to the likelihood of an underlying organic disorder often arise from the history and mental status examination. These basic tools, available to any clinician, are cornerstones in the diagnosis of organic mental disorders. The accuracy of these tools relies, in part, on the cognitive abilities and cooperation of the patient. Because these may be limited, it is critical to utilize all resources available in obtaining a history. Family, friends, caregivers, and other key resources may be vital in providing an objective account of the recent changes in a person's mental status.

Although hundreds of organic illnesses can produce psychiatric symptoms, several types of illness stand out. The missed brain tumor dreaded by all clinicians is, in fact, quite rare. The most common causes of organic mental disorders are adverse drug reactions (intoxications, withdrawals, and side effects of prescribed and abused drugs), neurological disorders, electrolyte imbalances, infections, endocrine disorders (especially diabetes and thyroid disease), and nutritional deficiencies. Clues suggesting these specific disorders may be elicited during a thorough diagnostic interview.

The possibility of underlying serious medical illness necessitates a current or recent physical examination and laboratory evaluation. This second principle in assessment underscores the responsibility of the psychotherapist to request (or require) a physical examination as an integral part of the psychological evaluation. Medical screening forms filled out by the patient and medical physician are becoming widely used in psychiatric clinics. Medical evaluation may also be necessary later in treatment if new symptoms that suggest organicity develop. For patients aged 45 years or older, an annual physical check-up is recommended.

The third general principle is to recognize that the answer may be complex. Most presentations involving organicity are neither purely psychological nor organic, but mixed. Making a determination of one cause does not remove the need to consider and treat others. When a decision about this is made prematurely, the result is likely to be inadequate treatment. Foreclosure of diagnostic considerations can especially occur when a patient is difficult or unpleasant and evokes negative countertransference. In emergency room settings such patients are frequently labeled organic or psychiatric on the basis of a single symptom, one item of their history, or their previous diagnosis. This can occur despite the presence of known indicators of organic illness. In one emergency room study of organic brain syndrome, for example, 36% of the patients had significant findings on the initial physical examination or history suggestive of organic illness, yet were labeled medically cleared and referred for psychiatric evaluation.[3] Hence, even when the patient's symptoms have been labeled psychiatric, be skeptical!

The History (Table 9-1)

Any first episode of major psychiatric illness warrants a medical assessment to rule out a possible organic contribution. This is especially the case for psychotic symptoms that have their onset after the age of 40 years. Among the major disorders, schizophrenia rarely begins after the age of 40, and bipolar affective disorder has a mean onset at an age of about 30 years. Panic disorder or acute anxiety attacks usually begin before the age of 35 years. As a general rule, a first episode of psychosis or panic disorder in a person who is older than 40 years should be assumed to be organic until proven otherwise. Other disorders such as depression may initially occur at any age. The first appearance of depression, however, should also be carefully assessed. Depressed mood and many of the vegetative signs of depression are nonspecific symptoms that may represent early features of organic illness.

Acuteness of onset is a clue to possible organicity. Most psychiatric disorders have a prodome or set of symptoms, which are the subclinical precursors of the major illness. These initial symptoms develop and evolve over time into a major psychiatric syndrome. With the exception of those few disorders that have clear precipitants (such as acute grief reactions or brief reactive psychoses), an acute onset is highly suspect. In particular, the onset of a major psychiatric disorder over a period of hours or days in the context of a good premorbid personality and no clear precipitants warrants a full work-up for organic mental disorder.

Table 9-1
Clues to Organic Mental Disorder from the History

First episode of major psychiatric illness
Age of onset > 40
Acute onset (esp. weeks, days, or hours)
Medication history
Alcohol and substance-abuse history
Accompanying physical illness/new onset of physical complaints
Recent history of head trauma
Family history of inherited illnesses
Work/travel/sexual history

A thorough history of *medication, alcohol, and substance use,* as well as a basic *medical history*, often provides the answers to questions about organicity. There are literally hundreds of prescribed medications that can cause changes in mental status. Although the elderly are particularly at risk for toxic side effects of medications, this possibility should be considered for patients of any age. An evaluation of the patterns of medication usage is therefore critical. For example, one key question to be asked is, "Do you take your medications as prescribed?" It is surprisingly common for patients' actual medication use to differ from their prescribed schedule or dosage.

A comprehensive list of medications may also raise the question of toxicity secondary to polypharmacy. Multiple medications (sometimes from multiple sources) may interact or combine to produce life-threatening organic states. In addition to prescribed medication, it is important to ask about the use of over-the-counter medications and home remedies, which otherwise may not be mentioned by the patient. After this list of medications is obtained, an attempt should be made to identify any recent changes in the way they are used. Sometimes a change in mental status will correlate with a recent change in type or dosage of medications.

Alcohol and substances of abuse are a major cause of changes in mental status and should always be considered in a psychiatric evaluation. These changes may be acute, as in the case of intoxication or withdrawal states, or chronic, as in the cognitive and mood changes associated with dependency. Intoxication or withdrawal may be detected by attention to physical appearance, speech, and behavior. Physical manifestations including elevated vital signs and tremor may provide clues to a potentially life-threatening acute withdrawal state. In chronic dependency, the clues may be more subtle. They may require corroborative information from family members. A patient's report of alcohol or drug use should be considered with a high degree of skepticism because it may underestimate actual use. One factor that leads patients to underestimate their use of substances is denial. To avoid a fruitless confrontation with denial, it is often more productive to question less about the amount of alcohol consumed and focus instead on information about negative consequences of drinking (problems with relationships or self-esteem) and efforts to control or cut down on alcohol intake. This approach to obtaining history of alcohol use is exemplified by the questions from the CAGE mnemonic[14]:

- Have you ever Cut down on drinking?
- Do you get Annoyed when people criticize your drinking?
- Do you ever feel Guilty about your drinking?
- Do you ever have an Eye opener in the morning?

Other key aspects of taking a history of alcohol use include asking about unplanned drinking, drinking alone, arrests related to drinking, blackouts, withdrawal symptoms, and periods of sobriety. Also important are any past detoxifications or attendance at Alcoholics Anonymous.

A list of any long-standing or recent *known physical illnesses* is critical in the assessment of factors possibly contributing to changes in mental status. In particular, endocrine, metabolic, neurological, kidney, or heart diseases are commonly associated with psychiatric complaints. The worsening of a chronic thyroid condition, for example, may reveal itself first through a change in mood or personality. Any new onset of physical complaints such as severe headache or weakness should also be evaluated. In particular, it is important to inquire about any head trauma preceding the new onset of psychiatric complaints. Finally, a *family history of inherited medical illnesses* such as Huntington's disease may be pertinent to a comprehensive psychiatric evaluation.

The history is incomplete without a *work, travel, and sexual history*. Any decline of function should be noted with a comprehensive description of the deficits. A history of exposure to industrial toxins is also pertinent. A recent travel history which might arouse suspicion of exposure to infectious diseases or parasites may be significant. A sexual history also may be useful in assessing the possible exposure to venereal diseases. Current estimates are that 30% to 40% of AIDS patients show CNS dysfunction and it is recognized that depression may precede other signs or symptoms of AIDS.[15] The sexual history can also point toward organic disorder by eliciting data about sexual function, as impotence or anorgasmia may result from underlying medical illness. Impotence, for example, may be an early symptom of diabetes.

The Mental Status Examination

Appearance as well as mentation can be affected by an organic disturbance. Flushed, dry red skin, dilated pupils, and confusion may indicate anticholinergic medication toxicity, a state described by the mnemonic "dry as a bone, red as a beet, and mad as a hatter." A bodily infection may reveal its presence through warm skin that is damp from perspiration. Large or small pupils may be evidence of substance abuse or medication toxicity. Vomiting, drooling, excessive sweating, rapid or slow breathing, and dizziness each can signify serious medical illness. Pronounced weakness (especially if one-sided), tremor, incoordination, staggering gait, or slurred speech may indicate a major neurological disorder.

Sudden changes in *alertness or level of activity* may point to an organic illness. Fluctuating or altered levels of consciousness are a common sign of delirium. They may be evidenced by restlessness or agitation alternating with drowsiness. Episodes of violent, bizarre, or uncharacteristic behavior may alternate with lethargic, somnolent, or lucid periods. This may also be reflected in a marked disturbance of the sleep/wakefulness cycle, which may become completely reversed or severely fragmented. Bizarre, exceptionally disorganized, or disoriented behavior (such as getting lost in familiar surroundings) may also be a clue to organic illness. Catatonia (mutism, posturing, rigidity, stereotypic movements, negativism, waxy flexibility, stupor or extreme excitement, and combativeness) is mistakenly considered by some to be a hallmark of schizophrenia, yet one-sixth of catatonia is secondary to organic mental disorder.[16] Many medical etiologies of catatonia, such as encephalitis, toxic or drug-induced psychoses, alcohol withdrawal, or seizure disorders, are life-threatening.[17]

Extreme lability of *affect*, especially over a brief span of time, should be closely assessed. Patients may abruptly switch from euphoria or sadness to hostile, threatening, or violent behavior. Depressed, manic, or anxious moods are not diagnostic in themselves of any disorder. Each can represent an organic mental disorder at times.

Slurred or incoherent *speech* or difficulty in word-finding or recalling names points to diffuse or focal cerebral dysfunction. Extreme difficulty focusing or sustaining *attention* or inability to *concentrate* is typical of organic mental states. Patients may require repeated instructions and lose their train of thought in mid-sentence. In addition, extreme distractibility may occur so that outside stimuli such as extraneous noises are incorporated into thinking. *Thinking* may be especially concrete or stereotyped with an absence of abstraction.

Perceptual disturbances are common in people with organic mental disorders. Visual, tactile, or olfactory hallucinations should be considered organic in etiology until proven otherwise because they are rare in functional disorders. Visual hallucinations are frequently associated with toxic/withdrawal states or seizure disorders. Perceptual distortions or illusions may also occur. In one outpatient clinic study, 20% of medically induced psychiatric disorders were accompanied by visual hallucinations, distortions, or illusions. In comparison, only 0.5% of nonorganic psychiatric disturbances were associated with these symptoms. Withdrawal states and olfactory hallucinations are often associated with temporal lobe epilepsy (TLE).

Any and all *cognitive* deficits suggest the possibility of organic illness and must therefore be clinically investigated. Tests of orientation, memory (short- and long-term), concentration, calculation, general information, similarities, abstraction, insight, and judgment are all part of a general cognitive examination. Clear deficits of orientation or memory are *not* a typical part of functional psychiatric disorders. If cognitive deficits are found on the mental status examination, the burden is on the clinician to rule out potential organic disturbances.

Several brief and easily administered instruments are available for rough quantification of cognitive impairment. These are generally used in the assessment of dementia, yet can also be used as adjuncts in general clinical assessment of suspected organicity. The Mini Mental State Exam (see Table 9-2) provides a measure of general cognitive impairment in less than ten minutes.[18] Out of a possible 30 points, patients with a score of 12

Table 9-2
Mini Mental State Examination

Assess level of consciousness: (Vigilant)(Alert)(Drowsy)(Stupor)

Maximum Score	Score	
		Orientation
5	( )	What is the (year) (season) (day) (month)?
5	( )	Where are we (state) (county) (town) (hospital) (floor)?
		Registration
3	( )	Name 3 objects: 1 second to say each. Ask patient for all 3 after you have said them. 1 point given for each correct answer. Then repeat until patient learns all 3. Count trials and record: _____.
		Attention and Calculation
5	( )	Serial 7's: 1 point for each correct answer. Stop after five answers. Alternatively, spell "world" backwards.
		Recall
3	( )	Ask for 3 objects repeated above. 1 point for each.
		Language
2	( )	Name a pencil, a watch. 1 point for each.
1	( )	Repeat the following: "No ifs, ands, or buts." 1 point.
3	( )	Follow a 3-stage command: "Take a paper in your right hand, fold it in half, and put it on the floor." 3 points.
1	( )	Read and obey the following: "Close your eyes." 1 point.
1	( )	Write a sentence. Must contain subject and verb and make sense. 1 point.
		Visual-Motor Function
1	( )	Copy 2 intersecting pentagons. All 10 angles must be present and 2 must intersect. 1 point.
30		

Total score: _____

Adapted from Folstein MF, Folstein SE, McHugh PR: "Mini-Mental state," a practical method for grading the cognitive state of patients for the clinician. *J Psychiatric Res* 1975;12:189–198. Parts reproduced by permission from Pergamon Press.

or less have a high likelihood of an organic impairment (such as dementia) and need a thorough medical evaluation. This test is an especially useful assessment because it tests several distinct brain areas including the frontal, parietal, and temporal lobes. In addition to orientation, memory, concentration, and calculation, it also tests *dysgraphias* (impaired writing — among the most useful simple tests of organicity), *agnosia* (impaired ability to name objects), *apraxia* (impaired ability to draw or copy shapes), *aphasia* (impaired comprehension or expression of language), and *visuospatial deficits*.

Another screening test for dementia is the set test, recalled by the acronym FACT.[19] In this examination, the patient is asked to name 10 Fruits, 10 Animals, 10 Colors, and 10 Towns. With a maximum score of 40, a score of 14 or less has been shown to be consistent with severe dementia.

In summary, the history and mental status examination are critical tools in the assessment of organic mental disorder. In the event that clues of possible underlying organicity are found, the therapist must immediately pursue further medical evaluation. The first step in further evaluation, when possible, is to obtain vital signs. The presence of abnormal vital signs provides important additional information and underscores the urgency of referral for further medical assessment. When organicity is suspected, a timely referral for medical assessment is among the most important interventions that a therapist can make.

It is no secret that patients with forms of organic mental disorder may be extremely difficult to assess and to manage. For example, the intoxicated, verbally abusive patient brought by police into the emergency room may be pejoratively labeled a *GOMER* (the acronym for "Get out of my emergency room!"). Countertransference issues may complicate the assessment of organic factors in such a patient, as demonstrated in the following example:

> Case 1. A middle-aged alcoholic homeless man is evaluated for alcoholism and paranoid psychosis. After initial placement in the city jail for drunken and disorderly conduct, he is sent to a prominent teaching hospital emergency room for assessment of "bizarre behavior." He is disoriented, verbally abusive, and uncooperative. He is quickly "examined" by an emergency room

physician, declared "medically cleared," and sent by ambulance to the local state hospital.

On admission there he is acutely intoxicated (reeking of alcohol) and complains that he was "beat-up" while in jail. On inquiring further about these physical assaults, he reports that he "blacked-out" when he was thrown against the wall. Since that time he has had "the worst headache in my life."

As the admission interview proceeds, he appears progressively more "drunk." His speech becomes more slurred, and he has more difficulty keeping awake. His diagnosis: a life-threatening subarachnoid (brain) hemorrhage.

MAJOR PSYCHIATRIC SYNDROMES AND MEDICAL DISORDERS WHICH CAN IMITATE OR CAUSE THEM

In this section the major categories of psychiatric syndromes are addressed, with a focus on the more common medical disorders that may produce similar symptoms or signs. The major categories to be discussed are psychoses, mood disturbances, anxiety disorders, and personality syndromes. Each of these entities has an equivalent DSM-III-R organic mental disorder subtype (see Table 9-3).[20]

Organic Causes of Psychosis: Delirium, Dementia, and Other Organic Psychotic Syndromes

Delirium

Case 2. A 41-year-old Haitian woman was admitted to the hospital with a chief complaint of having been placed under a "curse" by her sister-in-law. The patient worked for several years as a secretary at a local business. She was well liked by her supervisors, who described her as "responsible" and "a hard worker." Two weeks prior to her admission she began to have significant difficulty sleeping and was noted to be preoccupied and disorganized at work. Two days prior to her admission she failed to show up at work and made phone calls to family members complaining that demons were threatening to kill her because of a "voodoo curse" placed on her by an estranged sister-in-law. On the day of admission she was brought to the outpatient clinic by her family, with a request for medication to help her sleep. Only after extensive negotiation with patient and family was the out-

Table 9-3
Major Psychiatric Syndromes and Organic
Disorders Which Can Imitate or Cause Them[*]

Functional Disorders	DSM-III-R Organic Imitators[20]
Psychosis	Delirium
	Dementia
	Organic amnestic syndrome
	Organic hallucinosis
	Organic delusional syndrome
Depression/mania	Organic mood syndrome
Anxiety disorders	Organic anxiety syndrome
Personality disorders	Organic personality syndrome

[*] In addition, "imitators" common to each functional diagnosis are substance intoxication and withdrawal.

patient clinician able to arrange that she be admitted for further observation and examination.

In the hospital the patient was at times lucid. At other times, she would lapse into trance-like states. During these episodes she became acutely disoriented and paranoid, and sometimes appeared to be responding to "visions" of demons coming to attack her. Nursing staff reported that the patient appeared to "act as if" she couldn't hear what people were trying to say to her, and impulsively throw herself on to the floor and act bizarrely — sometimes posturing. During her lucid intervals she was fully oriented and appropriate, although she could quickly become irritable and demanding. Findings on physical examination and laboratory data were essentially normal.

On the second day after admission the patient was placed on low-dose haloperidol (2–4 mg) with little effect. Episodes of lucid behavior and speech alternated with periods in which the patient lay mute or sleeping. On the third day after admission the patient's family secretly performed a "faith-healing" ceremony in the patient's room. Shortly thereafter the patient assaulted a nurse and required physical restraint.

Haloperidol was increased to 40 mg/d, but the patient became even more withdrawn and demonstrated increased posturing. At this point the patient's vital signs became mildly elevated with a pulse of 100 and a temperature of 99.4° F. Medical consultation was obtained and found the patient "grossly intact," and attributed the patient's condition to "psychiatric causes." The patient's family requested a meeting with the patient's clinician, insisting that they had seen this type of condition in Haiti and demanded that the patient be discharged to their care so that a proper healing ceremony occur in an appropriate cultural setting.

This case demonstrates many of the features of organic mental disorder described earlier in this chapter. Review the section on the history and mental status examination and see how many of these clues you can identify. If you were the responsible clinician, would you accept the assessment of the medical consultant without question? Is this a first onset of schizophrenia? Or is it a hysterical conversion reaction? Considerable effort was required to obtain further medical assessment. Finally a lumbar puncture was performed, and this revealed dramatically abnormal cerebrospinal fluid. Her final diagnosis? A florid and life-threatening encephalitis (infection of the brain).

This patient was suffering from a delirium caused by an infectious process. A delirium is a transient organic brain syndrome characterized by acute onset, global impairment in cognitive functions (including thinking, perception, and memory) as well as widespread derangement of cerebral metabolism (see Table 9-4). This is the equivalent of acute brain failure and represents a potentially life-threatening emergency. In patients who are older than 65 years this is perhaps the most common mental disorder and among the most serious. Fifteen to thirty

Table 9-4
DSM-III-R Criteria for Delirium

A. Clouding of consciousness with decreased ability to shift, focus, and sustain attention
B. Disorganized thinking
C. At least two of the following:
   1) Reduced level of consciousness
   2) Perceptual disturbances: misinterpretations, illusions, or hallucinations
   3) Disturbance of the sleep-wake cycle
   4) Increasing or decreased psychomotor activity
   5) Disorientation
   6) Memory impairment
D. Clinical features that develop acutely (hours to days) and fluctuate over the course of a day
E. Demonstration of an etiological organic factor, or the disturbance cannot be accounted for by a nonorganic disorder

Reprinted with permission from the *Diagnostic and Statistical Manual of Mental Disorders, third edition, revised.* Copyright 1987. American Psychiatric Association.

percent of geriatric patients with a delirium deteriorate to stupor, coma, and death.[13]

Although delirium may resemble functional psychosis, it is often a life-threatening medical emergency and requires prompt recognition and action. Many of the most common medical causes of delirium are *potentially fatal* but *reversible*.

Among the most common causes of delirium are alcohol or substances.[21,22] Life-threatening effects of alcohol or substances may be due to either toxicity or withdrawal. Toxicity may occur unintentionally, during recreational use, or intentionally, during a suicide attempt. It may also occur accidentally with use of prescribed or over-the-counter medications. Alternatively, acute withdrawal states may also present a life-threatening emergency. Alcohol or sedative drugs are the most dangerous in terms of withdrawal. Although withdrawal from heroin or other narcotics is extremely uncomfortable, it is not lethal. An additional alcohol-related cause of delirium (and dementia) is Wernicke's encephalopathy. This disorder results from the nutritional deficiencies often found in chronic alcoholics and may sometimes be reversed by administration of thiamine.

Although substances of abuse, medications, and alcohol are responsible for many presentations of organic psychosis or delirium, there are several other important but potentially reversible causes. Infectious processes (as described in the case example) may affect thinking by direct infection of the brain (encephalitis or meningitis) or through the toxic effects of systemic infection (sepsis). Hemorrhages of the brain may be spontaneous (cerebrovascular accidents or strokes) or traumatic secondary to head injuries. Various locations and tissues of the brain may be involved. Hemorrhages can be epidural (outside of the protective layer of tissue covering the brain), subdural (beneath the tissue), or intracranial (within the brain substance).

Metabolic abnormalities affecting blood electrolyte levels (especially sodium, potassium, or calcium) or acid-base balance may profoundly affect cognitive functioning. Endocrine (hormonal) abnormalities may also represent potentially life-threatening yet potentially reversible causes of severe delirium. Extreme thyroid hormone excess ("thyroid storm"), diabetic states ("ketoacidosis"), and low levels of body-produced cortisone (adrenal insufficiency) are examples of endocrine disorders that can severely impair cognition. Severe derangements of blood oxygenation (hypoxia) directly affect brain function and may result from various causes including anemia, poor lung function, or heart failure. Finally, severely high blood pressure may also result in acute confusional states in the form of hypertensive encephalopathy. Almost *any* organ failure (heart, lung, kidney, liver, adrenal, pancreas, thyroid, and so on) may result in an encephalopathy (see Table 9-5).

Dementia

Case 3. A 76-year-old woman was referred for evaluation of rapidly progressing forgetfulness and withdrawal. For the last five to six years she had mild difficulty in recalling names, remembering appointments, and locating possessions, yet she had largely been able to compensate for this and to live happily with her husband in their home. Several months after the sudden death of her husband her memory and function precipitously worsened. Her house was in disarray and she sometimes forgot to turn off running water. She had significant difficulty with names and often forgot to take her medications unless reminded. She lost weight and said she no longer cooked hot meals since her husband's death.

Only after obtaining a thorough and negative medical evaluation was she started on a tricyclic antidepressant. Within five weeks her memory improved dramatically and she returned to her prior level of independent function. With the encouragement of her case-worker, she moved to elderly housing, became involved in the senior center, and progressively became less withdrawn.

In contrast to delirium, a chronic and persistent decline in mental capacity is termed dementia. Especially in the assessment of the elderly patient, dementia may underlie apparent presentations of psychosis, anxiety states, or depression. In the example just described, an astute clinician considered the possibility of a reversible dementia. In this instance, the psychomotor retardation, withdrawal, diminished self-care, and impaired concentration of a major depression produced the symptoms of dementia. With treatment of the depression, the patient resumed her prior level of function. It is worth noting that this case is somewhat atypical, since depression is a relatively infrequent cause of dementia. Like depression, however, many organic causes of dementia are treatable.

Dementia is characterized by a loss of previously attained intellectual abilities that is severe enough to interfere with social

Table 9-5
Organic Disorders That Produce Delirium or Organic Psychosis

I. Drugs
  A. Toxicity
    1. Prescribed medications: lithium, tricyclic antidepressants, anticholinergic meds, sedative-hypnotics, steroids, antihypertensive and antiarrhythmic meds, digitalis, anticonvulsants, anti-inflammatory drugs, cimetidine
    2. Over-the-counter medications: Esp. anticholinergic meds (benadryl/allergy meds, steroid preparations)
    3. Abused substances: alcohol, PCP (phencyclidine), cocaine, hallucinogens, stimulants, sedatives, narcotics
    4. Poisons: Organic solvents, insecticides, heavy metals
  B. Withdrawal
    1. Prescribed: sedative-hypnotics
    2. Abused: alcohol, sedative-hypnotics

II. Metabolic disorders
  A. Elevated or lowered levels of sodium, potassium, calcium, glucose, magnesium
  B. Acid-base: acidosis, alkalosis
  C. Failure of major organs: kidney, liver, lung, pancreas

III. Neurological
  A. Head trauma
  B. Cerebrovascular: cerebrovascular accident (stroke, hemorrhage)
  C. Space-occupying lesions: tumor, subdural hematoma, hydrocephalus, abscess, aneurysm
  D. Seizure disorders (including TLE)
  E. Degenerative disorders: Alzheimer's disease, multiple sclerosis

IV. Infectious: encephalitis, meningitis, systemic infection, AIDS

V. Endocrine:
  A. Hyperthyroidism (thyrotoxicosis), hypothyroidism
  B. Cushing's syndrome, adrenal insufficiency
  C. Hypoparathyroidism, hyperparathyroidism
  D. Diabetes or hyperinsulinism

VI. Cardiovascular/Hematological
  A. Myocardial infarction, arrhythmias, congestive heart failure, hypertensive encephalopathy
  B. Anemia, polycythemia

VII. Nutritional
  A. Wernicke's encephalopathy: thiamine deficiency (often associated with severe alcoholism)
  B. Other: folate, nicotinic acid, B_{12}

Adapted from Beresin EV: Delirium, in Sederer LI (ed): *Inpatient Psychiatry: Diagnosis and Treatment,* ed. 2. Baltimore, Williams and Wilkins, 1986, p 133.

or occupational functioning. In addition, DSM-III-R criteria require that there be memory impairment and no clouding of consciousness, a suspected organic etiology, and one or more of the following: impaired abstraction, impaired judgment, aphasia, agnosia, constructional difficulty, or personality change (see Table 9-6).

The hallmark of dementia is significant memory impairment without the clouding of consciousness or profound fluctuations in levels of alertness classically found in delirium. Unlike delirium the onset of dementia is often insidious and gradual rather than acute. The course is often chronic (when untreated) rather than brief as in delirium. In dementia, attention and concentration may remain grossly intact, yet they are almost always impaired in delirium. Finally, perceptual disturbances are absent or minimal in dementia and thinking is often impoverished or concrete. In delirium, hallucinations, florid thought disorders, and delusions are common.

The most common cause of dementia is Alzheimer's disease. This disorder, like other degenerative brain diseases, is currently considered irreversible. This is not the case for all causes of dementia, though! It is vitally important to recognize that some forms of dementia are treatable and even reversible (see Table 9-7). Deficiencies of thiamine or folate, for example, may result

Table 9-6
DSM-III-R Criteria for Dementia

A. Impairment in short- and long-term memory
B. At least one of the following
　1. Impairment in abstract thinking
　2. Impaired judgment
　3. Other disturbances of higher cortical function
　　(eg, aphasia, apraxia, agnosia, constructional difficulty)
　4. Personality change
C. The disturbance in A and B significantly interferes with work, social activities, or interpersonal relationships
D. The disturbance doesn't occur exclusively during delirium
E. Either there is evidence of a specific etiological organic factor or the disturbance cannot be accounted for by any nonorganic mental disorder

Reprinted with permission from the *Diagnostic and Statistical Manual of Mental Disorders, third edition, revised.* Copyright 1987. American Psychiatric Association.

Table 9-7
Frequent (and Potentially Reversible) Causes of Dementia

1. Degenerative disorders — Alzheimer's disease, Pick's disease, Parkinson's disease, Huntington's disease
2. Metabolic disorders — hypothyroidism*, hypoparathyroidism*, Cushing's syndrome*, Wilson's disease, hepatic or renal insufficiency*
3. Vascular disorders — Multi-infarct dementia, vasculitis*
4. Hypoxia (low-oxygenation states) — anemia*, heart failure*
5. Neurological — normal pressure hydrocephalus*, seizures*
6. Nutritional deficiency states — Deficiencies of thiamine*, B_{12}*, folate*, or niacin*
7. Toxic states* — alcohol, medications, drugs of abuse, heavy metals
8. Tumors* — of the central nervous system, lungs, and other organs
9. Post-traumatic states
10. Infection — post-infectious states (post-encephalitis), slow-virus infections (Creutzfeldt-Jakob syndrome), AIDS
11. Psychiatric — "pseudo-dementia" of depression*

* Potentially reversible.
Adapted from Jenike MA: Alzheimer's disease and other dementias, in *Handbook of Geriatric Psychopharmacology*. Littleton, MA, PSG Publishing, 1985, p 119.

in severe dementias, which may quickly be reversed with appropriate treatment. Endocrine disorders such as hypothyroidism or Cushing's syndrome (excessive cortisol production) may also produce gradual deterioration of cognitive function, which is reversible with appropriate treatment. In patients who demonstrate the clinical triad of progressive confusion, ataxia, and urinary incontinence, a potentially treatable buildup of fluid in the brain (termed *normal pressure hydrocephalus*) may be responsible. Finally, the syndrome of major depression may produce a so-called pseudodementia. Especially in the elderly, the impaired concentration, attention, psychomotor retardation, and withdrawal of a severe depression may be easily mistaken for a progressive dementing process. When this is the case, an appropriate antidepressant may dramatically alter the course of an apparently hopeless cognitive deterioration.

Other Organic Syndromes Which Produce Psychotic Symptoms

In addition to delirium and dementia, two other organic syndromes produce symptoms of psychosis or thought disorder: organic hallucinosis and organic delusional syndrome.[26,27] *Organic delusional syndrome* is characterized by delusions that are caused by a physical factor. There is no change in the level of consciousness as with delirium and no intellectual deficits as with dementia. Hallucinations are not a prominent feature of this syndrome. Patients with this syndrome frequently report persecutory delusions which may be either fixed or fluctuating. Associated hallucinations, when they occur, are more often visual than auditory, yet differentiating this diagnosis from chronic paranoid schizophrenia may nonetheless be extremely difficult. One of the most common causes of organic delusional syndrome is drugs, either prescribed or abused. Amphetamines are particularly associated with drug-induced paranoid states. In addition, complex partial seizures (temporal lobe epilepsy) and certain cerebrovascular accidents (strokes) can lead to an organic delusional syndrome.

Organic hallucinosis is a syndrome of persistent or recurrent hallucinations caused by a physical factor. As with organic delusional syndrome, there is neither an associated clouding of consciousness nor a loss of intellectual functioning. In addition, prominent disturbances of mood or prominent delusions exclude the use of this diagnosis. Patients with this syndrome most commonly experience visual or auditory hallucinations because of drugs, alcohol, seizure disorders, or sensory deprivation. Chronic hallucinogen abuse may result in episodic visual flashbacks. Prolonged alcohol abuse may result in alcoholic hallucinosis, an unusual syndrome of vivid auditory hallucinations usually occurring within the first 48 hours of abstinence. Hallucinations may also be produced by focal seizures, especially those occurring in the limbic system or occipital cortex. These hallucinations can be olfactory, auditory, or visual. In the elderly, especially, loss of hearing or vision may produce a sensory deprivation state leading to hallucinosis.

Organic Causes of Memory Impairment: Organic Amnestic Syndrome

Organic amnestic syndrome is characterized by disturbed short- and long-term memory without impairment of consciousness (as in delirium), intellectual functioning (as in dementia), or deficits in immediate recall. Patients with this disorder have a relatively circumscribed memory impairment without additional signs of organic brain disease. They are able to repeat information that has just been provided (such as measured by testing digit span), yet have difficulty in learning new information or recalling information that has been learned in the past. Causes of this syndrome include thiamine deficiency (associated with deficient intake of vitamins as seen in chronic alcoholics who neglect their nutrition), head trauma, post-surgical amnestic states, some forms of cerebrovascular accidents (strokes), encephalitis (brain infection), anoxia (oxygen deprivation), and brain tumors.

Organic Causes of Depression and Mania:
Organic Mood Syndrome

Case 4. A 28-year-old teacher came to an outpatient clinic with symptoms of depression and marital problems. She sought counseling on one prior occasion for depression and anxiety, yet abruptly terminated her treatment over a "disagreement" with her psychiatrist. She did not sign a release of information because she "wants a new start" with an unbiased therapist. Although she reported that "years ago" she had an "alcohol and drug problem," she reported drinking only on weekends at the current time. She denied other use of drugs or medication, although she occasionally found diazepam useful during severe anxiety in the past.

The patient cited her marital difficulties as the reason for her depression. Recently, her husband threatened to "move out if things don't change around here." She complained that she did not know what her husband wanted from her and how she could change to please him. She stated that they argue "all of the time now," and she was feeling increasingly hopeless. She was having difficulty at work because of poor concentration, "forgetfulness," and recurrent headaches. There were times when she felt that she experienced "memory lapses" and periods of "confusion." She reported a poor appetite and had lost ten pounds. She complained that she had severe difficulty falling and staying asleep, yet "feels tired all of the time."

The principal issued her a "warning" based on her deteriorating performance and multiple recent missed work days. She became angry at the suggestion of a couples meeting and insisted that she will "have a nervous breakdown" if she doesn't "get something for sleep."

Making a diagnosis of organic mood syndrome (see Table 9-8) is especially difficult when specific clues of organicity are absent. In the case just described, the patient had many of the classic symptoms of a major depression including depressed mood, poor concentration, decreased appetite with weight loss, impaired sleep, and low energy. Yet she also reported physical complaints such as headaches. Although these should be seriously considered, the presence of physical symptoms or complaints is to be expected in functional or nonorganic depression. Patients with true depressive illness regularly have a high incidence of somatic symptoms such as weakness, dizziness, headaches, and abdominal discomfort. For example, as many as 82% of female inpatients with depression report a distressing level of somatic discomfort or complaints.[28]

The history of alcohol and substance abuse in conjunction with the presence of periods of confusion and memory lapses should raise suspicion of an organic illness in the patient in case 4. Shortly after this evaluation she was brought to the hospital in an acute delirium secondary to withdrawal from alcohol and diazepam. Following detoxification and outpatient treatment the symptoms of depression entirely resolved. Her denied overuse of drugs and alcohol had been a major factor in her depression.

Symptoms of depression may appear organic and organic illness may present as depression. The distinction between functional and organic depression is further complicated by the extensive and varied list of organic disorders associated with depression. At least 25 medical illnesses frequently induce depression, at least 23 medical disorders are associated with reactive depression, more than 20 causes of dementia can mimic

Table 9-8
DSM-III-R Criteria for Organic
Mood Syndrome

A. Prominent and persistent depressed, elevated, or expansive mood
B. There is evidence from the history, physical examination, or laboratory tests of a specific organic factor (or factors) judged to be etiologically related to the disturbance
C. Not occurring exclusively during the course of delirium

Reprinted with permission from the *Diagnostic and Statistical Manual of Mental Disorders, third edition, revised.* Copyright 1987. American Psychiatric Association.

depression, and at least 75 medical illnesses are capable of presenting with depressive symptoms.[29,30]

Organic disease can also present with a manic syndrome, as in the following example:

> Case 5. A 17-year-old boy's first psychiatric admission occurred in the midst of an apparent acute psychotic episode. He was a bright and outgoing young man who ran away from a troubled home situation at the age of 15 years and spent a year living on the streets. During this time he became involved in drugs and prostitution. Over the past two years he moved in with an older male lover and sporadically attended school.
>
> Approximately one month prior to his psychiatric admission, he reported that he began to feel "depressed" and "run-down." This immediately followed a brief episode of pneumonia. Shortly thereafter, he began to experience auditory hallucinations and paranoid fears that prevented him from leaving his apartment.
>
> On admission to the psychiatric inpatient unit, he had a mixed and inconsistent set of symptoms. Although he claimed to be "depressed," his affect was labile and at times he was expansive and even euphoric in mood. He had difficulty sleeping, yet no other vegetative symptoms of depression. He was well liked and socially engaged on the ward, although he claimed to have felt "paranoid and confused" outside of the hospital. His description of auditory hallucinations seemed vague and even his history had inconsistencies. A diagnostic debate, which included consideration of manic-depressive illness, malingering, and sociopathy, ensued. In the context of this debate and a failure to respond to several different treatments including antipsychotic medication, he signed himself out of the hospital. Two months later he was readmitted to the medical floor with a fatal pneumocystis pneumonia and a diagnosis of AIDS.

A psychotherapist would suspect organic affective disorder in patients such as the one just described by maintaining a high index of suspicion of organicity; taking a careful history for substance abuse, medical illness, medication use, or family history of heritable illnesses; and reassessing after poor response to psychosocial interventions. The therapist should beware of assuming that symptoms such as sleep disturbance, appetite and weight changes, fatigue, weakness, or anxiety represent depression. These symptoms are nonspecific signs of many physical disorders as well and may appear before the medical illness is more

Table 9-9
Factors Causing Organic Mood Syndrome

Exogenous Substances
  amphetamine withdrawal
  reserpine
  mononucleosis
  methyldopa
  cocaine
  lead poisoning
  steroids
  oral contraceptives
  digitalis toxicity
  alcohol
  barbiturates
  bromides
  opiates
  other sedatives
  carbon monoxide
  carbon disulfide
  propranolol
  antabuse
  heavy metals
Degenerative Diseases
  Parkinson's disease
  Huntington's disease
  Alzheimer's disease
  other CNS degenerative disorders
  multiple sclerosis

Infectious Diseases
  brucellosis
  tuberculosis
  meningitis
  syphilis
  postencephalitic states
  encephalitis
  hepatitis
  AIDS
Tumors
  carcinoma of the pancreas
  primary cerebral tumor
  cerebral metastasis
Miscellaneous Conditions
  Meniere's disease
  arthritis
  pancreatitis
  lupus
  chronic pyelonephritis
  seizure disorders
  post-concussion syndrome
  multi-infarct dementia
  cerebral hypoxia
  normal pressure hydrocephalus

Metabolic Disturbances and Endocrine Disorders
  hyperthyroidism
  hypothyroidism
  hyponatremia
  hypokalemia
  Cushing's disease
  Addison's disease
  diabetes
  uremia
  hypopituitarism
  porphyria
  carcinomatosis
  hepatic disease
  hyperparathyroidism
  pernicious anemia
  pellagra
  Wernicke-Korsakoff syndrome
  Wilson's disease

Adapted from Anderson WH: Depression, in Lazare A (ed): *Outpatient Psychiatry: Diagnosis and Treatment.* Baltimore, Williams and Wilkins, 1979, p 259.

clearly manifest. Atypical presentations of depression should be especially suspect. Examples include weight gain occurring with a decreased appetite (suggesting hypothyroidism) or vegetative symptoms of depression (weight loss, low energy, and insomnia) occurring in the absence of subjective sadness.

A wide range of organic etiologies can induce a manic or depressive syndrome (see Table 9-9). In general, common imitators of mania are similar to those causing delirium and include adverse drug reactions (including intoxication and withdrawal), neurological disorders, electrolyte imbalances, infections, and endocrine disorders.[31] Frequent organic causes of depressive symptoms include medications (especially antihypertensive, cardiac, and tranquilizing medications), alcohol and sedative abuse,[14] hypothyroidism,[32] Parkinson's syndrome,[33] Alzheimer's disease,[24] and cancer.

Organic Causes of Anxiety: Organic Anxiety Syndrome

Case 6. A 32-year-old clinical psychologist was in private practice. Her friends knew her to be a quick-witted, fast-talker with unlimited stores of energy. On social occasions, her capacity to drink and to consume large quantities of food was legendary. On "good days" she was charismatic and witty, but on "bad days" she was irritable and tempestuous. She quickly became impatient and argumentative and recently alienated many old friends.

Because of these issues she entered into treatment with a prominent local analyst, first in twice weekly psychotherapy, and eventually in analysis. After two years of treatment she felt that she developed some degree of insight into key dynamic issues, yet complained that her symptoms only worsened. At times she was so "on-edge" that she was literally unable to sit still, pacing back and forth while she spoke. Friends told her to "calm down and stop being so 'hyper'."

At work she began to open her office windows between patients because she felt so "hot." She ended the day drenched in sweat. Her patients increasingly complained that she was impatient, distracted, and "nervous." When she was especially anxious a fine tremor developed. In spite of a ravenous appetite, she lost weight and was sleeping poorly.

In this case, the limited response to intensive treatment should in itself have prompted a diagnostic re-evaluation. Several additional clues suggest that this patient had an organic disorder.

In addition to her emotional lability and anxiety she had physical symptoms of significant hyperarousal including sweating, pacing, tremor, and an increased appetite with weight loss. Although some of these symptoms are consistent with the physiological activation which occurs in contexts of fear or acute anxiety reactions, the continued and regular presence of these symptoms and their increase over time clearly warrants a medical workup.

After two years of psychoanalysis this patient sought out a medical physician who immediately diagnosed hyperthyroidism. A simple medication quickly alleviated the vast majority of her symptoms, although the delay in treatment resulted in a permanent change in physical appearance including protruding or bulging eyes.

Anxiety is one of the most nonspecific and basic of emotions. In the form called the fight-or-flight response, it is the key biological reaction that protects a person in the context of certain life-threatening situations. In readiness for a perceived assault, the sympathetic nervous system becomes highly activated and stimulates different organ systems. The heart beats faster, breathing rate increases, pupils dilate, and blood is shifted to vital internal organs causing the skin to become pale, cool, and moist. Muscle tone increases (sometimes to the point of shaking), digestion stops, and the body eliminates waste with increased urination and, at times, diarrhea. Anxiety in this role can be life-saving for a mammal on the run from predators; often, however, it is experienced as a signal not of external danger but rather of internal psychodynamic conflicts. A third source of anxiety occurs, as in the patient just described, when physical disturbances affect the body in relatively subtle ways that may not attract notice except in respect to nonspecific symptoms of anxiety (see Table 9-10). The most common causes of such organically based anxiety are endocrine, metabolic, toxic, cardiac, and neurological disturbances (see Table 9-11).[34,35]

Excesses of certain hormones commonly produce anxiety. Hyperthyroidism is an excess of thyroid hormone. The range of clinical presentation extends from symptoms of mild anxiety to a life-threatening thyrotoxicosis which may look like a florid manic psychosis or a major depression. In appearance, patients with this disorder develop a goiter as well as a staring gaze, protrud-

**Table 9-10
DSM-III-R Criteria for Organic Anxiety Syndrome**

A. Prominent, recurrent panic attacks or generalized anxiety
B. There is evidence from the history, physical examination, or laboratory tests of a specific organic factor (or factors) judged to be etiologically related to the disturbance.
C. Not occurring exclusively during the course of delirium

Reprinted with permission from the *Diagnostic and Statistical Manual of Mental Disorders, third edition, revised.* Copyright 1987. American Psychiatric Association.

ing eyes, and fine, thin hair. Signs of hyperthyroidism include nervousness, palpitations, irritability, fine tremor, and diarrhea. These patients often report that they have lost a significant amount of weight despite increased appetite and food intake. Their skin is warm and moist and they complain that they have difficulty tolerating heat. The increased appetite with weight loss and warm, moist skin distinguish hyperthyroidism from anxiety,

**Table 9-11
Organic Factors that Cause Organic Anxiety Syndrome**

1. Endocrine
   Hyperthyroidism
   Pheochromocytoma (rare, yet clinically similar to panic attacks)
   Hypoglycemia (rare!)
   Cushing's syndrome
   Hypoparathyroidism
2. Cardiopulmonary
   Angina
   Cardiac arrhythmias
   Mitral valve prolapse
   Recurrent pulmonary emboli
3. Toxic/Metabolic
   Medication/substance abuse (including caffeinism)
   Withdrawal states
4. Neurological
   Post-concussion syndrome
   Complex partial seizures

Adapted from Dietch JT: Diagnosis of organic anxiety disorders. *Psychosomatics* 1981;22:662.

in which appetite and weight go hand-in-hand and skin is cold and clammy.

Other pertinent endocrine disorders include Cushing's syndrome, hypoglycemia, and pheochromocytoma. Cushing's syndrome is caused by an excess of steroids secreted by the adrenal gland, which results in physical changes: a round moon-shaped face, a buffalo-hump on the back of the neck, and obesity of the mid-section with thin extremities. The same symptoms can occur when a patient takes large amounts of prescribed steroids by pill, injection, or topical ointment. Hypoglycemia is a condition of low blood sugar which is frequently considered, yet extremely rare. Pheochromocytoma is also a rare condition caused by a tumor secreting adrenalin into the blood stream. These patients have profound and acute onset of rushes of anxiety, headaches, sweating, and tremor.

Among the toxic causes of organic anxiety syndrome are nicotine, cocaine, amphetamines, and other psychostimulants (including certain decongestant nasal sprays or drops). Caffeine-induced anxiety may occur at doses in excess of 250 mg/day of caffeine. A 5-oz serving of brewed coffee contains 90 to 120 mg, a cup of instant coffee or tea contains 70 mg, and a serving of cola contains 20 mg. Over-the-counter pain medications may contain as much as 30 to 60 mg of caffeine per tablet.[30] Caffeinism is diagnosed by symptoms of overstimulation, high intake of caffeine, and withdrawal symptoms which include headache, nausea, depression, and anxiety occurring about 18 hours after the last dose of caffeine. The withdrawal of a CNS depressant drug such as alcohol or a sedative/hypnotic may produce anxiety symptoms that can progress to a life-threatening delirium. Among prescribed medications, the most prone to produce anxiety are thyroid preparations, over-the-counter cold and allergy preparations (with ephedrine or pseudoephedrine), asthma medications (aminophylline, antihistamines), amphetamines, and L-dopa. Antipsychotic drugs sometimes induce a restlessness called *akathisia*, which can be difficult to distinguish from anxiety from other causes.

Many cardiac conditions may present with anxiety. A middle-aged or older adult with a first attack of severe anxiety with sweating, chest tightness, nausea, and shortness of breath may be in the midst of a myocardial infarction or heart attack. In the event that these symptoms are recurrent, angina pectoris (pain from inadequate oxygen to the heart) may be present. Palpitations, dizziness, and shortness of breath may be due to irregular heart rhythms (arrhythmias). Feelings of anxiety and panic have been associated with mitral valve prolapse, a common and usually not dangerous disorder in which the mitral valve of the heart flops back into the wrong chamber. Acute onset of cardiac symptoms (especially in any patient over the age of 45 years) warrants a referral to a physician for assessment.

Among neurological disorders that can present as anxiety, post-concussion syndrome is an important consideration. In any intake or evaluation process for a recent change in mental status the question of recent (past year or two) head injury should be raised. The most common presenting symptom of post-concussion syndrome is anxiety. Other symptoms are irritability, fatigue, difficulty concentrating, insomnia, headache, and extreme sensitivity to noise, light, or heat. Persistent headaches which worsen on changes of head position (such as in bending over or making sudden changes) can indicate a brain injury. Memory loss for the events surrounding the trauma commonly accompanies episodes of unconsciousness. Although a loss of consciousness occurring with the head trauma should increase the clinician's concern, post-concussion syndrome can occur with more minor injuries in which consciousness is not lost. Any patient with onset of anxiety (or other mental status changes) following an episode of head trauma should therefore be referred to a physician for examination. Another neurological cause of anxiety is temporal lobe seizures. This should be ruled out by neurological assessment in patients whose anxiety episodes are brief, spontaneous, and associated with other seizure-like symptoms such as an aura, a post-ictal confused or amnestic state, olfactory or other hallucinations, or motor automatisms.

Organic Causes of Personality Disorders:
Organic Personality Syndrome

Case 7. A 55-year-old woman sought couples counseling because of increasing marital strife. While the marriage had long been difficult, it had recently become increasingly troubled as she developed episodic temper outbursts which seemed unprovoked and had become nearly intolerable to her husband. In addition, this intelligent and thoughtful woman had experienced a general alteration of her personality that her husband attributed to depression. She had become more serious and absorbed in religion, spent increasing amounts of time writing in her diary, showed labile fluctuations of her mood, and appeared increasingly disinterested in sex. Though never previously psychotic, she had begun intermittently to notice an orb of light which appeared at her left side and was sometimes accompanied by an odor of garlic and a feeling of inexplicable irritation. At times there was also a strange physical sensation of stomach fullness, which bubbled up and spread through her limbs. Her temper outbursts often followed these odd experiences. When the patient medicated her severe occasional migraine-like headaches with a phenobarbital-containing medication, her temper also seemed to gain stability. An astute couples counselor wondered whether the personality change, with its accompanying episodic altered thinking, perception, and somatosensory function, might represent complex partial seizures with ictal rage attacks and interictal personality changes. An EEG confirmed the presence of a limbic seizure disorder. Careful neurological assessment was done to screen for a progressive or life-endangering cause of the illness. Anticonvulsant treatment and education about her seizure disorder proved helpful adjuncts to the couple's counseling.

Organic personality syndrome (see Table 9-12) is marked by significant changes in personality, which result from an organic cause. New onset of affective lability (sudden outbursts or irritability), impulsivity, apathy, or paranoia may each be organically caused. The most common types of organic personality changes are the frontal lobe personality syndromes and the temporal lobe epileptic interictal personality changes.[1] Table 9-13 offers a more comprehensive list of physical disorders producing personality change.

Brain injury, hemorrhage, or tumor affecting the frontal lobes may each have dramatic effects on personality. Depending on their location, the resulting personality change may be toward increased dullness and blunting (pseudodepressed) or bizarreness and impulsivity (pseudopsychopathic). In the deficit state of pseudodepression, there is a constricted affect, lack of initiative or spontaneity, and vacuous facial expression. In spite of the appearance of depression, sad mood is not present. Alternatively, frontal lobe pseudopsychopathic syndrome is characterized by a picture of global disinhibition. Instead of being dulled or blunted, thinking and emotions are disinhibited. Hyperactivity,

Table 9-12
DSM-III-R Criteria for Organic Personality Syndrome

A. A persistent personality disturbance, either lifelong or representing a change or accentuation of a previously characteristic trait, involving at least one of the following:
 1. Affective instability; eg, marked shifts from normal mood to depression, irritability, or anxiety
 2. Recurrent outbursts of aggression or rage that are grossly out of proportion to any precipitating psychosocial stressors
 3. Markedly impaired social judgment; eg, sexual indiscretions
 4. Marked apathy and indifference
 5. Suspiciousness or paranoid ideation

B. There is evidence from the history, physical examination, or laboratory tests of a specific organic factor (or factors) judged to be etiologically related to the disturbance.

C. This diagnosis is not given to a child or adolescent if the clinical picture is limited to the features that characterize attention deficit–hyperactivity disorder

D. Not occurring exclusively during the course of delirium and does not meet the criteria for dementia

Reprinted with permission from the *Diagnostic and Statistical Manual of Mental Disorders, third edition, revised.* Copyright 1987. American Psychiatric Association.

impulsivity, labile affect, poor judgment, and inappropriate verbal and sexual behavior occur.

Patients with temporal lobe epilepsy (complex partial seizure disorder) often go undiagnosed because their seizures may consist of episodes of repetitive behaviors, dissociative states, or aggressive and violent behavior. As demonstrated in the case example, interictal (between seizure) personalities may be marked by

Table 9-13
Causes of Organic Personality Syndrome[1,27]

Complex partial seizures	Multiple sclerosis
Head trauma (brain injury)	Huntington's disease
Cerebrovascular accident	PCP or heavy metal poisoning
Brain tumor	
Neurosyphilis	
Post-encephalitic states	
AIDS?	
Toxic exposures or substance abuse	

changes in sexual behavior, hyperreligiosity, hypergraphia (excessive writing), irritability, paranoia, and profound humorlessness. Other causes of organic personality syndrome include PCP poisoning, neurosyphilis, multiple sclerosis, Huntington's disease, and postencephalitic states.

Patients with organic personality syndrome may easily be mistaken for borderline, schizoid, paranoid, antisocial, or narcissistic personalities. In particular, the diagnosis of dissociative disorder (or hysterical neurosis, dissociative type) should be made only with great care. Dissociative states and bizarre behavior suggesting multiple personalities may be the primary symptoms of temporal lobe epilepsy. Of clinic patients with temporal lobe epilepsy, 33% exhibit dissociative phenomena.[36] A psychosocial explanation of conversion symptoms also requires careful medical evaluation, since studies of patients with the diagnosis of conversion hysteria who were reexamined ten years later revealed one-fourth to one-half to have an organic basis for what had been defined as hysterical.[37,38] In conversion hysteria, the burden of proof lies with the clinician to rule out organicity.

Guidelines in the detection and diagnosis of organic personality syndrome include maintaining a high index of suspicion when symptoms of personality change are acute and marked by extreme lability, impulsivity, bizarre behavior, outbursts, paranoia, severe apathy, flat affect, or loss of ability to think abstractly. These symptoms should arouse particular medical concern when there is any history of major medical illness or disorder (especially recent head trauma, unconsciousness, cerebrovascular accident, or symptoms suggestive of seizures), substance or alcohol abuse, or nonresponse to psychosocial treatment of conversion hysteria or dissociative episodes.

SUMMARY

Any psychiatric symptom may be duplicated or exacerbated by an underlying physical illness. The means for detecting or suspecting organic mental disorder are available to any conscientious, trained clinician. The question of possible organicity should be asked, even if momentarily, in the process of any psychological evaluation.

The history and mental status examination are the cornerstones of this assessment. Acuteness of onset, age of onset, premorbid functioning, medication and substance history, and medical history are key areas of inquiry. Any unusual or atypical symptoms or signs should be carefully assessed. The mini mental state examination is especially useful in screening for cognitive deficits which, if present, must be evaluated further. In addition, unusual symptoms such as visual, olfactory, or tactile hallucinations, altered or fluctuating levels of consciousness, catatonia, extreme lability of affect, or extreme changes in personality are suggestive of underlying organic illness.

Patients who are difficult, unpleasant, or uncooperative often receive inadequate medical and psychological assessments, and hence are especially at risk for suffering an undetected organic disorder. The patient who fails to improve with appropriate treatment and represents a treatment failure also warrants careful reconsideration of the diagnosis and consultation. As a general principle, it is recommended that therapists request documentation of a medical assessment from all patients beginning or continuing in treatment.

The missed diagnosis of organic mental disorder may lead to months and even years of inappropriate treatment and unnecessary suffering. For the patient, the stakes are high. In some cases, a thorough and thoughtful assessment may be the determining factor between life and death.

REFERENCES

1. Ellison JM: DSM III and the diagnosis of organic mental disorders. *Ann Emerg Med* 1984;13:521-528.
2. Dubin WR, Weiss KJ, Zeccardi JA: Organic brain syndrome. *J Am Med Assoc* 1983;249:60-62.
3. Leeman CP: Diagnostic errors in emergency room medicine: Physical illness in patients labeled "psychiatric" and vice versa. *Int J Psychiatry Med* 1975;6:533-540.
4. Hoffman RS, Koran LM: Detecting physical illness in patients with mental disorders. *Psychosomatics* 1984;25:654-660.
5. Hall RCW, Gardner ER, Popkin MK, et al: Unrecognized physical illness prompting psychiatric admission: A prospective study. *Am J Psychiatry* 1981;138:629-635.
6. LaBruzza AL: Physical illness presenting as psychiatric disorder:

Guidelines for differential diagnosis. *J Oper Psychiatry* 1981;12:24–31.
7. Roca RP, Breakey WR, Fischer PJ: Medical care of chronic psychiatric outpatients. *Hosp Community Psychiatry* 1987;38:741–745.
8. Farmer S: Medical problems of chronic patients in a community support program. *Hosp Community Psychiatry* 1987;38:745–749.
9. Koranyi EK: Morbidity and rate of undiagnosed physical illnesses in a psychiatric clinic population. *Arch Gen Psychiatry* 1979;36:414–419.
10. Marshall H: Incidence of physical disorders among psychiatric inpatients. *Br Med J* 1949;2:468–470.
11. Davies WD: Physical illness in psychiatric outpatients. *Br J Psychiatry* 1965;11:27–37.
12. Hall RCW, Popkin MK, Devaul RA, et al: Physical illness presenting as psychiatric disease. *Arch Gen Psychiatry* 1978;35:1315–1320.
13. Weddington, WW: The mortality of delirium: An underappreciated problem? *Psychosomatics* 1982;23:1232–1235.
14. Bean-Bayog M: Alcoholism treatment as an alternative to psychiatric hospitalization. *Psychiatric Clin N Am* 1985;8:501–512.
15. Faulstich ME: Psychiatric aspects of AIDS. *Am J Psychiatry* 1987;144:551–556.
16. Abrams R, Taylor MA: Catatonia: Prediction of response to somatic treatments. *Am J Psychiatry* 1977;134:78–80.
17. Stoudemire A: The differential diagnosis of catatonic states. *Psychosomatics* 1982;23:245–252.
18. Folstein MF, Folstein SE, McHugh PR: "Mini-Mental state," a practical method for grading the cognitive state of patients for the clinician. *J Psychiatric Res* 1975;12:189–198.
19. Issacs B, Kennie AT: The set test as an aid to the detection of dementia in old people. *Br J Psychiatry* 1973;23:467–470.
20. *Diagnostic and Statistical Manual of Mental Disorders*, ed 3, revised. (DSM III-R). Washington, DC, American Psychiatric Association, 1987.
21. Kulick AR, Ahmed I: Substance-induced organic mental disorders. *Gen Hosp Psychiatry* 1986;8:168–172.
22. DiSclafani A, Hall RCW, Gardner ER: Drug-induced psychosis: Emergency diagnosis and management. *Psychosomatics* 1981;22:845–850.
23. Beresin EV: Delirium, in Sederer LI (ed): *Inpatient Psychiatry: Diagnosis and Treatment*, ed. 2. Baltimore, Williams and Wilkins, 1986, pp 126–149.
24. Jenike MA: Alzheimer's disease and other dementias, in *Handbook of Geriatric Psychopharmacology*, Littleton, MA, PSG Publishing Company, Inc, 1985, pp 113–142.
25. Jenike MA: Alzheimer's disease: Clinical care and management. *Psychosomatics* 1986;27:407–416.

26. Wells CE: Organic syndromes: Amnestic syndrome, in Kaplan HI, Sadock BJ (eds): *Comprehensive Textbook of Psychiatry*, ed. 4. Baltimore, Williams and Wilkins, 1985, pp 870–872.
27. Wells CE: Other organic brain syndromes, in Kaplan HI, Sadock BJ (eds): *Comprehensive Textbook of Psychiatry*, ed. 4. Baltimore, Williams and Wilkins, 1985, pp 872–875.
28. Wittenborn JR, Buhler R: Somatic discomforts among depressed women. *Arch Gen Psychiatry* 1979;36:465–471.
29. Hall RCW: Depression, in Hall RCW (ed): *Psychiatric Presentations of Medical Illnesses.* New York, SP Medical and Scientific Books, 1980, pp 37–63.
30. Dietch JT, Zetin M: Diagnosis of organic depressive disorders. *Psychosomatics* 1983;24:971–979.
31. Krauthammer C, Klerman GL: Secondary mania. *Arch Gen Psychiatry* 1978;35:1333–1339.
32. Gold MS, Pearsall HR: Hypothyroidism — or is it depression? *Psychosomatics* 1983;24:646–656.
33. Harvey NS: Psychiatric disorders in Parkinsonism. *Psychosomatics* 1986;27:91–103.
34. Mackenzie TB, Popkin MK: Organic anxiety syndrome. *Am J Psychiatry* 1983;140:342–344.
35. Dietch JT: Diagnosis of organic anxiety disorders. *Psychosomatics* 1981;22:661–665.
36. Schenk L, Bear D: Multiple personality and related dissociative phenomena in patients with temporal lobe epilepsy. *Am J Psychiatry* 1981;138:1311–1316.
37. Slater ETO, Glithero E: A followup of patients diagnosed as suffering from "hysteria." *J Psychosomatic Res* 1965;9:9–13.
38. Watson CG, Buranen C: The frequency and identification of false positive conversion reactions. *J Nerv Ment Disord* 1979;167:234–237.

10

Interactions of Alcohol, Street
Drugs, and Prescribed Medications

Michael L. Johnson
James M. Ellison

Concurrent use of alcohol, street drugs, and prescribed medications is a common yet dangerous practice among psychiatric patients. By many mechanisms, recreational drugs can interfere with the effects of prescribed medications or produce toxic interactions. Beyond the direct interactions, drug abuse may produce physiological changes in the abuser that alter the actions of prescribed medications. The thoughtful patient may ask for information about the interactions of medications with recreational drug use. A responsible physician will make a point of discussing these matters while educating a patient about a prescribed medication. Polysubstance abuse, however, is widespread. The informed use of medications and the awareness of their interactions with recreational drugs or alcohol remain all too infrequent.

Physicians consider a knowledge of drug interactions and the bodily effects of drug abuse essential to safe prescribing practices. For nonphysician clinicians, too, an awareness of these potential treatment hazards is valuable. This chapter discusses the prevalence of substance abuse among psychiatric patients, explores some current biological explanations of this widespread problem, and reviews some common pitfalls in mixing drugs of abuse with prescribed medications.

SUBSTANCE ABUSE AMONG GENERAL AND PSYCHIATRIC POPULATIONS

Among the general population, the lifetime prevalence of substance abuse approaches 15%.[1] The acute and chronic effects of this abuse cost society dearly. Alcohol, for example, is involved in half of the 21,000 homicides committed annually in this country.[2] Half of the annual 46,000 driving fatalities are attributable to alcohol.[2] About one-third of the yearly 30,000 suicide deaths involve significant alcohol use.[2] One-third of the half million currently imprisoned felons are known to have drunk heavily before committing crimes against persons.[2]

Concurrent use of alcohol with other drugs of abuse is frequent. Schuckit and Bogard found concurrent drug abuse in 20% of 500 consecutive patients admitted for alcohol abuse.[3] Half of the polydrug abusers in this sample admitted to abusing intravenous drugs. An even higher figure was reported by Hesselbrook and colleagues, who found that 43% of patients admitted for inpatient alcohol treatment reported additional substance abuse.[4]

In recent years, cocaine has increasingly added to the casualties of drug abuse. In a recent survey, 17% of high-school seniors admitted to trying cocaine.[5] In the country at large, six million use cocaine at least once each month and three million are dependent on the drug.[5] More than 1 thousand deaths in 1986 were attributed to its use.[6] In its free-based form, crack, it is obtainable for as little as $10 to $15 a "rock."[7] Because of its rapid onset and intense intoxication and withdrawal effects, crack has been characterized by cocaine abuse experts as an "almost instantaneous addiction."[7]

Though widespread among the general population, drug abuse is even more frequent among the mentally ill. A 1986 report from the Alcohol, Drug Abuse and Mental Health Administration (ADAMHA) documented the abuse of illicit drugs and alcohol by at least 50% of the almost 2 million Americans with chronic mental illness.[8] These "dual diagnosis" patients require hospital admission at an earlier age.[8] Their more severe course of illness is evidenced by their higher rates of hospital readmission and of suicide.[8] When hospitalized, they tend to need longer inpatient stays than single diagnosis patients need.[8] The presence of substance abuse, however, is often missed or not reported in the formal discharge diagnosis.[8]

Clinicians continue to wonder why individuals with impaired reality testing seek drug experiences that apparently increase their difficulties. The use of hallucinogens or stimulants by psychotic patients remains baffling. Use of cocaine, with its depressive withdrawal phases, seems puzzlingly self-destructive among individuals already suffering from depression. When individuals impaired by depression or impulsivity continue to abuse alcohol or narcotics, their motivations are often obscure to the clinicians who seek to understand them. Recent theoretical work has attempted to explain these seemingly incongruous behaviors.

NEUROCHEMICAL BASES OF SUBSTANCE ABUSE

One model that has emerged from the attempt to understand substance abuse among the mentally ill is called the self-medication hypothesis. Khantzian, the articulator of this theory, stated that "Clinical work with narcotic and cocaine addicts has provided us with compelling evidence that the drug an individual comes to rely on is *not a random choice*."[9] On the contrary, "... addicts are attempting to medicate themselves for a range of psychiatric problems and painful emotional states."[9] Khantzian (personal communication, February 1988) proposes that abuse of sedative-hypnotics, including alcohol and the benzodiazepines, permits the relaxation of superego and ego boundaries to allow a "fusion" experience. These substances therefore become drugs of choice for those whose boundaries are too limiting. Many opiate abusers, according to Khantzian's theory, are attempting to calm intense, violent, aggressive affects. These painful affects, originating in backgrounds of chaos and abuse, are unbearable. As superego and ego boundaries in this group have "holes," unsoothed affects are acted out, sometimes very destructively. Opiates provide relief and solace. Khantzian (personal communication, February 1988) sees the cocaine abuser as treating depressive "anergia." The effects of the drug are to relieve anergia or dysphoria, even if only briefly, and to help focus undifferentiated, often uncontrolled energy. If the self-medication hypothesis is correct, many drug abusers are driven by an underlying and often treatable psychiatric disorder. Recognition and treatment of these disorders may allow many individuals to be spared the ravaging effects of long-term drug abuse.

Recent research findings offer external confirmation of this viewpoint by demonstrating a high prevalence of mood disorders among cocaine abusers seeking treatment. These mood disorders apparently preceded the cocaine abuse for many individuals. Bipolar affective disorder or its less severe relative, cyclothymic disorder, has been found among half of these treatment seekers.[10] Others have shown evidence of unipolar depression.[10] One in 20 cocaine abusers are seen with an adult form of attention deficit disorder, an impairment of attention and impulsivity.[11] Some of the bipolar individuals show greater mood stability and a decreased craving for cocaine when medicated with lithium or carbamazepine.[11] Some unipolar patients have responded to antidepressant treatment with improved mood and decreased cocaine craving.[11] Methylphenidate has been reported to beneficially affect personality and drug abuse in some patients with adult attention deficit.[11] Thus the recognition of an underlying psychiatric disorder and appropriate pharmacologic intervention can reduce both primary symptoms and drug abuse behavior. While medications alone should never be considered a sole intervention in treating drug abuse, many patients who switch from uncontrolled substance abuse to controlled use of medication become more receptive to psychotherapy and other psychosocial treatments. Many pharmacotherapists have come to consider medication to be an essential component of treatment in selected cases.

The self-medication hypothesis has been extended in an attempt to understand drug-seeking behavior as a manifestation of subsyndromal neurochemical differences among individuals. It is possible that such differences, whether hereditary or acquired, may account for subtle psychopathology that predisposes to drug abuse behavior. Applied to the problem of cocaine addiction, this approach has led to the "dopamine depletion hypothesis" of Dackis and Gold.[12] In the view of these investigators, cocaine addicts find special relief in the use of cocaine because it amplifies the effects of a specific neurotransmitter, dopamine, which may be present in inadequate amounts. A similar line of reasoning was developed by Cloninger in an attempt to divide alcohol abusers into subpopulations with differing clinical presentations.[13] He proposes subtypes that "result from various combinations of response biases in brain systems" which are based on neurochemical differences. Cloninger postulates a type-1 alcoholic whose illness typically begins after the age of 25 years. Such an individual is less impulsive in alcohol seeking, has fewer alcohol-related fights and arrests, and manifests substantial psychological dependence and guilt about alcohol use. Type-1 alcoholics are low in novelty-seeking behavior, high in harm avoidance, and high in reward dependence. In contrast, in type-2 alcoholics, their illness develops before the age of 25, they show greater impulsivity in alcohol use, and they have frequent fights and arrests while drinking. They manifest less psychological dependence and less guilt about alcohol abuse. Their personality style is characterized more by high novelty seeking, low harm avoidance, and low reward dependence.

Cloninger cites neurophysiologic studies that support the subtyping of alcoholics. Type-1 and type-2 alcoholics respond differently to ingestion of alcohol even during a period of abstinence. Type-1 alcoholics, for example, demonstrate an increase in alpha EEG activity and report a sense of calm upon ingesting a small amount of alcohol. Abstinent type-2 alcoholics, after drinking a similar amount of alcohol, report an increased capacity to focus attention. The type-2 alcoholic's EEG shows a pattern of diminished amplitude in reactance in response to alcohol. Both groups use alcohol to self-treat brain states based on underlying neurochemical response bias. In a later extension of this work, Cloninger proposed that differences such as these may be linked to individual variations in neurotransmitter availability.[14]

NEUROTRANSMITTER EFFECTS OF ALCOHOL AND STREET DRUGS

Subtle neurochemical differences among individuals may at least in part predispose to drug or alcohol abuse. Abused drugs, in turn, alter brain levels of neurotransmitters. An understanding of the acute and chronic effects of abused drugs on these neurotransmitters may help to explain how drugs are both appealing and destructive to abusers. To further develop the point, however, it is necessary to briefly review the roles played by neurotransmitters.

Neurotransmitters are chemicals that are released between brain cells to communicate from one cell to the other. They act by changing the electrical potential or facilitating a chemical reaction within the receiving cell. Specific neurotransmitters are associated with specific pathways from one part of the brain to another. Cell bodies having high concentrations of dopamine, for example, are found connecting parts of the brain that affect emotion and involuntary muscular activity. Other brain pathways, with other neurotransmitters, facilitate different functions. Although a wide variety of amino acids and neuropeptides are putative neurotransmitters,[15] our understanding of psychiatric disorders has focused on the functioning of a small number of these endogenous chemical messengers. Of particular importance in recent research have been five neurotransmitters: dopamine (DA), serotonin (5HT), norepinephrine (NE), gamma-aminobutyric acid (GABA), and acetylcholine (ACh).

Dopamine's importance has been noted especially in schizophrenia, a disorder hypothesized to arise from an excess of dopamine activity.[16] Medications used in the treatment of schizophrenia block dopamine activity.[17] In mood disorders and obsessive-compulsive disorder, serotonin has been postulated to play an important role.[18] Each of these conditions is linked by research evidence to relative deficiency or inefficiency of serotonin neurotransmission.[19] An inefficiency of norepinephrine neurotransmission has been invoked to explain the biochemical basis of some mood disorders and attention deficit disorder.[20] Some types of anxiety may be linked to disturbances of GABA system functioning, since some powerful antianxiety medications seem to act through enhancing GABA activity.[21] Acetylcholine appears to be important in the functioning of memory[22] and regulation of certain automatic body functions.[31] For further discussion of neurotransmitters and how medications act upon their activity, see chapter 7.

Though conclusions from research remain far from complete, it has become clear that neurotransmitters are significantly affected by alcohol and street drugs. Many of the findings have derived from studies of animal brains or postmortem human brain tissue. Some drugs have been more easily understood than others. Research on the effects of alcohol, for example, has been complicated by issues of dosage and duration of use.[23] Common marijuana is a crude compound containing a large number of cannabinoid derivatives, a fact that has complicated marijuana research.[24] In contrast, amphetamine, LSD, and PCP have lent themselves well to basic research in organic chemistry.[25] The neurotransmitter effects of traditional pharmaceuticals such as opiates and antianxiety drugs have been explored in a substantial body of basic and clinical research.[26,27]

Reported alcohol effects on neurotransmitters have depended on dosage (high versus low) or duration of use (acute versus chronic).[23] Single low doses of ethanol stimulate both norepinephrine and dopamine.[23] Higher doses and chronic use generate depletion states in both neurotransmitters.[23] Acute, low-dose use of ethanol affects serotonin in a biphasic pattern: an initial increase is followed by a decrease in activity.[23] High-dose and long-term ethanol effects on serotonin are unclear.[23] GABA activity seems to be reduced after an acute low dose.[23] Alcohol competes with GABA at brain receptor sites.[23] The antianxiety drugs of the benzodiazepine group also compete for GABA receptor sites. This explains the similarity of behavioral effects between alcohol and benzodiazepines and provides the neurochemical explanation for benzodiazepines' effectiveness in treating alcohol withdrawal.

Marijuana acts to increase the synthesis and turnover of norepinephrine and dopamine.[24] In addition it tends to block reuptake of these neurotransmitters.[24] Specific cannabis compounds decrease receptor site binding of dopamine antagonists (agents that block dopamine effects) or enhance dopamine agonists (agents that act like dopamine).[24] This competition for dopamine receptor sites is of particular clinical importance when a medicated schizophrenic patient abuses marijuana. The commonly observed exacerbation of psychosis is probably due to stimulation of dopamine activity and competition with the dopamine-blocking antipsychotic medication. Acute marijuana ingestion probably also stimulates serotonin activity. Chronic marijuana use, however, seems to result in a net reduction of activity. Cocaine is a catecholamine reuptake blocker which increases the synaptic activity of norepinephrine and dopamine.[12] In addition, it directly stimulates release of norepinephrine.[12] Availability of both dopamine and norepinephrine is reduced, however, after acute dosage or during chronic use.[12] Neuroleptics probably increase cocaine craving by further blockade of the dopamine receptor.[12] For the chronic patient who abuses cocaine but continues to take prescribed antipsychotic medication, the result can be a vicious cycle of dopamine stimulation and blockade. Cocaine effects on serotonin are less well studied but the drug appears to reduce serotonin activity.[25] Amphetamines and other stimulants have effects similar to those of cocaine, although the mechanism of action is different.[25] Chronic use of cocaine and stimulants clearly intensify mood disorders and this seems at least partially due to depletion of catecholamine activity. The subjective experiences of catecholamine depletion are anergia, impairment of concentration, and depression.[12]

LSD, PCP, and related hallucinogens significantly increase dopamine activity, moderately stimulate norepinephrine, and reduce serotonin in the central integrative pathways.[25] Norepinephrine and serotonin activity and turnover are increased.[25] The acute and chronic effects of abused drugs on neurotransmitters are summarized in Table 10-1.

These aspects of drug and neurotransmitter interactions help explain how alcohol and street drugs are used in an effort to self-medicate. From studies of cocaine abusers and from subtyping studies of alcoholics it has become apparent how subjective drug effects may differ on the basis of underlying individual neurochemical characteristics. The short-term effects of abused drugs on psychiatric symptoms are often sought for their palliative subjective effects, even though the long-term effects may intensify illness. As noted in the ADAMHA report, drug-seeking behavior is further enhanced by peer group support for drug abuse and a lack of peer approval for medication compliance.[8] Miami vices have greater sex appeal than medication use.

Table 10-1
Neurotransmitter Effects of Recreational Drug Use*

	Norepinephrine	Dopamine	Serotonin	GABA
Alcohol				
Acute; low dose	↑	↑	Biphasic	↓
Chronic; high dose	↓	↓	?	↓
Marijuana				
Acute	↑	↑↑	↑	?
Chronic	↓	↓	↓	?
Cocaine, amphetamine				
Acute	↑↑	↑↑	↓	?
Chronic	↓↓	↑	↓	?
LSD, PCP	↑	↑↑↑	↓	?
MDMA	↑	↑	↑↑↑	?
Narcotics	↑	↑↑	↓	?

*? means "unknown."

INTERACTIONS BETWEEN ALCOHOL AND PRESCRIBED MEDICATIONS

Beyond the effects just noted, medications and abused drugs may interact through a variety of pharmacologic and physiologic mechanisms. We review some of these effects, first for alcohol and then for other drugs of abuse.

A common effect of combining alcohol with a prescribed drug is *potentiation*, a term used to describe a synergistic combination of drug effects that exceed that of alcohol or the prescribed medication alone.[28] Alcohol depresses the activity of the CNS, an effect shared for example with most antidepressant medications.[28] The combination of alcohol with one of these drugs may produce drowsiness that is excessive and dangerously interferes with activities such as driving a car. Barbiturates and more current antianxiety medications, antihistamines, and antipsychotic medications also are CNS depressants which can combine adversely in this way with alcohol.[28] Sedating antidepressants, particularly amitriptyline and nortriptyline, are especially potentiated by alcohol.[28] Alcohol combined with high-dose benzodiazepines, in overdose for example, can be fatal.[28] Long-acting benzodiazepines, like diazepam and chlordiazepoxide, are more strongly potentiated by alcohol than are short-acting benzodiazepines such as lorazepam.[28] The sedating effects of antihistamines such as diphenhydramine, commonly found in over-the-counter cold remedies, are potentiated by alcohol and may in combination cause dangerously unacceptable sedation.[28]

In addition, alcohol affects liver metabolism in a way that undermines the effects of many drugs.[28] There are molecules within liver cells called microsomal enzymes.[28] These enzymes metabolize food and drug products. Consumption of alcohol stimulates the liver to produce an increased level of these enzymes, which results in more rapid deactivation of alcohol and also of concurrently taken medication. Larger doses of these medications are then required to produce the same therapeutic effects. Alcoholics may require, for example, higher doses of antidepressants than nonalcoholics to achieve the same therapeutic effects.[29] Another example of the result of increased microsomal activity in alcoholics is their need for higher doses of antianxiety medications in the treatment of anxiety or alcohol withdrawal.[30] When individuals with seizure disorders combine alcohol with the use of anticonvulsants such as phenytoin or carbamazepine, the resulting enhancement of liver deactivation of these drugs can increase the risk of having a seizure.[28]

Alcohol can also reduce the liver's metabolic activity. Because the liver is the chief site of metabolic deactivation for many prescription drugs, this impairment of function can dangerously elevate blood levels of these compounds. A patient taking an anticoagulant, for example, has an increased risk of hemorrhaging if liver function is impaired. Alcohol use over a long period is also associated with impairment of cardiac function, which can potentiate toxic effects of prescribed medications.

The interactions of wine and beer with MAO inhibitors have been noted in chapter 7. Chianti wine, especially, is high in tyramine and should be avoided by patients taking MAO-inhibiting antidepressants.[28] Most wines and champagnes contain tyramine in low amounts and should be used with caution.[28] Imported beers and ales contain higher amounts of tyramine than domestic beer.[28] A dose of 10 to 25 mg of tyramine, the amount contained in two glasses of Chianti, is sufficient to produce a serious increase in blood pressure.[28] An equivalent amount of tyramine can be obtained from two pints of ale.[28] While white wine and distilled liquors contain too little tyramine to produce a hypertensive reaction when they are taken in moderate amounts, they still can produce other toxic interactions with antidepressants such as potentiation of sedation.

Several final miscellaneous interactions of alcohol with prescribed medications deserve mention. When combined with antipsychotic medications such as chlorpromazine or haloperidol, alcohol increases the risk of dystonia, which is an involuntary tightening of muscles.[28] In combination with beta-adrenergic blockers such as propranolol, alcohol is known to cause memory impairment and unpredictable impairment of driving.[28] Clonidine and alcohol are a particularly unsafe combination with respect to driving ability.[28] The combination of lithium and alcohol has also been reported to have an unpredictable effect on driving.[28]

INTERACTIONS BETWEEN STREET DRUGS AND MEDICATIONS

Cocaine's interactions with prescribed medications are quite different from those of alcohol. Before reviewing these, however, special mention must be made of the combination of cocaine with alcohol. Alcohol abuse intensifies the depression experienced following cocaine use. Alcohol, however, is used commonly to "cool off" a cocaine binge. Users of alcohol combined with cocaine demonstrate a higher suicide risk than alcoholics, perhaps because an intensified depression after cocaine use can more easily be directed toward suicidal behavior when an individual is disinhibited by the use of alcohol.[32]

Whether taken with or without alcohol, cocaine has potent physical effects that can interact with those of prescribed medications. The cardiotoxic effects of cocaine have received considerable recent attention.[33] Cardiac deaths of prominent sports and entertainment figures have highlighted this concern. Although cocaine itself can produce dangerous disturbances of the heart's functioning, the danger may be further increased when cocaine is combined with medications that affect cardiac activity. Antidepressants vary in the degree to which they affect the heart, but virtually all of them have cardiovascular effects.[17] The risk of dangerous rhythm disturbances or myocardial infarction may be increased by this combination.

Recent reports of the effectiveness of desipramine in

reducing cocaine craving have encouraged clinicians to prescribe this antidepressant to drug abusers attempting to maintain abstinence.[11] Patients treated with desipramine for cocaine abuse commonly report cocaine craving during the early stages of adjusting the desipramine dose.[1] These patients often experiment with cocaine to reduce their craving and test its effects with desipramine. Anecdotal reports of the interaction effects describe an extremely unpleasant subjective state with dysphoria, clouding of awareness, and an increase in heart rate and cardiac palpitations. It is unusual for cocaine to break through the effects of desipramine to produce the usual cocaine euphoria, particularly if desipramine is being used in the range of 150 to 200 mg a day.[11] Lithium also seems to nullify the euphoric effects of cocaine and amphetamine.[11]

Since cocaine affects neurotransmitter activity similarly to tricyclic antidepressants, it is probable that the combination of cocaine with an MAO inhibitor would result in a hypertensive reaction. Currently, MAO inhibitors are being recommended by many clinicians especially for the treatment of atypical depression, a syndrome which often features periods of fatigue and anergia, sometimes associated with stimulant or other drug abuse. Patients with a history of substance abuse and atypical depression, for which MAO inhibitors are currently considered potentially superior to other antidepressants, therefore represent a special clinical risk that warrants explicit warning and education. Antipsychotic medications, like antidepressants, vary in their cardiac effects. Thioridazine, a strongly anticholinergic antipsychotic drug, has particularly prominent effects on cardiac rhythm.[17] A patient who abuses cocaine while taking thioridazine may increase the risk of cardiac arrhythmias. Also, as noted, cocaine craving can be intensified by the use of antipsychotic medications.[12]

One of the effects of high-dose or high-potency cocaine is to stimulate seizures in vulnerable patients. The effects of cocaine on limbic seizure activity have recently been reported.[36] Cocaine's interactions with medications used in the treatment of epilepsy, such as carbamazepine and phenytoin, await description.

As noted, the interaction of prescribed medications with cannabis or hallucinogens can lead to intensification of psychotic symptoms and can diminish the effectiveness of antipsychotic treatment.[24]

Particular mention should be made of a compound called ecstasy, known chemically as MDMA. This compound has enjoyed recent popularity for its alleged consciousness-expanding properties. A recent survey of seniors at a prominent West-coast university indicated that one-third had tried MDMA. MDMA has a molecular structure somewhere between LSD and amphetamine.[37] It seems to be a powerful stimulus for serotonin activity.[25] Following use there is a period of serotonergic depletion.[25] Antidepressant users who may make use of MDMA should be warned that it may potentiate toxic effects of MAO-inhibitor antidepressants. In particular, in combination with MAO inhibitors it may be capable of causing the sometimes fatal syndrome of serotonergic crisis. This state is characterized by agitation, psychosis, and cardiac symptoms and usually requires hospitalization.

The depletion stage of MDMA use may be particularly risky for individuals prone to obsessional or depressed states, as illustrated in the following example.

Case 1. A young, intelligent, well-organized author of one book and a frequent contributor to popular general interest magazines had spent almost one year in psychotherapy and on medication, recovering from feelings of rejection by an obsessively loved woman. Though not overtly troubled by obsessions or compulsions, he was impaired by a ruminative cognitive style. During mid-winter, he went on a camping trip into the mountains in the Southwest with his new girlfriend, a fitness enthusiast. Believing that a shared drug experience would intensify their closeness, they took MDMA together. Although they shared several hours of intense altered sensual experience, he then became irritable and despondent during the depletion stage and decided there was no future in the relationship. On returning to the Northeast, he continued to feel low and marked insomnia developed. He re-entered treatment "to talk things over." One of his immediate concerns was to learn more about the neurochemical effects of MDMA.

Had the patient ingested MDMA while taking medication, the outcome would have been even more complicated. The patient, a science writer, knew something about the pharmacology of MDMA but managed to deny his own risk of toxic effects.

Before concluding this discussion of interaction effects, the opiates require consideration. Opiates, like alcohol, are CNS depressants. Synergism with alcohol, barbiturates, benzodiazepines, antidepressants, and antipsychotics can therefore pose problems. Respiratory depression is a potential risk when these drugs are taken in combination.[28] Methadone maintenance patients and opiate abusers, therefore, require education about interaction effects. In addition, patients taking benzodiazepines, antidepressants, or antipsychotics need to be cautioned about concurrently prescribed opiate analgesics or cough suppressants.

A narcotic/medication interaction of particular danger occurs when meperidine (Demerol) is taken in combination with a MAO inhibitor.[28] This interaction is probably another manifestation of the serotonergic crisis previously mentioned, and is characterized by fever, agitation, sweating, and coma. Serious respiratory depression and shock may occur, requiring emergency medical treatment.[28]

SUBSTANCE ABUSE AND THE LABORATORY

Medical laboratories can now provide considerable assistance to a mental health treatment team. There are now reliable qualitative assays for most substances of abuse, to facilitate spot checks and contingency contracting by therapists.[34] Cocaine abuse can be well followed by laboratory testing, especially when the presence of its main metabolite, benzoylecgonine, is monitored.[34] Quantitative analysis for serum levels of alcohol, barbiturates, benzodiazepines, most antidepressants, and a few antipsychotics is reliable.[34] Routine measures of blood cell counts, liver functions, and kidney function support patient assessment by the psychopharmacologist. ECGs are routinely ordered in prescribing antidepressants for patients at risk, especially cocaine abusers and patients taking MAO inhibitors. EEGs and brain-imaging technologies such as tomography or nuclear magnetic resonance spectroscopy are chiefly used for diagnostic purposes, but may help to assess long-term effects of substance abuse, especially when combined with neuropsychological test batteries.

SUMMARY

Psychotherapists see an increasing number of clients who use alcohol and street drugs with or without concurrently prescribed medications. The psychotherapist can aid a substance-abusing patient by helping to identify an underlying, potentially medication-responsive disorder. In treating a substance abuser taking medication concurrently, the therapist can increase the patient's safety and enhance the efficacy of their pharmacologic treatment by learning about the interactions of abused drugs with prescribed medications.

REFERENCES

1. Robins LN, Helzer JE, Weissman MM, et al: Lifetime prevalence of specific psychiatric disorders in three sites. *Arch Gen Psychiatry* 1984;41:949–958.
2. Gerstein DR: Alcohol use and consequences, in Moore MH, Gerstein DR (eds): *Alcohol and Public Policy: Beyond the Shadow of Prohibition*. Washington, DC, National Academy Press, 1981, pp 182–224.
3. Schuckit MA, Bogard B: Intravenous drug use in alcoholics. *J Clin Psychiatry* 1986;47:551–554.
4. Hesselbrock MN, Meyer RE, Keener JJ: Psychopathology in hospitalized alcoholics. *Arch Gen Psychiatry* 1985;42:1050–1055.
5. Johnston LD, O'Malley PM, Bachman JG: *National Trends in Drug Use and Related Factors among American High School Students and Young Adults: 1975–1986*. Washington, DC, National Institute of Drug Abuse, 1987, pp 26–46.
6. MacDonald DI: From the alcohol, drug abuse, and mental health administration: Cocaine heads ED drug visits. *J Am Med Assoc* 1987;258:2029.
7. Johnson TE, Carroll G, Agrest S, et al: Kids and cocaine. *Newsweek* March 17, 1986, pp 57–65.
8. Ridgely MS, Goldman HH, Talbott JA: *Chronic Mentally Ill Young Adults with Substance Abuse Problems*. Baltimore, University of Maryland School of Medicine Mental Health Policy Studies, 1986.
9. Khantzian EJ: The self-medication hypothesis of addictive disorders: Focus on heroin and cocaine dependence. *Am J Psychiatry* 1985;142:1259–1264.

10. Dackis CA, Gold MS: Pharmacological approaches to cocaine addiction. *J Subst Abuse Treat* 1985;2:139–145.
11. Gold MS, Dackis CA: New insights and treatments: Opiate withdrawal and cocaine addiction. *Clin Ther* 1984;7:6–21.
12. Dackis CA, Gold MS: New concepts in cocaine addiction: The dopamine depletion hypothesis. *Neurosci Biobehav Rev* 1985;3:469–477.
13. Cloninger CR: Neurogenetic adaptive mechanisms in alcoholism. *Science* 1987;436:410–416.
14. Cloninger CR: A systematic method for clinical description and classification of personality variants. *Arch Gen Psychiatry* 1987;44: 573–588.
15. Snyder SH: Basic science of psychopharmacology, in Kaplan HI, Sadock BJ (eds): *Comprehensive Textbook of Psychiatry IV*. Baltimore, Williams and Wilkins, 1985, pp 42–54.
16. Meltzer HM, Stahl SM: The dopamine hypothesis of schizophrenia: A review. *Schizophrenia Bull* 1976;2:19–76.
17. Baldessarini RJ: *Chemotherapy in Psychiatry*. Cambridge, Harvard University Press, 1985.
18. Grosser BI: Serotonin: A reappraisal. *J Clin Psychiatry* 1987; 48(suppl):3–4.
19. Zohar J, Insel TR: Obsessive-compulsive disorder: Psychobiological approaches to diagnosis, treatment, and pathophysiology. *Biol Psychiatry* 1987;22:667–687.
20. Potter WZ: Introduction: Norepinephrine as an "umbrella" neuromodulator. *Psychosomatics* 1986;27(suppl):5–7.
21. Lloyd KG, Morselli PL: Psychopharmacology of GABAergic drugs, in Meltzer HY (ed): *Psychopharmacology: The Third Generation of Progress*. New York, Raven Press, 1987, pp 183–195.
22. Schneck MK, Reisberg B, Ferris SB, et al: An overview of current concepts of Alzheimer's disease. *Am J Psychiatry* 1982;139:165–173.
23. Hunt WA, Majchrowicz E: Alternations in neurotransmitter function after acute and chronic treatment with ethanol, in Majchrowski E, Noble EP (eds): *Biochemistry and Pharmacology of Ethanol*, vol 2. New York, Plenum Press, 1987, pp 167–182.
24. Bloom AS: Effects of cannabinoids on neurotransmitter receptors in the brain, in Augrell S, Dewey WL, Willette RE, et al (eds): *The Cannabinoids: Chemical, Pharmacologic and Therapeutic Aspects*. Orlando, Academic Press, 1984.
25. Hamon M: Common neurochemical correlates to the action of hallucinogens, in Jacobs BL (ed): *Hallucinogens: Neurochemical, Behavioral and Clinical Perspectives*. New York, Raven Press, 1984, pp 143–169.
26. Tallman JF, Paul SM, Skolnick P, et al: Receptors for the age of anxiety: Molecular pharmacology of the benzodiazepines. *Science* 1980;207:274–281.
27. Jaffe JH, Martin WR: Opioid analgesics and antagonists, in Gilman

AG, Goodwin LS (eds): *The Pharmacological Basis of Therapeutics*. New York, Macmillan, 1985, pp 491–531.
28. Stockley IH: *Drug Interactions*. Oxford, Blackwell Scientific Publications, 1981, pp 1–59, 345–384.
29. Ciraulo DA, Jaffe JH: Tricyclic antidepressants in the treatment of depression associated with alcoholism. *J Clin Psychopharmacol* 1982;2:2–7.
30. Jaffe JH: Drug addiction and drug abuse, in Gilman AG, Goodwin LS (eds): *The Pharmacological Basis of Therapeutics*. New York, Macmillan, 1985, pp 532–581.
31. Weiner N, Taylor P: Neurohumoral transmission: The autonomic and somatic motor nervous systems, in Gilman AG, Goodwin, LS (eds): *The Pharmacological Basis of Therapeutics*. New York, Macmillan, 1985, pp 66–99.
32. Smith DE: Cocaine-alcohol abuse: Epidemiological, diagnostic and treatment considerations. *J Psychoactive Drugs* 1986;18:117–129.
33. Duke M: Cocaine, myocardial infarction and arrhythmias — A review. *Conn Med* 1986;50:440–442.
34. Poklis A: Toxicology and therapeutic drug monitoring, in Bauer JD: *Clinical Laboratory Methods*. St. Louis, CV Mosby, 1982, 630–673.
35. Lowenstein DH, Massa SM, Rowbotham MC, et al: Acute neurologic and psychiatric complications associated with cocaine abuse. *Am J Med* 1987;83:841–846.
36. Lesse H, Collins JP: Effects of cocaine on propagation of limbic seizure activity. *Pharmacol Biochem Behav* 1979;11:689–694.
37. Shulgin AT, Nichols DE: Characterization of three new psychotomimetics, in Stillman RC, Willette RE (eds): *The Psychopharmacology of Hallucinogens*. New York, Pergamon Press, 1978, pp 74–83.

11

ADHD, CEBV, FM, PMS, Etc: Controversial Syndromes at the Psychiatry/Medicine Interface

Eliot Gelwan

> This afternoon, in bright sunlight, I saw a young woman waiting for a streetcar, accompanied by her body.
>
> Rene Magritte

With zeal and fascination, the popular press seizes upon partially characterized medical syndromes and turns them into household acronyms. News of these conditions, gleaned from the television or press, can greatly influence patients' attitudes about their physical and emotional health. Because the medical basis and exact clinical picture of many of these syndromes are poorly understood, their descriptions usually include a broad range of somatic and psychological symptoms that catch the interest of affected and unaffected individuals. This chapter discusses a number of partially understood syndromes of recent interest, including chronic Epstein-Barr virus (CEBV) infection, adult attention deficit–hyperactivity disorder (adult ADHD), fibromyalgia (fibromyositis, FM), and premenstrual syndrome (PMS), which is included in the DSM-III-R under the label of "late luteal phase dysphoric disorder" or LLPDD.

For psychotherapists, the importance of understanding these faddish diagnoses is both medically and psychodynamically based. Familiarity with these syndromes allows assessment of the need for medical consultation. It also aids the psychodynamic assessment of a patient's interest in considering such an explanation for his or her symptoms. Conceptualizing one's problems as having a medical basis is sometimes accurate; at other times, it can provide an opportunity for resistance, a focus for concern over real or projected stigmatization, or a comforting legitimization of suffering as well as a sense of belonging to a community of similarly afflicted individuals. Locus of perceived control over one's distress and responsibility can thus be shifted in either productive or unproductive ways.

What the syndromes discussed in this chapter share, and what distinguishes them from other medical disorders, is both their uncertain medical validity as causes of psychological symptoms and the unsystematized way in which knowledge of them has spread. The attention given at a particular time by our culture as a whole, or the subculture of the mental health community, to any of these disorders is reflected in such diverse forms as press emphasis, increasing medical research, word-of-mouth discussion among patients, the establishment of self-help organizations, the promotion of nutritional and other lifestyle solutions by the health-food and holistic health establishments, and even (as in the case of CEBV) congressional subcommittee hearings. Diminished responsibility because of PMS has been used as the basis of successful legal defenses in criminal proceedings, even while its inclusion in DSM-III-R has been only provisional, following extended controversy within the psychiatric community about its scientific validity and its potential impact on gender bias. The complexity of these issues will become more apparent through discussion of the individual syndromes.

ADULT ADHD

In an October 1987 issue of the *New York Times Magazine*, a free-lance photographer and editor described how at the age of 30 years he was diagnosed with attention deficit–hyperactivity disorder, a syndrome which until recently was only associated with childhood.[1] In the article the author included his own, rather idiosyncratic list of the disorder's clinical features. Since that time, at least some psychiatrists have noticed a significant increase in consultation requests from patients wishing to know whether they have adult ADHD. These requests come especially from people troubled by nonspecific self-esteem problems or under-achievement and interpersonal difficulties such as were portrayed in the article. These requests raise the issue of whether a spectrum for a disorder such as ADHD exists from the situations of more unequivocal psychopathology in which a diagnosis is usually made, through *formes frustes* where it accounts for much subtler difficulties and dissatisfactions.

Childhood ADHD is a common behavioral syndrome that underwent several changes of name (including hyperactivity and minimal brain dysfunction [MBD]) prior to its current description in DSM-III-R under the name of attention deficit–hyperactivity disorder (ADHD). Such relatively recent agreement on definition has probably been an important factor in the dramatic explosion of journal articles about the disorder. One reviewer counted more than 7,000 citations in the three-year period of 1977 to 1980 as contrasted with only 31 in 1957 to 1960.

The behavior pattern characteristic of childhood ADHD involves inattention (with impersistence and distractibility), impulsivity, lability and anger, and low self-esteem, which presumably results from the other deficits. There may or may not be hyperactivity and difficulty keeping still. The symptomatology varies with time and setting — it is worse in more structured and socially demanding situations — and is often unrecognized before a child begins school, though its earlier harbingers will often be evident retrospectively. Stimulant medications, such as amphetamine, methylphenidate (Ritalin), and pemoline (Cylert), and tricyclic antidepressants have been shown to be effective in ameliorating both the attentional and the behavioral components of the disorder, presumably by actions on the biological substrates of the disordered attention in subcortical and frontal brain areas.

The administration of psychostimulants for an indefinite length of time to children, especially when parents fear the medications will stunt the child's growth or lead to abuse, tends to provoke strong feelings both in the public and among caregivers. Furthermore, the facts of the developmental and neurological maturation of adolescence have led to theoretical speculation and some observations that at least some ADHD symptoms might spontaneously resolve over time. Such concerns have stimulated curiosity about the natural history and adult outcome both of ADHD and of long-term exposure to its medications. It took, of course, ten to fifteen years after the codification of the diagnosis in DSM-III for a cohort of children who had been reliably diagnosed with ADHD to reach late adolescence and early adulthood. For that reason, longitudinal investigation of the speculation that ADHD might persist into adulthood is relatively recent.[2]

Ever since its inception in the mid-1970s, longitudinal follow-up has demonstrated that, as they age, a significant proportion of MBD or ADHD children continue to demonstrate concentration and attention difficulties, overactivity, and impulsivity both by self-report and on objective measures.[3] The dramatic motor hyperactivity that characterizes the ADHD subgroup with pronounced hyperactivity does appear to drop out of the picture, supporting the idea that attentional problems are the primary deficit. Retrospective studies of patients with complaints of inattention, irritability and impulsivity in adulthood suggest that a substantial proportion would have met criteria for the childhood diagnosis of ADHD.[4-6] A smaller proportion of ADHD children go on to develop substance use disorders, sociopathy or delinquency problems, and dyscontrol syndromes.[7] Delinquent or conduct-disordered adolescents and antisocial young adults show more ADHD-like symptoms in childhood than either control subjects or their nondelinquent siblings in several studies.[8,9]

Family studies have also shown that the parents of hyperactive children have an increased incidence of sociopathy and other character disorders, alcoholism, and substance abuse and that a significant proportion of them had themselves demonstrated hyperactivity or ADHD symptoms in childhood.[10,11] A family association with pathological gambling has also been reported. Where ADHD children have been adopted away, it is the biological parents and not the adoptive ones who demonstrate such trends, suggesting a heritable influence.[12]

Beginning in 1976, the notion that ADHD might persist into adulthood as a dysfunctional behavior pattern has led to trials with agents that are effective in treating the childhood disorder.[12]

Wender and colleagues examined adults with prominent complaints of impulsivity, irritability, restlessness, and emotional lability and, after excluding those with organic or functional major mental disorders, selected patients who had reported childhood ADHD symptoms. The target symptoms were significantly responsive to methylphenidate or imipramine. In a subsequent replication, to address criticisms that the methylphenidate used in the original study had produced a nonspecific euphoric effect, patients responded equally well to pemoline,[13] a stimulant that does not produce euphoria.[14] Subsequently, responses to various tricyclic and MAO-inhibitor antidepressants have been demonstrated, sometimes at doses lower than those used to treat depression. When patients have been treated with effective medications, a tendency has been observed for them to underestimate their improvement on self-report in comparison to ratings by clinicians or family members.

Patients with ADHD demonstrate a so-called paradoxical response to stimulants, consisting of calming; increased task persistence; decrease in activity, racing thoughts, and talkativeness; decreased temper; and better stress-tolerance. In short, their function is improved and they use their stimulation productively. Like hyperactive children but unlike adult stimulant abusers, adult ADHD patients do not develop tolerance (a need for higher and higher doses with time to maintain the same pharmacological response) and they respond well to pemoline, a drug of little interest to stimulant abusers. In fact, a clue to the diagnosis of adult ADHD may be a history of such paradoxical past reactions to stimulants, including amphetamines, cocaine, stimulating antidepressants, and even nicotine or caffeine. Khantzian and coworkers[15,16] and others[17] suggested that a subset of abusers of cocaine and other stimulants may in fact be self-medicating themselves with the drugs of abuse in order to achieve the paradoxical calming effect.

These patients may present to the mental health system with a variety of prior diagnoses including anxiety disorders, substance and alcohol abuse, minor affective disorders, or legal difficulties. Clues to their recognition (see Table 11-1) include a history of birth or other head trauma; delayed milestones, childhood learning difficulties, conduct problems, or ostracism (if not a

Table 11-1
Clues to the Recognition of Adult ADHD

Dysattention, distractibility	Family history:
Irritability, labile moods	ADHD/hyperactivity
Impulsivity or dyscontrol syndrome	Alcoholism
	Sociopathy
Delinquent or sociopathic activities	Paradoxical calming from stimulants
Alcohol abuse, substance abuse	Neurological soft signs
Hyperactive, learning- or conduct-disordered as children	Delayed developmental milestones

frank diagnosis of MBD, ADHD, or hyperactivity); eye-hand coordination problems or clumsiness; diffuse irritability, anxiety, or dysphoria; rapidly labile mood since childhood; prominent temper or impulse dyscontrol; prominent complaints of restlessness, difficulty concentrating, or distractibility; rapid speech with frequent shifts of subject; and the characteristic family history just reviewed. When lithium has been prescribed during prior treatment, a negative response is consistent with ADHD. A number of studies have found that, among adults presenting with this clinical picture, stimulant response can be expected only in those with a plausible childhood history of ADHD.[13,18–20] Emphasis is thus placed on the value of a detailed childhood history, corroborative history from family members or clinicians who saw the patient in childhood, and review of documented evidence such as school records.

Generally, the disorder is diagnosed when the characteristics just mentioned are prominent enough to disrupt job and marital stability, and when they occur in individuals whose low achievements seem to belie their apparent intelligence. Recognition may be more difficult when the attentional impairment is mild or has been compensated for by advantages in upbringing, other characterological strengths or supports offered by chosen careers or relationships. Because response to effective medications will generally be rapid and unequivocal, an empirical trial may be of use when the diagnosis seems plausible. Recently, however, even pemoline has apparently been taken by a number of generally intellectually-minded recreational substance users who claim it to be a general cognition-enhancer. Insufficient study of its clinical effects in control subjects makes these claims, and thus the specificity of ADHD's responsiveness to a pemoline trial, hard to evaluate. Similarly, response to an antidepressant may represent treatment of an underlying affective disorder.

Special attention has been paid to the association between adult ADHD and alcohol abuse. Tarter and others suggest that a subset of adult alcoholics with an apparent earlier onset, fewer precipitants for their alcoholic drinking, more severe drinking, and poorer treatment outcome are more likely to report childhood ADHD symptoms than other alcohol abusers, and that a family history of alcoholism also clusters in this so-called primary alcoholic subset.[21,22] Primary alcoholics show more psychopathology on their Minnesota Multiphasic Personality Inventory (MMPI) scales, have more interpersonal difficulties on several measures, and are more likely to admit that their drinking is for purposes of altering their mood; they more frequently abuse other substances along with alcohol.[23] Primary alcoholics in one study did more poorly on several neurocognitive measures, reflecting either the sequelae of their more severe drinking histories or the possible premorbid deficits in cognitive functioning consistent with their possible greater tendencies toward ADHD.[24] Moreover, primary alcoholics are more likely to meet the criteria for antisocial personality disorder (ASP). As previously mentioned, an individual or family history of ASP has also been shown to be related to ADHD.

Other studies have found that the retrospective diagnosis of childhood ADHD may be made anywhere from three to ten times more frequently in alcoholics than in nonalcoholics, even without consideration of the primary/secondary alcoholic distinction.[21,25,26] It has been suggested that treatment for ADHD may enhance compliance with alcohol rehabilitation, though the potentially liver-damaging effects of pemoline and the abuse potential of the other stimulants complicate treatment in these ADHD individuals. In light of a recent theory correlating left-handedness, history of developmental learning disability, and autoimmune disease, a report of increased correlation between left-handedness in alcoholic men and familial alcoholism is of interest.[27] Chronic diarrhea has been noted to be a precursor of both irritable bowel disease (IBD) and ADHD in children; in one study adults with IBD were found to show a greater proportion of ADHD symptoms than controls without IBD.[28]

At least one study found an increased prevalence of ADHD history in narcotics abusers.[29] Results from a number of investigations implied that a treatment-resistant subset of patients with chronic psychotic illness diagnosed as chronic schizophrenia can be demonstrated to have a childhood history of ADHD symptoms and may respond to stimulants.[30–32] This may represent one "organic" subgroup among schizophrenics. Several case reports describe stimulant-responsive adult ADHD presenting as manic disorder and thus support an association with major affective disorder.[33,34] A subgroup of patients with borderline personality disorder who had a history of ADHD may also be distinguishable.[35] In short, ADHD may be implicated as an imitator or as a neurological underpinning of a variety of symptom patterns in adulthood. A recent report approaches this question by reviewing the range of stimulant applications in psychiatry.[36] ADHD may underlie a range of the atypical stimulant applications reviewed.

A patient with a history and presentation consistent with the features discussed here could profitably be referred for structured neuropsychological assessment of attentional processes and/or a psychiatric consultation to evaluate the efficacy of treatment for ADHD. ADHD may exist in milder or more severe forms, complicating recognition in the psychotherapy patient with other reasonable explanations of distractibility, underachievement, or difficulties in regulating self-esteem.

CHRONIC EPSTEIN-BARR VIRUS (CEBV) INFECTION

The Epstein-Barr virus is a human virus in the herpes family. It is lymphotropic, which means that it infects lymphocytes, one subclass of white blood cells involved in immune function. Over the past 20 years, it has been identified as the causative agent in most cases of infectious mononucleosis (IMN) and it is implicated in several malignant and pre-malignant diseases. The virus is ubiquitous, infecting as many as 60% of people before the age of

10 years and as many as 100% by the age of 40. Most primary infections with EBV are subclinical or asymptomatic; there is usually no clear history of IMN in people who test positive (indicating exposure) for the antibodies to the virus. In a sense, all EBV infection is probably chronic. After the virus is contracted, it colonizes lymphoid tissue and resides within our bodies ever after. Like other herpes viruses, it can integrate itself into the genetic material of human cells and either lie dormant indefinitely or replicate actively, making its carrier a source for infection of others.

Because convalescence from IMN is characterized by a prolonged neurasthenia (fatigue, low energy, subjective feelings of weakness, anxiety, boredom, and depression) and occasionally persistent neurological symptoms, attention has turned to the possibility that EBV plays a role in the more widespread chronic neurasthenic conditions, which have perennially resisted medical attention and are often termed depressive equivalents or dismissed as malingering. In general there has been a growing medical appreciation that diverse viruses, previously considered to cause only acute infections, may also lead to chronic infections.[37] Further interest in the role of EBV has been sparked by evidence that lymphocytes and neurons have similar surface antigens (molecules on the cell's surface which serve as the viral binding sites), suggesting that certain lymphotropic viruses may also be neurotropic; ie, they may also infect brain or nerve cells. New antibody testing techniques for EBV infection now allow diagnosis of persistent infection. This has facilitated studies which demonstrate that EBV infection may, in some individuals, follow a chronic or recurrent course.

In 1985, for example, the Center for Disease Control received a report of 134 cases of chronic fatigue and lethargy, many with sore throat and swollen glands, around Incline Village, Nevada.[38] EBV antibody testing had been performed on all. Their antibody levels were found to correlate with their degree of debility, as measured by persistence of symptoms, amount of missed work, and degree of reduction in daily activity. This and similar studies have been publicized and support groups have sprung up throughout the country. Patients who recognize themselves in the press descriptions and seek out these groups have typically experienced a great sense of relief at finding an explanation and a name for their distressing and confusing chronic condition, which previously may have been the cause of blame and stigmatization. Even though no medical treatment has been proven to be effective for CEBV infection, the relief of diagnosis can be of great value to an affected individual.

The proportion of patients whose chronic fatigue and related complaints may be referable to CEBV remains controversial. Some medical practitioners deny that the antibody test findings represent active EBV infection; others propose that the findings are incidental rather than causal.[39] In a recent study 21% of 500 unselected patients seen at a primary care practice complained on screening of a chronic-fatigue-like syndrome, usually cyclical, fitting CEBV descriptions.[40] While the level of antibodies to several EBV antigens was higher than that in matched controls, the differences were not significant and the authors doubted that CEBV infection was related to the complaints of the patients.

A 1988 review of chronic fatigue by Holmes and colleagues[41] concluded that, to judge from thousands of inquiries which the Center for Disease Control (CDC) had received from patients diagnosed with the syndrome and from physicians diagnosing it, many physicians' diagnoses of CEBV have been based on little more than the detectable presence of EBV titers. Because of the nonspecific nature of the diagnosis and the lack of confidence in a diagnostic test, the CDC authors assembled a working group of epidemiologists, clinicians, and biomedical researchers to devise a case definition as a basis for standardization and comparative evaluation of research on chronic fatigue syndrome (CFS); they offered this as an alternative name to avoid the etiologic suppositions of calling it CEBV syndrome. Their proposed criteria are listed in Table 11-2.

It should be noted that a reliable case definition for the CEBV syndrome per se might be derived by requiring the serological pattern for chronic or reactivated EBV infection along with the criteria for CFS. Descriptions of the proposed CEBV syndrome emphasize that the recurrent viral syndromes, which resemble episodes of IMN but are less intense, assume less prominence than the ennervation and the neurological complaints, which wax and wane in severity. The latter generally

Table 11-2
Proposed Case Definition for the Chronic Fatigue Syndrome (CFS)

Major criteria
1. "New onset of persistent or relapsing, debilitating fatigue or easy fatiguability in a person without prior history of such symptoms, that does not resolve with bedrest, and that is severe enough to reduce or impair average daily activity below 50% of the patient's premorbid activity level for a period of at least 6 months."
2. The exclusion by thorough evaluation of other clinical conditions that produce similar symptoms. (A lengthy exclusion list is presented.) A recommended evaluation should include serial weights and temperatures, a variety of laboratory blood tests, urinalysis and chest x-ray, and psychiatric history. While an abnormal finding on any such measure does not rule out CFS, the burden is on the physician to search for another underlying explanation for the abnormality before concluding that CFS is the cause.

Minor criteria
  Symptom criteria
   1. Mild fever
   2. Sore throat
   3. Painful axillary or cervical lymph nodes
   4. General muscle weakness
   5. Myalgias (muscle aches)
   6. Decreased exercise tolerance or easy fatiguability
   7. Generalized headaches
   8. Migratory arthralgias (joint pains) without joint inflammation
   9. One or more neuropsychological symptoms including photophobia, transient visual scotomata, forgetfulness, excessive irritability, confusion, difficulty thinking, inability to concentrate, or depression
   10. Sleep disturbance (hypersomnia or insomnia)
   11. Onset over a few hours to a few days
  Physical criteria (documented by physician on at least two occasions more than 1 month apart)
   1. Low-grade fever
   2. Nonexudative pharyngitis
   3. Palpable or tender cervical or axillary lymphadenopathy

[*] Both of the major criteria are necessary; of the minor criteria, at least 8 of 11 symptom criteria, or at least 6 of 11 symptom criteria *and* at least 2 of 3 physical criteria are required as well.

From Holmes GP, Kaplan JE, Gantz NE, et al: Chronic fatigue syndrome: a working case definition. *Ann Intern Med* 1988;108:387–389.

becomes the basis of the sufferer's debilitation. A history of severe acute viral illness preceding the changes in mental status, if not an episode of frank IMN, can often be elicited. In the chronic case, however, the results of the heterophil antibody test (Monospot) used to diagnose acute IMN will remain negative. Indeed, results of most prior workups have been negative, and patients often report a long frustrating history of knowing something is wrong but having their complaints dismissed by medical practitioners.

A history of childhood allergy has been associated with CEBV infection and may point toward the immunological vulnerability thought to underlie these patients' inability to resolve their CEBV infection as the rest of us do. Supporting this presumption, at least one case of familial susceptibility to CEBV, with persistent infection in two members of the same family, has been reported.[42] In another report, three children with long-standing CEBV infection were studied immunologically. Each was shown to have an individual disturbance of immune function, suggesting that heterogeneity may underlie vulnerability to the infection.[27] Further studies of the relationship with allergy have shown that CEBV patients are more severely reactive to a greater number of allergens than comparison groups without CEBV.[44,45] A higher-than-chance association with juvenile rheumatoid arthritis has also been observed, further supporting the idea of an underlying immune defect.[46]

The antibody test panel used for the diagnosis of EBV, which is fairly expensive, consists of four separate tests whose overall pattern distinguishes between prior acute, current acute, or chronic infection patterns. The literature suggests that latent EBV infection can be reactivated by immunosuppression due to either disease or congenital immunodeficiency, so that findings of EBV antibody positivity should stimulate a thorough medical workup for underlying (possibly treatable) medical disorders.

Both theoretically and empirically based hypotheses regarding mechanisms by which chronic EBV infection could cause or contribute to a neurasthenic syndrome have been made. One hypothesis emphasizes the virus's neurotropism, speculating that CNS infection could directly affect brain function. Another theory attributes fatigue and depression to the relentless systemic effects of a persistent viral infection. Chronic lymphocyte infection may impair immune function and allow debilitating secondary viral infections. Activated by chronic infection, lymphocytes and other cells of the immune system may secrete substances into the bloodstream which have CNS effects either directly or via hormonal mediation. Because depression from any cause has been observed to suppress some aspects of immune function, depression may be both an effect of CEBV and itself the cause of further debilitation. These hypotheses require investigational clarification. Even if they suggest no cure for CEBV, they may point the way to alleviation of target symptoms. Suggested CEBV treatments will require careful examination, since placebo responses may be increased in patients with a disorder with such vague and subjective symptomatology. With this in mind, it is notable that most of the CEBV clinical studies reported to date are not double-blind or placebo-controlled.

Because immunity to EBV is so widespread in the general population, gamma globulin injections (which represent a fraction of blood from pooled sources containing antibodies) have been tried, with some success in double-blind trials, in CEBV patients. Two children with CEBV have shown a response to thymostimulin, a hormone which invigorates the body's immune response.[47] Small numbers of CEBV sufferers treated with the anti-herpes drug acyclovir have been reported to achieve a reduction in flare-ups.[48,49] The general applicability of this treatment is unclear, as the extent to which active viral replication plays a part in the clinical manifestations of the CEBV syndrome is not known.

One interesting report described a series of chronically depressed patients diagnosed with CEBV in whom remissions were induced with histamine blockers (cimetidine and ranitidine), a class of agents usually employed to suppress gastric acid secretion in patients with ulcer disease.[50] The theoretical justification for this treatment involves the hypothesized importance of circulating substances with CNS effects, whose secretion by lymphocytes activated by EBV infection can be suppressed by medications that bind to the histamine receptors demonstrated to be present on lymphocyte surfaces.

Antidepressants have also been used to treat some CEBV

sufferers, with improvement in mood, energy, and concentration. It may be that CEBV infection impairs these through the same sorts of effects on CNS neurotransmitter activity that are seen in patients with functional depression. An alternate explanation would be that the complaints represent depressive equivalents, which are ameliorated by the antidepressants. Alexithymia, literally "no words for feelings," is a term that has been used to describe a hypothesized psychological structure characterized by the tendency to experience unpleasant affects as bodily states instead of emotions. This structure may underlie some patients' use of a somatic methaphor for distress they cannot recognize as emotional in nature.[51] They may be particularly susceptible to publicity about CEBV or for that matter some of the other syndromes to be described. Choice of treatment, from among a spectrum which includes antiviral agents, immune modulators, antidepressants, and psychosocial support or therapy, will depend on a thoughtful assessment which locates a patient somewhere along the continuum from clear-cut physical illness (unequivocal laboratory findings and definite viral-syndrome symptoms) to distress which seems primarily emotional, sustained by secondary gain. Neuropsychological assessment should play an important part in detecting possible subtle CNS effects that may accompany symptoms that look more functional.

FIBROMYALGIA/FIBROMYOSITIS (FM)

This syndrome of chronic fatigue, muscle aches, insomnia, and mood disturbance has recently attracted much interest within medicine. Although some clinicians believe that FM is not a discrete condition, it has reportedly become one of the most common diagnoses in rheumatological practices. Recent estimates place its prevalence at 3 to 6 million in the United States.[52]

Because no specific microscopic tissue changes, radiological abnormalities, or laboratory findings have been demonstrated, many authors designate the disorder as psychogenic, especially since complaints of depression and anxiety are prominent among the other symptoms. During the past decade, however, a growing number of investigators have claimed that FM can be differentiated from purely psychogenic complaints. The hallmark, they report, is the consistent finding of reproducible localized tenderness at specific trigger points when palpated by an experienced examiner. The advent of electron microscopy and new biochemical tests has offered confirmatory demonstrations of nonspecific tissue changes in biopsies of muscle tissue from tender points.[53] A leading theory suggests that the muscle changes follow from chronic spasm and resultant alterations in blood supply to the affected muscles, perhaps because of tension and stress.[53,54] Low tissue oxygenation at trigger points has been demonstrated. The syndrome may be a final common musculoskeletal response to a variety of insults.

The manifestations of this syndrome (see Table 11-3) include chronic fatigue, long-standing diffuse aches and pains, morning stiffness, disturbed and nonrestorative sleep with intensification of symptoms on awakening, irritable bowel symptoms, and the presence of multiple characteristic tender points, or trigger points (soft-tissue regions which cause radiating pain, numbness, or tingling either spontaneously or when direct pressure is applied). Arguing against psychogenic causes is the fact that patients are generally unaware of the presence or location of these trigger points until an experienced examiner locates them in expectable sites.[55]

Table 11-3
Clues to the Recognition of Fibromyalgia

Long-standing chronic fatigue
General malaise
Diffuse muscle aches, morning stiffness
"Trigger points" (of which patient may be unaware)
Numbness or tingling extremities
Sleep disturbance:
    Nonrestorative sleep
    Intermittent awakening
Diurnal variation of symptoms
    Worst in morning and at end of day
Mood disturbance:
    Depression, dysthymia, dysphoria, anxiety
Irritable bowel symptoms
Family history of affective disorder
Multiple past medical evaluations without diagnostic findings

Symptoms are characteristically modulated by predictable factors including weather, activity, quality of sleep, time of day (worst as the day begins and again at the end of the day), and stress levels. The typical FM sufferer is a woman between 20 and 50 years old, although the syndrome has also been reported in men and children. The diagnosis depends on exclusion of the clinical findings of other diseases such as rheumatoid arthritis (RA) with similar symptoms. A so-called secondary FM syndrome associated with other connective tissue or rheumatologic diseases has been reported; however, it responds to treatment of the underlying disease. In primary FM, three distinct patterns of natural history have been proposed: a remitting-intermittent, a fluctuating-continuing, and a progressive subtype. FM, however, is not degenerative or deforming and causes no serious secondary complications.

Research directed toward the etiology of FM has linked it variously to sleep disorders, neurological abnormalities, immune disorders, and muscle disease. Even though it is probably not psychogenic in nature, many findings support the central role of psychological and psychobiological factors in the etiology, perception, and course of this syndrome. FM shares many manifestations with acknowledged psychosomatic disorders such as irritable bowel, chronic lower-back pain, and tension headache. The diurnal variation in symptom severity and the sleep disturbance are suggestive of depressive disorders. In contrast to patients with RA, FM patients have higher rates of affective disorders and of family history of affective disorders than the general population.[56] In one study, however, there was no excess depression rating on the Zung Self-Rating Depression scale in FM patients, compared with RA patients. MMPI profiles have shown approximately equal proportions of FM patients with "normal," "chronic pain," and "psychologically disturbed" patterns.[57] Patients with FM express more intense feelings of being ill and show higher scores than RA patients on several ratings of stress. FM has a higher-than-chance association with past hypothyroidism, but patients generally have normal thyroid function at the time of onset of the FM.

Anecdotal reports have linked FM with viral illnesses including IMN, which may not be surprising in terms of the overlapping symptoms of FM and CEBV. A recent study, however, failed to find higher levels of antibodies to EBV in 50 FM patients who reported the onset of the FM symptoms after a viral illness and had complaints which appeared more typically in CEBV patients, including recurrent fevers, sore throats, rash, and swollen glands.[58]

Neurophysiological studies show that the fatigue reported by FM patients is at least partly central in origin rather than localized to their muscles. EEG studies in FM patients during sleep have shown disturbed non-REM sleep, and many FM symptoms can be reproduced by selectively depriving normal volunteers of non-REM sleep.[54] Similar sleep patterns have been reported in patients with other chronic pain syndromes including post-accident pain, clouding the issue of whether the chronic pain or the sleep disturbance is primary in FM patients. Some investigators have attempted to link FM with the perimenopausal period and estrogen deficit,[59] but therapeutic benefits of estrogen replacement have not, it appears, been investigated.

FM is a poorly recognized syndrome, so patients have frequently been seen by many prior physicians who have failed to give them an adequate diagnosis despite sometimes invasive investigations. Sufferers may have had their symptoms dismissed as imaginary or told that they heralded more severe disorders such as lupus or multiple sclerosis.[52] For these reasons, an important component of treatment is a good alliance with a physician who can give a patient a definite diagnosis, explanations about possible mechanisms, and ongoing reassurances about the benign course of FM.[55] Reviews of treatment approaches show that most treatments have been found only partially effective. In one study, more than 60% of a group of 39 patients had moderate to severe recurrent symptoms at two-year follow-up regardless of prior treatments[60]; in another, over 90% remained symptomatic at follow-up after three years of treatment compliance.[52] Anti-inflammatory medications including aspirin, non-steroidals, and steroids have generally been ineffective although there are suggestions that steroid injections to trigger points may provide temporary relief; narcotic analgesics seem of little use and carry the risks of abuse and dependence.

Current treatment strategies are directed at modification of the factors that modulate the severity and course of FM. A sleep disorder can be treated symptomatically and stress reduction attempted. In an open trial, biofeedback aimed at tension reduction was effective in 56% of patients who had not responded to more than one year of medication treatment; the subgroup that did not respond was the more psychopathological.[61] These findings were strengthened by a controlled study comparing "true-" with "pseudo-biofeedback" training.[61] Cardiovascular fitness (aerobic) training has been demonstrated to be effective when compared with a program of nonaerobic flexibility exercises only, as have various forms of physical therapy. In one double-blind study of 62 patients with FM, amitriptyline taken at much lower doses than used in the treatment of depression surpassed either placebo or anti-inflammatory medication in ameliorating almost all parameters of the syndrome.[62] Acupuncture seems not to have been investigated in the treatment of FM, though it would seem to be a natural candidate.

In summary, FM is a diagnosable syndrome and patients derive clinical benefit from receiving the diagnosis when it is appropriate. Treatments are ineffective if considered in isolation, but a multimodal approach involving lifestyle changes, physical therapy, treatment of underlying psychological issues, medical reassurance, counselling, and sometimes the judicious use of medications can have an impact on quality of life. It is likely, given the growing recognition and popularity of this syndrome, that increasing numbers of psychotherapy patients will request evaluation for FM. Only a proportion will be found to have the diagnostic "trigger points," but all can benefit from an exploration of their concerns and symptoms.

PREMENSTRUAL SYNDROME (PMS) OR LATE LUTEAL PHASE DYSPHORIC DISORDER (LLPDD)

PMS (termed LLPDD in the DSM-III-R) comprises a variety of emotional, behavioral, and physical symptoms with cyclical occurrence in menstruating women and severity ranging from mild to incapacitating. Its manifestations are worst during the days prior to the menses, the late luteal phase in biological terms.

After onset of menses, there is definite improvement or resolution. PMS has become a controversial battleground of notions about the relationship between biological and psychological variables. A number of women accused of serious crimes have relied successfully on a plea of innocence using PMS as the basis of diminished responsibility.[63] Other women and men denounce the concept of the disorder as a sexist medical fabrication. These are the extreme ends of a spectrum of viewpoints about the extent to which PMS may influence mood and behavior.

It has been estimated that 20% to 40% of women of childbearing age have some degree of PMS, and in 5% to 10% of them it is so severe as to disrupt domestic, occupational, or social functioning.[64,65] Psychological testing during various phases of the menstrual cycle has shown premenstrual cognitive disturbances in women who complain of PMS symptoms but not in asymptomatic women,[66] although the evidence has been somewhat contradictory.

A wide range of reported symptoms has been attributed to PMS, including cramps, irritability, anxiety, tension, fluid retention, weight gain, abdominal distention, bloating, headache, skin disorders, breast swelling and tenderness, emotional lability, depression, and fatigue. Affected women are more often young and nulliparous and have lower educational background and socioeconomic status, longer menstrual cycles, and heavier or longer menstrual flow. They tend to cycle so regularly that they can predict the arrival of their next menstrual period.[67]

Theories of the mechanisms behind PMS implicate a variety of hormonal imbalances, metabolic factors, and psychosocial variables. Various authors implicate alterations in estrogen/progesterone balance, pyridoxine (a vitamin) deficiency, prostaglandin imbalance, increased aldosterone (a hormone involved in regulation of the body's fluid balance), deficits in trace dietary constituents, and imbalances in endogenous opiates.[68]

There is mounting evidence that the syndrome may be heterogeneous in etiology and presentation, and that it may be the final common pathway of diverse interacting causative factors.[69] Inconclusiveness or irreproducibility of clinical findings, which has led to controversy about the very existence of the syndrome, may thus be the result of broad diagnostic criteria and heterogeneous patient populations. One emerging schema (see Table 11-4) proposes subtypes presenting with predominance of: (a) anxiety, irritability, tension; (b) bloating, water retention, and weight gain; (c) breast tenderness and swelling; and (d) depression, memory, and concentration difficulties.[70]

Various theories attribute PMS to the unopposed action of either estrogen or progesterone because of its excess or the relative deficit of its antagonist during the premenstrual (luteal) phase. Researchers have found seemingly contradictory evidence for both excess premenstrual estrogen and excess premenstrual progesterone.[64] Although it is doubtless an oversimplification, one hypothesis proposes that unopposed estrogen, which is stimulatory, underlies PMS characterized by anxiety, hostility, irritability, or tension. Unopposed progesterone is proposed as the basis of depressive PMS. Consistent with this hypothesis, progesterone has been found useful in treating anxious or irritable PMS in some patients. Estrogen has been reported to have some effectiveness in treating depressive PMS,[71] whereas progesterone has been ineffective.

The premenstrual administration of danazol, a synthetic androgen and gonadotropin inhibitor used for the treatment of fibrocystic breast disease and endometriosis, has been investigated by several authors.[72-74] Some benefits have been found, particularly in patients in whom breast tenderness and swelling are the primary symptoms. Virilizing side effects, a major limiting factor in their use, have been avoided when low doses (100-200 mg/day) or intermittent dosing schedules were employed.

Initial interest in the role of pyridoxine (vitamin B_6) in treating PMS was based on the concept that pyridoxine deficiency in laboratory animals impaired estrogen metabolism. More recently, attention has turned to the role of this vitamin as a facilitator of certain enzyme reactions in the synthesis of dopa-

Table 11-4
Symptoms of PMS Grouped by Proposed Subtypes

Anxiety, irritability, tension
Bloating, water retention, weight gain
Breast tenderness, swelling
Depression, memory and concentration difficulties

mine and serotonin, two CNS neurotransmitters important in the regulation of mood and behavior. Premenstrual estrogen-induced deficits in pyridoxine supplies may lead to neurotransmitter imbalances. In both open and double-blind trials, pyridoxine in doses varying between 50 and 500 mg/d has been found useful in alleviating symptoms including headache, bloating, depression, and irritability. Despite such promising evidence, pyridoxine must be used cautiously in light of recent reports that in large doses it can be neurotoxic.[75]

There are some reports that the hormone prolactin is elevated premenstrually. Interest in its involvement in PMS has centered on its role as a regulator of fluid balance in some animals. It is probably also involved in the feedback regulation of some CNS neurotransmitters involved with mood and behavior. Premenstrual levels of prolactin have been demonstrated to correlate with the severity of PMS symptoms. The drug bromocriptine, which inhibits prolactin secretion in the CNS and has some actions on fluid balance at the level of the kidney, has been shown to be effective in reducing breast tenderness in many open and controlled trials,[76] usually in doses of 2.5 mg twice a day.

Premenstrual fluid retention and electrolyte imbalance have long been assumed to play an important part in PMS distress, suggesting a role for diuretic treatment. Careful investigations, however, yielded contradictory results and failed to confirm the link between fluid retention and PMS symptoms. Findings with a variety of diuretics have been equivocal, but results of a number of studies favored the use of spironolactone, generally in doses of 25 mg four times a day, when bloating and distention are the major discomforts. An improvement in the underlying psychological symptoms has also been noted with diuretic treatment.[77]

The prostaglandins (PGs) are a group of fatty acids with diverse and potent biological actions that affect cell function in every organ system. Their importance to metabolic processes has been appreciated only recently in medical science. Their effects on the reproductive system, where they occur in high concentrations, are currently being studied intensively. They have both CNS and end-organ effects on the ovulatory cycle and its hormones. Their involvement in the regulation of fluid balance, endocrine activity, modulation of CNS neurotransmitter effects, and the inflammatory response may also be pertinent to PMS.

It has been proposed that a relative premenstrual decrease in one of the PGs (PGE_1) may cause abnormal sensitivity to prolactin effects. A fatty acid precursor of PGE_1 found in evening primrose oil (generally sold in health food stores) has been found effective against a wide variety of PMS symptoms in three controlled and two open studies.[78] Many substances which have played a part in the dietary approaches to PMS — magnesium, zinc, niacin, ascorbic acid (vitamin C), pyridoxine among them — share an ability to enhance the body's production of PGE_1.

There has been considerable interest in the relationship between PMS and conventional psychiatric disorders. In one study it was reported that when women with PMS were misled about where in their menstrual cycle they were, their complaints correlated better with their belief that they were premenstrual than with the hormonally defined phase.[79] Psychiatric screening of PMS patients has revealed a significantly higher proportion of psychiatric morbidity than in the general population,[80,81] although there are methodological problems in these studies.[82] Different subtypes of premenstrual discomfort appear to correlate differently with lifetime psychiatric history,[83] and PMS should be considered especially in the differential diagnosis of any woman of childbearing age with fluctuating psychiatric symptoms.[84] Dysthymia, phobias, obsessive-compulsive disorder, alcohol abuse, substance abuse, psychosis, bulimia, and anxiety disorders have all been found in increased proportion among women with PMS.[85] Significantly, somatization disorder has not been detected to a greater extent in women with PMS than in controls.[86] Various conceptual models for the relationship between premenstrual and psychiatric symptoms have been suggested. Do these symptoms represent coexistence or common underlying causality of PMS and psychiatric morbidity? Does PMS unmask or exacerbate psychopathology? Or does psychiatric morbidity worsen or predispose to PMS?

The most consistent relationship seems to be with the affective disorders. On psychological testing, a significant subgroup of women with PMS have evidence of continuing depression regardless of phase of the cycle and level of superimposed PMS symptoms.[87] In one study, women reporting PMS symptoms were more likely to have received mental health services and a diagnosis of affective disorder.[88] A case report described three women with a history of premenstrual affective symptoms in whom full mood disorders developed and suggested that they may represent a genetically predisposed subgroup of PMS patients who are also at risk for postpartum depression or psychosis.[89]

Partial sleep deprivation, a treatment approach to depression as well, has been reported to be effective in treating premenstrual depression.[90] Parry and colleagues reported the case of a patient with PMS symptoms only in fall and winter who obtained relief from treatment with bright artificial light, an accepted treatment for seasonal affective disorder.[91]

Some authors have considered PMS to be a variant or relative of rapid cycling bipolar affective disorder. In one study, 25 rapid-cycling patients had an increased tendency to have PMS symptoms, compared with matched controls. When present, the PMS was more severe than that of the non-rapid-cyclers. Moreover, those rapid-cyclers with PMS had more severe bipolar cycling than rapid cyclers without PMS.[92] However, a number of studies have shown no or equivocal benefits from lithium in comparison with placebo in treating PMS.[64] There is a case report of a postpartum psychosis in a woman (with a strong family history of schizophrenia), which resolved with treatment but recurred premenstrually every month and was responsive to danazol.[93]

OTHER SYNDROMES

Several popular difficult-to-diagnose syndromes deserve briefer mention here. Hypoglycemia, currently of less interest, has often been suggested by patients as an explanation for depressive or anxiety states. A body of medical research has discredited this suggestion, by showing that reactive hypoglycemia is a rare condition and that, when it occurs naturally or is induced, changes in mental status are not typical.[94] To link anxiety with hypoglycemia in a specific patient, it would be necessary to demonstrate a low glucose level and to show that symptoms are maximal at the glucose nadir and relieved by the administration of glucose.[95] A variety of other notions of dietary influence on mood and behavior appear from time to time. Suggested mechanisms of the influence of dietary factors on psychiatric symptoms have included cerebral allergy, hypersensitivity to additives, reaction to vasoactive substances in food (akin to the substances that must be restricted in patients taking an MAO-inhibitor antidepressant), neurotransmitter alterations due to ingestion of natural precursors in the diet, and food addiction or withdrawal reactions.[96] Interest in proposed allergies with cerebral consequences, either to food or to environmental substances, has led some individuals to consult a controversial new type of clinician specializing in clinical ecology. A clinical ecologist might be likely to attribute behavioral symptoms to allergies and suggest dietary alternations and challenge testing to determine and treat sensitivities.

A "pan-allergic disease," "multiple allergy syndrome," or "twentieth-century disease" involving sensitization to multiple food and environmental substances, contaminants, and additives and responsible for diverse vague and troubling complaints has been proposed. Fatigue, nonspecific aches and pains, and dysphoric or depressive feelings, which may be conceptualized as a patient's reaction to apparent incurability, are said to characterize patients with this condition. A particular proposed offender of recent interest is *Candida albicans*, the ubiquitous yeastlike organism responsible for vaginal candidiasis (moniliasis), oral thrush, and other opportunistic infections.[97] It is claimed that long-term use of antibiotics, cortisone, oral contraceptives, or refined sugar and alcohol upset the guest-host relationship and predispose an individual to be overrun by a proliferation of candida. Chronic vague systemic and constitutional complaints, sleep disturbance, mood and anxiety disorders, hormonal disturbances, skin problems including psoriasis, chronic gastrointestinal complaints, and even autoimmune disease and multiple sclerosis have been claimed to be caused or exacerbated by systemic candidiasis. Proponents have not made systematic distinctions in their own thinking between hypothesized toxic, allergic, autoimmune, and other infective mechanisms for the various proposed manifestations of this condition. Some authors on the subject will acknowledge that the mechanisms remain obscure. In any case, in some areas where exposure to these concepts is substantial and sympathetic practitioners of various backgrounds exist to give them guidance, a significant number of patients are pursuing dietary regimens (yeast-free, low-carbohydrate) to eliminate candida and invigorate the host responses to this organism. Some have even undergone treatment with the antifungal agent nystatin.

Reviewing these allergic/nutritional/ecological perspectives further is beyond the scope of this chapter other than to note that there is a dearth of controlled trials of such treatment approaches in the medical literature. Basic science research is proceeding in the laboratory on interactions, heretofore unappreciated, between the immune system and the CNS. This knowledge may conceivably converge with some of the more unorthodox clinical approaches.

The temporomandibular joint (TMJ) syndrome is another chronic pain syndrome in which behavioral and psychological factors are implicated in both etiology and sequelae.[98] Alteration of TMJ function due to trauma or psychogenic causes of muscular tension and spasm leads to diffuse radiating facial pain and distracting perception of joint noises. TMJ complaints may cause or exacerbate, be caused or exacerbated by, coexist with, or substitute for an anxiety or depressive disorder. Muscle relaxants, antianxiety agents, anti-inflammatory agents, joint injections, mechanical supports, behavioral interventions for stress management, and, as a last resort, surgical correction have been advocated in management. The possible efficacy of antidepressants, on the basis of roles in treating chronic pain and depression, needs study. The frequency of attributing emotional stress to TMJ, which coincided with significant press attention several years ago, seems to have declined along with that attention.

CONCLUSIONS

The conditions discussed here vary in terms of how credible they are as diagnoses, how much is known about each of their pathophysiologies and etiologies, and where the balance between the physiological and the psychodynamic seems to lie. What they have in common is the seductive interest each seems to hold for a subset of individuals who ask psychotherapists how much of their dysphoria or dysfunction might be explained in that way. Their seductiveness is also apparent in the faddish attention these syndromes receive in the lay press and through word-of-mouth.

Some individuals may be best understood as actually affected by one of these syndromes. They have often known that "something is terribly wrong," but have been unable to find a medical explanation. For others, a somatizing or dissociative style, or perhaps an alexithymic diathesis, underlies and is expressed in an attachment to one of these diagnoses. In still other cases, the appeal of a physical explanation for emotional distress may represent resistance emerging in the exploration of painful psychotherapy issues.

The complexities of mind-body interaction make it comprehensible that an organic pathophysiological process may not (yet) be recognized by such an accepted name in medical science because its influence on cognitive function, affect regulation, or other parameters of character structure is too subtle or indirect to characterize with current investigational techniques. Furthermore, there is a sociology of knowledge from which the structures of medical science are not exempt. Ideological influence on the recognition and classification of diseases is attested to, for example, by the continual revision process which the *Diagnostic and Statistical Manual* of the American Psychiatric Association undergoes. There will always be clinical presentations or syndromes which are interstitial or marginal to currently accepted classificatory structures. As ideology changes or knowledge expands, they will be accepted or discredited as entities, yet they will always be replaced by new marginal syndromes. It is probably no accident that many of these syndromes inhabit the fertile interface between the behavioral sciences and other disciplines: CEBV with infectious disease, ADHD with neuroscience, FM with rheumatology, and PMS with endocrinology.

The psychotherapist's familiarity with these conditions and with the generic phenomenon of the controversial syndrome can inform both the process of seeking medical consultation and that of working through the dynamic meaning of a patient's somatic concerns, whether the outcome of a specific workup is negative or positive.

REFERENCES

1. Wolkenberg F: Out of a darkness. *NY Times Mag* October 11, 1987.
2. Wood DR, Reimherr FW, Wender PH, et al: Diagnosis and treatment of minimal brain dysfunction in adults: A preliminary report. *Arch Gen Psychiatry* 1976;33:1453–1460.
3. Cantwell DP: Hyperactive children have grown up. What have we learned about what happens to them? *Arch Gen Psychiatry* 1985;42:1026–1028.
4. Gomez RL, Janowsky D, Zetin M, et al: Adult psychiatric diagnosis and symptoms compatible with the hyperactive child syndrome: A retrospective study. *J Clin Psychiatry* 1981;42:389–394.
5. Shelley EM, Riester A: Syndrome of MBD in young adults. *Dis Nerv System* 1972;33:335–339.
6. Quitkin F, Klein DF: Two behavioral syndromes in young adults related to possible minimal brain dysfunction. *J Psychiatr Res* 1969;7:131–142.
7. Gittelman R, Mannuzza S, Shenker R, et al: Hyperactive boys almost grown up. I. Psychiatric status. *Arch Gen Psychiatry* 1985;42:937–947.
8. Borland BL, Heckman HK: Hyperactive boys and their brothers: A 25-year followup study. *Arch Gen Psychiatry* 1976;33:669–675.
9. O'Neal P, Robbins LM: The relation of childhood behavior problems to adult psychiatric status: A 30-year followup study of 150 patients. *Am J Psychiatry* 1958;114:961–969.
10. Cantwell DP: Psychiatric illness in the families of hyperactive children. *Arch Gen Psychiatry* 1972;27:414–417.
11. Morrison JR, Stewart MA: A family study of the hyperactive child syndrome. *Biol Psychiatry* 1971;3:189–195.
12. Alberts-Corush J, Firestone P, Goodman JT: Attention and impulsivity characteristics of the biological and adoptive parents of hyperactive and normal control children. *Am J Orthopsychiatry* 1986;56:413–423.
13. Wender PH, Reimherr FW, Wood DR: Attention deficit disorder ('minimal brain dysfunction') in adults. A replication study of diagnosis and drug treatment. *Arch Gen Psychiatry* 1981;38:449–456.
14. Langer DH, Sweeney KP, Bartenbach DE, et al: Evidence of lack of abuse or dependence following pemoline treatment: Results of a retrospective survey. *Drug Alcohol Depend* 1986;17:213–217.
15. Khantzian EJ: The self-medication hypothesis of addictive disorders: focus on heroin and cocaine dependence. *Am J Psychiatry* 1985; 142:1259–1264.

16. Khantzian EJ, Gawin F, Kleber HD, Riordan CE: Methylphenidate (Ritalin) treatment of cocaine dependence — a preliminary report. *J Subst Abuse Treat* 1984;1:107-112.
17. Weiss RD, Pope HG, Mirin SM: Treatment of chronic cocaine abuse and attention deficit disorder, residual type, with magnesium pemoline. *Drug Alcohol Depend* 1985;15:69-72.
18. Arnold LE, Stroebel D, Weisenberg A: Hyperactive adults: study of the "paradoxical" amphetamine response. *JAMA* 1972;222:693-694.
19. Mann HB, Greenspan SI: The identification and treatment of adult brain dysfunction. *Am J Psychiatry* 1976;133:1013-1017.
20. Mattes JA, Boswell L, Oliver H: Methylphenidate effects on symptoms of attention deficit disorder in adults. *Arch Gen Psychiatry* 1984;41:1059-1063.
21. Tarter RE, McBride H, Buonpane N, et al: Differentiation of alcoholics: Childhood history of minimal brain dysfunction, family history and drinking pattern. *Arch Gen Psychiatry* 1977;34:761-768.
22. Goodwin DW: Familial alcoholism: a separate entity? *Subst Alcohol Actions/Misuse* 4:129-136, 1983.
23. Alterman AI, Tarter RE, Baughman TG, et al: Differentiation of alcoholics high and low in childhood hyperactivity. *Drug Alcohol Depend* 1985;15:111-121.
24. De Obaldia R, Parsons OA, Yohman R: Minimal brain dysfunction syndromes claimed by primary and secondary alcoholics: relation to cognitive functioning. *Int J Neurosci* 1983;20:173-181.
25. Wood D, Wender PH, Reimherr FW: The prevalence of attention deficit disorder, residual type, or minimal brain dysfunction, in a population of male alcoholic patients. *Am J Psychiatry* 1983;140:95-98.
26. Goodwin DW: Familial alcoholism: a separate entity? *Subst Alcohol Actions/Misuse* 1983;4:129-136.
27. London WP, Kibbee P, Holt L: Handedness and alcoholism. *J Nerv Ment Disord* 1985;173:570-572.
28. Wender PH, Kalm M: Prevalence of attention deficit disorder, residual type, and other psychiatric disorders in patients with irritable colon syndrome. *Am J Psychiatry* 1983;140:1579-1582.
29. Eyre SL, Rounsaville BJ, Kleber HD: History of childhood hyperactivity in a clinic population of opiate addicts. *J Nerv Ment Disord* 1982;170:522-529.
30. Bellak L: A possible subgroup of the schizophrenic syndrome and implications for treatment. *Am J Psychother* 1976;30:194-205.
31. Huey LY, Zetin M, Janowsky DS, et al: Adult minimal brain dysfunction and schizophrenia: a case report. *Am J Psychiatry* 1978;135:1563-1565.
32. Ciompi L: Is there really a schizophrenia? The long-term course of psychotic phenomena. *Br J Psychiatry* 1984;145:636-640.
33. Dvoredsky AE, Stewart MA: Hyperactivity followed by manic-

depressive disorder: two case reports. *J Clin Psychiatry* 1981;42:212–214.
34. Plotkin D, Halaris A, DeMet EM: Biological studies in adult attention deficit disorder: case report. *J Clin Psychiatry* 1982;43:501–502.
35. Andrulonis PA, Glueck BC, Stroebel CF, et al: Borderline personality subcategories. *J Nerv Ment Disord* 1982;170:670–679.
36. Chiarello RJ, Cole JO: The use of psychostimulants in general psychiatry: A reconsideration. *Arch Gen Psychiatry* 1987;44:286–295.
37. Berris B: Chronic viral diseases. *Can Med Assoc J* 1986;135:1260–1268.
38. Holmes GP, Kaplan JE, Stewart JA, et al: A cluster of patients with a chronic mononucleosis-like syndrome. Is Epstein-Barr virus the cause? *JAMA* 1987;257:2297–2302.
39. Merlin TL: Pitfalls in the laboratory diagnosis of chronic mononucleosis. *Hum Pathol* 1986;172–8.
40. Buchwald D, Sullivan JL, Komaroff AL: Frequency of "chronic active Epstein-Barr virus infection" in a general medical practice. *JAMA* 1987;257:2303–2307.
41. Holmes GP, Kaplan JE, Gantz NE, et al: Chronic fatigue syndrome: a working case definition. *Ann Intern Med* 1988;108:387–389.
42. Joncas JH, Ghibu F, Blagdon M, et al: A familial syndrome of susceptibility to chronic active Epstein-Barr virus infection. *Can Med Assoc J* 1984;130:280–284.
43. Kuis W, Roord JJ, Zegers BJ, et al: Heterogeneity of immune defects in three children with a chronic active Epstein-Barr infection. *J Clin Immunol* 1985;5:377–385.
44. Olson GB, Kanaan MN, Gersuk GM, et al: Correlation between allergy and persistent Epstein-Barr virus infections in chronic-active Epstein-Barr virus-infected patients. *J Allergy Clin Immunol* 1986;78:308–314.
45. Welliver RC: Allergy and the syndrome of chronic Epstein-Barr virus infection. *J Allergy Clin Immunol* 1986;78:278–281.
46. Schuchmann L, Neumann-Haefelin D: [Persistent (chronic active) Epstein-Barr virus infection and arthritis in childhood.] *Monatsschr Kinderheilkd* 1985;133:845–847.
47. Pernice W, Scheider H, Wais U, et al: [Improved immunocompetence in two children with chronic Epstein-Barr virus infection under treatment with a standardized thymus hormone preparation (thymostimulin).] *Arzneimittelforsch* 1985;35:869–870.
48. Schooley RT, Carey RW, Miller G, et al: Chronic Epstein-Barr virus infection associated with fever and interstitial pneumonitis. Clinical and serologic features and response to antiviral chemotherapy. *Ann Intern Med* 1986;104:636–643.
49. Wong KW, D'Amico DJ, Hedges TR III, et al: Ocular involvement associated with chronic Epstein-Barr virus disease. *Arch Ophthalmol* 1987;105:788–792.

50. Goldstein JA: Treatment of chronic Epstein-Barr virus disease with H2 blockers [letter]. *J Clin Psychiatry* 1986;47:572.
51. Krystal H: Alexithymia and psychotherapy. *Am J Psychother* 1979; 33:17–31.
52. Goldenberg DL: Fibromyalgia syndrome. An emerging but controversial condition. *JAMA* 1987;257:2782–2787.
53. Yunus MB, Kalyan-Raman UP, Kalyan-Raman K, et al: Pathological changes in muscle in primary fibromyalgia syndrome. *Am J Med* 1986;81:38–42.
54. Yunus MB: Primary fibromyalgia syndrome: Current concepts. *Compr Ther* 1984;10:21–28.
55. Yunus MB, Masi AT, Calabro JJ, et al: Primary fibromyalgia (fibromyositis): Clinical study of 50 patients with matched normal controls. *Sem Arthritis Rheum* 1981;11:151–171.
56. Hudson JI, Hudson MS, Pliner LF, et al: Fibromyalgia and major affective disorder: A controlled phenomenology and family history study. *Am J Psychiatry* 1985;142:441–446.
57. Ahles TA, Yunus MB, Riley SD, et al: Psychological factors associated with primary fibromyalgia syndrome. *Arthritis Rheum* 1984; 27:1101–1106.
58. Buchwald D, Goldenberg DL, Sullivan JL, et al: The 'chronic active Epstein-Barr virus infection' syndrome and primary fibromyalgia. *Arthritis Rheum* 1987;30:1132–1136.
59. Waxman J, Zatzkis FM: Fibromyalgia and menopause. Examination of the relationship. *Postgrad Med* 1986;80:165–171.
60. Bennett RM: Current issues concerning management of the fibromyositis/fibromyalgia syndrome. *Am J Med* 1986;81:15–18.
61. Ferraccioli G, Ghirelli L, Scita F, et al: EMG-biofeedback training in fibromyalgia syndrome. *J Rheumatol* 1987;14:820–825.
62. Goldenberg DL, Felson DT, Dinerman H: A randomized, controlled trial of amitriptyline and naproxen in the treatment of patients with fibromyalgia. *Arthritis Rheum* 1986;29:1371–1377.
63. Dalton K: Cyclical criminal acts in premenstrual syndrome. *Lancet* 1980;2:1070–1071.
64. Chakmakjian ZH: A critical assessment of therapy for the premenstrual tension syndrome. *J Reprod Med* 1983;28:532–538.
65. Logue CM, Moos RH: Perimenstrual symptoms: prevalence and risk factors. *Psychosom Med* 1986;48:388–414.
66. Posthuma BW, Bass MJ, Bull SB, et al: Detecting changes in functional ability in women with premenstrual syndrome. *Am J Obstet Gynecol* 1987;156:275–278.
67. Woods NF, Most A, Dery GK: Prevalence of perimenstrual symptoms. *Am J Public Health* 1982;72:1257–1264.
68. Smith MA and EQ Youngkin: Managing the premenstrual syndrome. *Clin Pharmacol* 1986;5:788–797.
69. Clare AW: Premenstrual syndrome: Single or multiple causes? *Can J Psychiatry* 1985;30:474–482.

70. Siegel JP, Myers BJ, Dineen MK: Premenstrual tension syndrome symptom clusters. Statistical evaluation of the subsyndromes. *J Reprod Med* 1987;32:395-399.
71. Abraham GE: Hormonal and behavioral changes during the menstrual cycle. *Senologia* 1978;3:33-39.
72. Watts JF, Butt WR, Logan ER: A clinical trial using danazol for the treatment of premenstrual tension. *Br J Obstet Gynaecol* 1987;94:30-34.
73. Sarno AP, Miller EF, Lundblad EG: Premenstrual syndrome: Beneficial effects of periodic, low-dose danazol. *Obstet Gynecol* 1987;70:33-36.
74. Day J: Danazol and the premenstrual syndrome. *Postgrad Med J* 1979;55(suppl 5):87-89.
75. Kendall KE, Schnurr PP: The effects of vitamin B6 supplementation on premenstrual symptoms. *Obstet Gynecol* 1987;70:145-149.
76. Kullander S, Svanberg L: Bromocriptine treatment of the premenstrual syndrome. *Acta Obstet Gynecol Scand* 1979;58:375-379.
77. Vellacott ID, O'Brien PM: Effect of spironolactone on premenstrual syndrome symptoms. *J Reprod Med* 1987;32:429-434.
78. Horrobin DF: The role of essential fatty acids and prostaglandins in the premenstrual syndrome. *J Reprod Med* 1983;28:465-468.
79. Ruble DN: Premenstrual symptoms: A reinterpretation. *Science* 1977;197:291-292.
80. DeJong R, Rubinow DR, Roy-Byrne P, et al: Premenstrual syndrome mood disorder and psychiatric illness. *Am J Psychiatry* 1985;142:1359-1361.
81. Kathol RG: Evaluation of psychiatric symptoms in patients presenting with symptoms of premenstrual tension syndrome. *Clin Obstet Gynecol* 1987;30:408-416.
82. Abplanalp JM: Psychological components of the premenstrual syndrome. Evaluating the research and choosing the treatment. *J Reprod Med* 1983;28:517-524.
83. Endicott J, Nee J, Cohen J, et al: Premenstrual changes: Patterns and correlates of daily ratings. *J Affect Disord* 1986;10:127-135.
84. Haskett RF, Steiner M: Diagnosing premenstrual tension syndrome. *Hosp Community Psychiatry* 1986;37:33-36.
85. Stout AL, Steege JF, Blazer DG, et al: Comparison of lifetime psychiatric diagnoses in Premenstrual Syndrome Clinic and community samples. *J Nerv Ment Disord* 1986;174:517-522.
86. Mackenzie TB, Wilcox K, Baron H: Lifetime prevalence of psychiatric disorders in women with premenstrual difficulties. *J Affect Disord* 1986;10:15-19.
87. Stout AL, Steege JF: Psychological assessment of women seeking treatment for premenstrual syndrome. *J Psychosom Res* 1985;29:621-629.
88. Wetzel RD, Reich T, McClure JN, et al: Premenstrual affective syndrome and affective disorder. *Br J Psychiatry* 1975;127:219-221.

89. Ghadirian AM, Kamaraju LS: Premenstrual mood changes in affective disorders. *Can Med Assoc J* 1987;136:1027–1032.
90. Parry BL, Wehr TA: Therapeutic effect of sleep deprivation in patients with premenstrual syndrome. *Am J Psychiatry* 1987; 144:808–810.
91. Parry BL, Rosenthal NE, Tamarkin L, et al: Treatment of a patient with seasonal premenstrual syndrome. *Am J Psychiatry* 1987; 144:762–766.
92. Price WA, diMarzio L: Premenstrual tension syndrome in rapid-cycling bipolar affective disorder. *J Clin Psychiatry* 1986;47: 415–417.
93. Dennerstein L, Judd F, Davies B: Psychosis and the menstrual cycle. *Med J Aust* 1983;1:524–526.
94. McFarland KF, Baker C, Ferguson SD: Demystifying hypoglycemia: When is it real and how can you tell? *Postgrad Med* 1987;82:54–65.
95. Leggett J, Favazza AR: Hypoglycemia: An overview. *J Clin Psychiatry* 1978;39:51–57.
96. Rippere V: Some varieties of food intolerance in psychiatric patients: An overview. *Nutr Health* 1984;3:125–136.
97. Truss CO: *The Missing Diagnosis*. Privately published by Dr. Truss, Birmingham, AL, 1983.
98. Bronstein SL: Update on temporomandibular joint problems: Diagnosis and treatment. *Resident Staff Phys* 1988;34:71–87.

Appendix: Use of the Laboratory in Pharmacotherapy

Pamela Marlink
James M. Ellison

In comparison to many other medical specialties, psychiatry suffers from a lack of diagnostic tests. Many patients, nonetheless, present to psychiatrists requesting diagnostic blood tests or other procedures. Some hope to find negative results to allay their fears that they are sick. Such patients may have a family member whose major mental illness has cast an alarming shadow over the patient's feelings of depression. Through laboratory testing, others seek to prove that their long-standing fatigue, low mood, anxiety, or other symptoms reflect a hidden medical illness. While a medical abnormality is sometimes found, very frequently the light shed on this question by laboratory results is simply too dim to reveal the cause of the patient's symptoms.

No infallible diagnostic laboratory tests for mental disorders exist at present, though new brain-imaging procedures and sophisticated EEG techniques hold out hope for the future. The laboratory, however, can play a useful role in diagnosis and treatment in several circumscribed areas. This appendix focuses on the use of the laboratory in ruling out medical disorders with behavioral manifestations (differential diagnosis); making certain that the patient is medically fit to take a prescribed psychotropic medication (medical clearance); making sure that the prescribed medication(s) are not harming the patient's body (monitoring of toxicity); and measuring whether an appropriate amount of medication is being taken (monitoring of serum level). In addition, new diagnostic techniques are mentioned briefly.

INITIAL LABORATORY EVALUATION AND MONITORING TESTS

1. The complete blood count (CBC) is routinely ordered prior to treatment with many psychotropic drugs. By estimating the numbers and proportions of several cell types in the blood, the CBC offers a general assessment of a patient's hematologic status. Many physical disorders (for example, blood loss or other systemic causes of anemia, infection, allergy, malnutrition, or vitamin deficiencies) reveal their presence through abnormalities of the CBC, so this test is useful in diagnosing organic illnesses that might be producing mental systems. Lithium, carbamazepine, and several other psychotropic drugs affect various blood cells. Establishing baseline measurements prior to treatment helps a clinician to assess the magnitude and potential danger of these drug effects.

2. Electrolytes in the blood include sodium, potassium, chloride, calcium, phosphate, magnesium, and bicarbonate. An excess or deficiency of one or more of these electrolytes can cause a range of changes in mental status, including seizures, coma, delirium, and even death. Lithium and carbamazepine affect certain electrolyte levels. Baseline electrolyte measurements are therefore useful in ruling out organic disorders and establishing norms with which later measurements can be compared. A further reason for assessing electrolytes is that several psychiatric conditions, for example anorexia, bulimia, and psychogenic water intoxication, can result secondarily in potentially dangerous electrolyte disturbances.

3. Thyroid function tests measure the activity of this highly important endocrine gland. Thyroid hormone, which affects many metabolic processes, is decreased in hypothyroidism and increased in hyperthyroidism. Either of these disorders can imitate a primary psychiatric illness. Furthermore, lithium can induce complicating abnormalities of thyroid function. Thyroid function tests, therefore, are initially obtained for many psychiatric patients and routinely followed in patients treated with lithium salts.

4. Serum chemistry profiles, such as the SMA 12 or SMA 20 panels, include tests of liver function, kidney function, and blood sugar. These tests help to rule out preexisting organic illness and provide baseline levels for monitoring drug effects. While the importance of lithium's effects on the kidney has remained controversial, most clinicians agree that periodic assessment is useful to detect at an early stage the decrease in function that occurs rarely during treatment. Antipsychotic drugs, antidepressant drugs, and the anticonvulsants can each induce liver damage, which would be noted through assessment of liver function tests. Blood sugar level is affected by MAO inhibitors. Though usually clinically unimportant, a baseline measurement is diagnostically useful when symptoms of hypoglycemia are initially present or develop later in treatment.

5. The ESR is a nonspecific serum test useful for detecting hidden autoimmune disease or following the progress of certain diseases. It may be ordered as part of a pretreatment medical evaluation.

6. The EEG measures the brain's electrical activity, as transmitted through the scalp. It is not routinely ordered prior to pharmacotherapy, but is requested when a patient is suspected of having structural or epileptic brain disease.

The EEG consists of a resting record of brain-wave functioning, followed by a number of activating procedures that attempt to exacerbate and measure any abnormality. Among the typical activating procedures are (1) rapid, deep breathing (hyperventilation); (2) powerful light stimulation to the patient's eyes; (3) sleep (natural or sedative-induced); (4) visual, auditory, or tactile stimulation with special measurement techniques; and (5) rarely, medication given intravenously to amplify a subtle EEG abnormality. An exciting recent advance in EEG technology allows patients to wear a portable device, which measures the EEG over a prolonged period, increasing the test's diagnostic sensitivity.

Prior to the EEG, a patient may be asked to prepare by abstaining from sedating medication or caffeine, as the normal EEG pattern can be modified by either of these substances. Abnormal wave activity that occurs intermittently or persistently may indicate organic illness. These findings may help to establish a diagnosis of epilepsy (all types), brain tumor, abscess, bleeding, cerebrovascular disease (such as a stroke), brain injury, or other disease processes that can alter alertness, sensation, cognition, or behavior.

7. Computerized axial tomography (CAT scan), introduced in 1973, uses a computer to integrate data obtained from a rotated series of radiographic views of the head or body. The collected data allow mathematical construction of high-resolution images that permit differentiation of bone, gray and white matter, cerebrospinal fluid, and pathological densities in the brain or other parts of the body. Additionally, contrast material may be injected intravenously. This allows for detection of certain types of lesions otherwise difficult to explore with radiographic techniques.

CAT scanning, because of its great usefulness, has become ubiquitous in psychiatry and neurology. It is not ordered routinely, however, to avoid unnecessary exposure of patients to radiation. Its expense, also, mitigates against unnecessary use.

Who then should be scanned? Current practice among many psychiatrists is to scan patients presenting with the recent new onset of psychosis, dementia, or severe personality changes or other severe psychiatric symptoms that have begun after the age of 40. Patients with symptoms of anorexia nervosa (which occasionally can be caused by the presence of a brain tumor), catatonic patients, and patients with involuntary movements are also potential candidates for a CAT scan.[1] While the brains of some schizophrenic patients show ventricular enlargement detectable on CAT scan, the degree of enlargement is often indistinguishable from the normal range in a specific individual. CAT scanning for the purpose of diagnosing schizophrenia, therefore, is not currently feasible.

8. Toxic screens (serum/urine) are useful in the diagnosis of drug-induced psychosis, depression, or anxiety. They are often useless in diagnosing withdrawal states, because an undetectable amount of drug may remain in the body by the time withdrawal symptoms begin. Specific drugs of abuse that can be detected chemically include marijuana, by measuring delta-9 tetrahydrocannabinol levels in blood or urine; opiates; amphetamines; cocaine; PCP; LSD; and of course alcohol. Some drugs are detected more easily in urine, others in serum. The optimal timing of the test and choice of body fluid for examination depend on the drug suspected. Some drugs, particularly cocaine, are metabolized so rapidly that screening for metabolites provides the only effective method of detection. One cocaine metabolite, however, remains in the body 20 hours or more after use.

False-negative results occur more often than false-positives, usually because a suboptimal body fluid has been sampled or the sample has been collected too long after use of the substance.

Toxic screens are also of use in verifying the presence of certain poisons when behavioral symptoms are suspected to represent toxicity. Environmental substances capable of inducing changes in mental status include the metals manganese, lead, and mercury. Along with careful history taking, serum measurements can confirm a diagnosis of toxic exposure.

9. Serum drug levels for medications such as tricyclic antidepressants, carbamazepine, and lithium have become increasingly valued in recent years. These drugs, in order to exert a clinically useful effect, must be present in the blood at levels above threshold. Many of them produce toxic effects when they are present above recommended levels. Optimal benefit, therefore, is obtained by adjusting dosage so that serum levels remain within a standardized therapeutic range. Serum drug level measurements are useful in verifying compliance, optimizing clinical response, and minimizing toxicity.[2]

INVESTIGATIONAL EXAMINATIONS

1. The dexamethasone test (DST), though less valued now than at the peak of its popularity a few years ago, may help to differentiate a true depressive illness from a depressive personality or certain other psychiatric diagnoses.

Research studies have determined that cortisol production is increased in patients with unipolar or bipolar depressive illness.[3,4] Furthermore, the regulation of serum cortisol levels is impaired.[3] The DST exploits this dysregulation as follows: a patient takes 1 mg of dexamethasone (an exogenous, synthetic corticosteroid) at 11 PM. This, under normal circumstances, would suppress endogenous cortisol production during the next day, an aberration which could be detected through serial cortisol measurements. In many depressed individuals, however, a nonsuppressed pattern of cortisol levels will be measured at the standardized sampling times of 4 PM and 11 PM. A positive result (ie, nonsuppression) strongly suggests a diagnosis of major depression, while a negative result is far less decisive. In other words, there is a 94% diagnostic confidence when the result is positive but only a 74% diagnostic confidence when the result is negative. A number of medical conditions, including anorexia nervosa, must be screened out clinically prior to performing a DST, as they may produce false-positive results.

2. The thyrotropin releasing hormone (TRH) response test exploits a similar dysregulation in hypothalamic/pituitary/thyroid regulation during depression. The TRH response test measures the increase in thyroid stimulating hormone (thyrotropin) following an infusion of TRH. Following an overnight fast, the patient reports for the test at 8 AM. An intravenous catheter is placed, usually in the arm, and baseline blood levels of thyroid hormones are measured. The patient is then infused intravenously with synthetic TRH and blood is drawn 15, 30, 60, and 90 minutes after the infusion. The baseline TSH value is subtracted from the highest (peak) level of TSH measured and the maximal change in TSH is recorded. Patients who are depressed will show less change in TSH than the average individual without thyroid disease, depression, or diseases that produce false-positive results. This test, therefore, is useful in confirming a diagnosis of depression or in determining hypothyroidism in patients whose normal results on thyroid screening tests seem to contradict clinical signs of thyroid disorder.

3. The measurement of urinary catecholamine metabolites such as 3-methoxy-4-hydroxyphenylglycol (MHPG) offers some hope of contributing one day to a biochemical standard for diagnosing depression. These substances represent breakdown products of the neurotransmitter norepinephrine. Some depressed individuals demonstrate decreased levels of urinary MHPG when measurements of their 24-hour collection of urine are compared with normal values. Manic patients can have elevated urinary MHPG levels. Because of overlap between pathological and normal ranges of levels, this test remains investigational at present.

4. Platelet MAO activity, similarly, is an investigational test, which may in time offer more valuable insights into the pathophysiology of mood disorders. MAO enzymatic activity in a collection of a patient's platelets is hoped to reflect the activity of this enzyme, a major deactivator of catecholamine neurotransmitters, in the brain. This test has also been proposed as useful in monitoring compliance with MAO-inhibitor antidepressant treatment, since proper use of MAO-inhibitors will inhibit the majority of both platelet and brain MAO enzymes. Finally, attempts have been made to link baseline MAO levels with aspects of behavior. Recent research, for example, has linked low levels of platelet MAO activity to a tendency toward thrill-seeking behavior.[5] A major

conceptual problem complicating the use of this test is that uncertainty remains as to how meaningfully platelet MAO activity relates to brain activity.

5. The lactate infusion test employs an intravenous injection of lactate, a substance considered harmless but known to induce panic attacks in vulnerable individuals. Ninety percent of panic disorder patients as compared with 10% of normal controls experience panic symptoms during this provocative maneuver. Patients with several other anxiety disorders, such as obsessive-compulsive disorder, generalized anxiety, or social phobia, fail to panic in response to lactate infusion.

REFERENCES

1. Weinberger DR: Brain disease and psychiatric illness: When should a psychiatrist order a CAT scan? *Am J Psychiatry* 1984;141:1521–1527.
2. Task Force on the Use of Laboratory Tests in Psychiatry: Tricyclic antidepressants — Blood level measurements and clinical outcome: An APA task force report. *Am J Psychiatry* 1985;142:155–162.
3. Gold MS, Kronig MH: Tests of the hypothalamic-pituitary-adrenal axis, in Gold MS, Pottash ALC (eds): *Diagnostic and Laboratory Testing in Psychiatry*. New York, Plenum Medical Book Company, 1986.
4. Sternberg DE: Biologic tests in psychiatry. *Psychiatr Clin N Am* 1984;7:639–650.
5. Gold MS, Pearsall HR: Platelet and trait markers, in Gold MS, Pottash ALC (eds): *Diagnostic and Laboratory Testing in Psychiatry*. New York, Plenum Medical Book Company, 1986.

INDEX

Acebutolol (Sectral), 189
Acetophenazine (Tindal), 164
Acetylcholine, 146-147, 245
Adjustment disorder with anxious mood, 127, 156
Adolescents. *See* Children and adolescents
Agnosia, 215
Agoraphobia, 19, 128
AIDS, 211
Akathisia, 163, 232
Akineton (biperiden), 187
Alcohol
  benzodiazepines and, 246, 248
  evaluation of usage, 210-211
  interactions with drugs, 248-250
  laboratory testing for, 253
  mortality from, 241
  neurotransmitters and, 244-247
  usage with drugs, 241, 250
  withdrawal from, 219
Alcoholics, type-1 and type-2, 244
Alpha blockers, 149
Alpha receptors, 148
Alprazolam (Xanax), 127, 155, 156, 178, 179
Alzheimer's disease, 222
Amoxapine (Asendin), 177-179
Amphetamines, 125, 224, 246, 259
Amytal interview, 153
Anergia, 242-243
Antianxiety drugs, 153-158. *See also specific drug*
Anticholinergics, 147, 186-188. *See also specific drug*
Anticonvulsants, 290
Antidepressants. *See also* Monoamine oxidase inhibitors; Tricyclic antidepressants
  blood levels of, 131
  for CEBV infection, 269-270
  mechanism of action, 169-170
  novel or second-generation, 178
  second-generation, 177
  side effects, 147, 290
  symptoms responsive to, 20
Antihistamines, 153-154, 248-249
Antipsychotic drugs
  alcohol and, 250
  dosages, 164-165
  indications for, 19, 160-161
  mechanism of action, 158-159
  for schizophrenia, 134-135
  side effects, 139, 147, 161-163, 166, 290
Anxiety
  caffeine-induced, 232
  gamma-aminobutyric acid and, 245
  organic causes of, 229-233
  pharmacotherapy for, 75, 126-130
  situational, 19
Anxiolytics, 129
Aphasia, 215
Apraxia, 215
Artane (trihexyphenidyl), 187
Asendin (amoxapine), 177-179
Atarax (hydroxyzine), 153
Atenolol (Tenormin), 188, 189
Ativan (lorazepam), 155, 248
Attention-deficit-hyperactive disorder
  adult, 258-264
  case illustrations, 198-201
  characteristics, in child, 259
  classification of, 194
  family studies of, 260
  norepinephrine and, 245
  pharmacotherapy, 139

Barbiturates, 125, 153, 253

295

Benadryl (diphenhydramine), 153, 248-249
Bench-warmer syndrome, 65
Benzodiazepines. *See also specific drug*
  addiction to, 156
  alcohol and, 246, 248
  for anxiety disorders, 127, 156
  dosages, 155
  for generalized anxiety, 129
  introduction of, 126
  laboratory testing for, 253
  mechanism of action, 154, 156
  side effects, 156-157
Benzoylecgonine, 253
Benztropine (Cogentin), 187
Beta blockers, 149, 188-190, 250. *See also specific blockers*
Beta receptors, 148
Biperiden (Akineton), 187
Bipolar affective disorder
  mood regulators for, 180-186
  pharmacotherapy, 133-134
  treatment of, 20
Blocadren (Timolol), 189
Brevital (methohexital), 153
Bromocriptine (Parlodel), 166
Bulimia, 138
Buspirone (BuSpar), 129, 158
Butyrophenones, 165. *See also* Haloperidol

Caffeine-induced anxiety, 232
Camphor injections, 125
Cannabis, 246, 251-252, 292
Carbamazepine (Tegretol)
  for bipolar disorders, 133, 139, 184-185
  blood electrolytes and, 290
  dosage, 182
  interactions with drugs, 151
  for mood disorders, 243
Catatonia, 212
CAT scan, 291-292
CBC (complete blood count), 290
CEBV (chronic Epstein-Barr virus), infection, 264-270

Centrax (prazepam), 155
Chemistry, blood, 290
Children and adolescents, 202-203
  critical care issues, 195-198
  DSM-III-R classifications for, 193-195
  evaluation process, 196
  evolution of pharmacotherapy, 192-193
  medication choice, 196-197
  parental disagreement over therapy, 197
  pharmacotherapy case illustrations, 198-202
  suicide risk and, 197-198
Children's Global Assessment Scale, 194-195
Chlorazepate (Tranxene), 155
Chlordiazepoxide (Librium), 126, 154, 155, 248
Chlorpromazine (Thorazine), 126, 135, 151, 164, 250
Chlorprothixene (Taractan), 165
Clomipramine, 129
Clonazepam (Clonopin), 127, 128, 156
Clonidine, 127, 130, 250
Clonopin (clonazepam), 127, 128, 156
Clozapine (Clozeril), 137, 159
Cocaine, 241-244
  interactions with drugs, 250-251
  laboratory testing for, 253
  neurotransmitters and, 247
Cogentin (benztropine), 187
Combined treatment
  absence of clinician and, 18
  advantages, 96-98
  disadvantages, 96-98
  disruption of, 107
  intertherapist conflict
    prevention, 107-109
    resolution of, 109-114
    sources of, 98-107
  nonrational factors and, 22-23, 48
  popularity of, 3-5

psychotherapist role, 18-19
referral for. *See* Referral
relationship between clinicians,
17-20
transference and, 79-94
treatment changes in, 18
Corgard (nadolol), 188, 189
Countertransference, 9, 215-216
Crack, 241
Cushing's syndrome, 223, 232
Cyclothymic disorder, 243
Cylert (pemoline), 259

Dalmane (flurazepam), 155,
157-158
Danazol, 276
Dantrolene (Dantrium), 166
Daxolin (loxapine), 165
Delirium, 216-220, 221
Dementia, organic causes of,
220-223
Demerol (meperidine), 253
Depakene (valproate; valproic
acid), 133-134, 182,
185-186
Dephenylbutylpiperidines, 165
Depression
in children, 191, 201-202
organic causes of, 225-229
of patient's spouse, 75
pharmacotherapy for, 19-20
with schizophrenia, 53
Desipramine (Norpramin), 200,
250-251
Desyrel (trazodone), 132, 138,
178, 179
Developmental impasse, 61, 62-63
Dexamethasone test (DST),
292-293
*Diagnostic and Statistical Manual
of Mental Disorders*,
193-194
child and adolescent disorders,
classification of, 193-195
delirium criteria, 218
organic anxiety syndrome
criteria, 231

organic personality syndrome
criteria, 235
Diazepam (Valium), 155
Dibenzoxazepines, 165
Diphenhydramine (Benadryl), 153,
248-249
Dopamine, 147-148, 243-245
Doriden (glutethimide), 129, 153
Drug(s). *See also specific drug or
drug class*
absorption of, 150-151
for adolescent, 72
behavioral effects of, 144-149
brain concentration of, 151-152
compliance with, 83-84
discontinuation of, 198
efficacy of, 19
elimination rates, 151
interactions of, 250-253
metabolism of, 150-151
nonpharmacologic effects, 152
placebo effect of, 92
potentiation of, 248-249
prn, 32-33
route of administration, 150
serum levels of, 292
transference to, 91-94, 106-107
transitional object role of,
92-94
trials of, 37-38
Dysgraphias, 215
Dysphoria, 243
Dystonic reactions, acute, 162-163

Eating disorders, 138
Ecstacy (MSMA), 252-253
Electrocardiogram (ECG), 253
Electroencephalogram (EEG),
244, 253, 291
Electrolytes, blood, 290
Empty nest syndrome, 73-75
Endocrine disorders, 223
Epidemiological Catchment Area
(ECA) study, 192-193
Epstein-Barr virus infection,
chronic (CEBV), 264-270
ESR, 291

Ethchlorvynol (Placidyl), 153
Extrapyramidal side effects, 163
Family
  adaptation during stress, 65–66
  development, 60–61
  developmental impasse and, 62–63
  hierarchy, 59, 72
  homeostasis, 59–60
  hospital admission and, 29
  life-cycle, 61
    adolescence, 72–73
    family with young children, 70–72
    launching, empty nest and aging, 73–75
    married couple, 68–70
    young adult, 66–68
  problem, symptoms as, 57–58
  responsibilities, reallocation of, 65–66
  structure, 59, 60
    deficit in, 61, 63–65
  symptoms in context of, 61
  with young children, implications of therapy, 70–72
Family history, 7
Family therapy, 52–54
Fatigue, chronic, 266, 267
Fibromyalgia/fibromyositis, 270–274
Fluoxetine (Prozac), 132, 178, 180
Fluphenazine (Prolixin), 135–136, 164
Flurazepam (Dalmane), 155, 157–158

GABA (gamma-aminobutyric acid), 149, 245, 246
Generalized anxiety disorder, 129, 156
Glutethimide (Doriden), 129, 153

Halazepam (Paxipam), 155
Halcion (triazolam), 155, 157

Haldol (haloperidol), 126, 137, 138, 165, 250
Hallucinogens, 242, 247, 251–252
Haloperidol (Haldol), 126, 137, 138, 165, 250
History of pharmacotherapy, 119–127
History-taking, 6–7, 13, 36
Hospitalization
  initial phase, 27–35
  middle phase, 35–43
  terminal phase, 43–47
Hospital staff, reductionism and, 40–42
Hydroxyzine (Atarax), 153
Hyperthyroidism, anxiety and, 230–231
Hypnotics, 154, 157–158
Hypoglycemia, 232, 279–280, 290

Imipramine, 128
Inderal (propranolol), 188, 189, 250
Informed consent, 11
Insulin shock, 125
Isocarboxazid (Marplan), 176

Juvenile rheumatoid arthritis, 268

Kemadrin (procyclidine), 187

Labetalol (Normodyne; Trandate), 189
Laboratory tests, 253–254, 289–294. See also specific tests
Lactate infusion test, 294
Late luteal phase dysphoric disorder (LLPDD), 274–279
Librium (chlordiazepoxide), 126, 154, 155, 248
Lithium
  alcohol and, 250
  for bipolar affective disorders, 133
  blood electrolytes and, 290
  formulations, 181, 182

indications, 181
  for mood disorders, 54-55, 131, 243
  side effects of, 20, 181, 183-184, 290
  therapeutic effects, 180-181
Liver enzymes, 151, 290
Liver metabolism, alcohol and, 249
Lopressor (metoprolol), 189
Lorazepam (Ativan), 155, 248
Loxapine (Daxolin; Loxitane), 165
LSD, 246, 247
Ludiomil (maprotiline), 132, 178, 179-180

Malarial fever therapy, 125
Malpractice, 10
Mania, organic causes of, 225-229
MAO inhibitors. See Monoamine oxidase inhibitors
Maprotiline (Ludiomil), 132, 178-180
Marijuana, 246, 251-252, 292
Marital conflict, mood disorders and, 54-56
Marplan (isocarboxazid), 176
Medical history, 6-7
Medical illness, in psychiatric patients, 206-212
Medication. See Drug(s); *specific drugs*
Mellaril (thioridazine), 164, 251
Memory impairment, organic causes of, 224-225
Meperidine (Demerol), 253
Meprobamate (Miltown), 129, 153
Mesoridazine (Serentil), 164
Methadone, 253
Methaqualone (Quaalude), 129, 153
Methohexital (Brevital), 153
3-Methoxy-4-hydroxyphenylglycol (MHPG), 293
Methylphenidate (Ritalin), 243, 259, 261
Metoprolol (Lopressor), 189

Miltown (meprobamate), 129, 153
Mind-body interaction, 205-206, 282
Mini Mental State Exam, 213, 214
Molindone (Moban), 165
Monoamine oxidase inhibitors
  antidepressant activity of, 169
  for anxiety disorders, 127, 128
  blood sugar levels and, 290
  with cocaine, 251
  dosages, 176
  for eating disorders, 138
  efficacy, 173
  interactions with foods and drugs, 132, 174, 249-250
  mechanism of action, 173-174
  monitoring of compliance, 293-294
  for mood disorders, 131
  side effects, 175, 177
Mononucleosis, chronic, 264-268
Mood disorders
  biological markers for, 130-131
  cocaine and, 243
  literature review, 54-55
  norepinephrine and, 245
  pharmacotherapy for, 126, 130-134
  serotonin and, 245
Mood regulators, 180-186
Morphine, 125-126
MSMA (ecstacy), 252-253
"Multiple allergy syndrome", 280-281

Nadolol (Corgard), 188, 189
Narcotics, 253
Nardil (phenelzine), 128, 129, 176
Navane (thioxanthene), 138, 165
Nembutal (pentobarbital), 153
Neuroleptic malignant syndrome, 166
Neuroleptics, 138-139, 159
Neurological disorders, anxiety from, 233
Neurons, 145
Neurotransmitters

Neurotransmitters *(cont'd)*
  alcohol and drug usage and, 244–248
  synthesis, release and destruction in synapse, 145–146
Noncompliance
  anticipation of, 68
  after discharge, 44–45
  discovery of, 34–35
  displaced feelings and, 92–93
Noradrenaline, 148–149, 245
Norepinephrine, 148–149, 245
Normodyne (labetalol), 189
Norpramin (desipramine), 200, 250–251

Obsessive-compulsive disorder, 129–130, 245
Opiates, 242, 253
Orap (pimozide), 137, 165
Organic amnestic syndrome, 224–225
Organic anxiety syndrome, 229–233
Organic delusional syndrome, 224
Organic hallucinosis, 224
Organic mental disorders, 215–217. *See also specific disorders*
  evaluation for, 212–216, 237
Organic mood syndrome, 225–229
Organic personality syndrome, 233–236
Oxazepam (Serax), 155
Oxoindolones, 165

Pan-allergic disease, 280–281
Panic disorder, 19, 127, 156
Paranoid reactions, 75
Parentification, 65
Parents, aging, 73–75
Parkinsonism, 147, 163
Parlodel (Bromocriptine), 166
Parnate (tranylcypromine), 139, 176
Partial sleep deprivation, 279
Patient
  ambivalence about hospitalization, 37–38
  child or adolescent, family implications and, 72–73
  identified, 57–58
  during intertherapist conflict, 101
  questions about medication, 20
  requests of, 4, 9, 107
  transference to pharmacotherapist, 81–87
  young adult, family implications and, 66–68
Paxipam (halazepam), 155
PCP, 246, 247
Pemoline (Cylert), 259
Pentobarbital (Nembutal), 153
Perphenazine (Trilafon), 164
Personality disorders, 138, 233–236
Pharmacotherapeutics
  history of, 119–127
  intervention for developmental impasse, 62–63
  irrationality in, 22–23
Pharmacotherapist
  choice as consultant, 11–12
  combined treatment and, 97–98
  competence of, 108
  ideological stance of, 108
  psychotherapist and, 108–109
  transference to medication, 94
Pharmacotherapy
  consultation
    indications for, 5–8
    preparation for, 8–13
    refusal of, 10
  disorders responsive to, 126–127
  for eating disorders, 138
  evolution of, 119–127
  family structure and, 63–65
  for personality disorders, 138
  request for, 14–15
Phenelzine (Nardil), 128, 129, 176
Phenothiazines, 138, 164
Pimozide (Orap), 137, 165
Pindolol (Visken), 189

Placidyl (ethchlorvynol), 153
Platelet MAO activity, 293-294
PMS (premenstrual syndrome), 274-279
Polysubstance abuse, 240
Postconcussion syndrome, 233
Post-traumatic stress disorder, 130
Prazepam (Centrax), 155
Pregnancy, drug usage during, 157, 162, 171
Premenstrual syndrome (PMS), 274-279
Procyclidine (Kemadrin), 187
Prolactin, 277
Prolixin (fluphenazine), 135-136, 164
Propranolol (Inderal), 188, 189, 250
Prostaglandins, 277-278
Prozac (fluoxetine), 132, 178, 180
Pseudodementia, 223
Psychoanalytic/psychodynamic model, 98-99, 102
Psychosis, organic, 219, 221
Psychostimulants, 259-260
Psychotherapeutic relationship, 81
Psychotherapist
    combined treatment and, 97
    family structure and, 75-76
    motivation for referral, 8-9
    psychopharmacologist and, 20-21
    role of, 18-19, 51
Psychotherapy
    biological perspective, 52
    biopsychosocial perspective, 52
    evaluation, directive component in, 6
    exploration of patient's attitude about referral, 9-10
    family systems approach, 52
    indications for evaluation, 5-8
    integrated perspective vs. clinical ideology, 52
    models of, disparity with pharmacotherapeutic models, 98-107
    psychoanalytic model, 52
    termination of, 18
Psychotropic drugs, 4, 75, 119, 144-149. *See also specific drugs or class of drugs*

Quaalude (methaqualone), 129, 153

Referral
    early discussion for, 12-13
    family implications of, 66-68
    indications for, 5
    motivation for, 8-9
    from psychopharmacologist to psychotherapist, 16-17
    refusal of, 10
    request form for, 14-15
Restoril (temazepam), 155, 157
Ritalin (methylphenidate), 243, 259, 261

Sanguinaria extract, 124
Schizophrenia
    beta blockers for, 188
    brain structure and, 205
    dopamine and, 245
    literature review, 53-54
    pharmacotherapy for, 126, 134-138
    relapse in, 53-54
    sleep treatment for, 125
Sectral (acebutolol), 189
Selective serotonin reuptake blockers, 132
Self-psychology, 99
Serax (oxazepam), 155
Serotonin, 149, 245, 246
Shock therapies, 125
Spironolactone, 277
Spouse, treatment and, 55-57, 69
Stelazine (trifluoperazine), 164
Stimulants, 166-169
Substance abuse
    evaluation of, 210-211
    incidence of, 241-242
    laboratory evaluation, 253-254

Substance abuse *(cont'd)*
  neurochemical bases of, 242–244
Suicide, 241, 250
Sulpiride, 137
Symptoms
  in family context, 61
  from family structural deficit, 63
  indications for psychiatric consultation, 8
  target, 19
Syphilis, 125

Taractan (chlorprothixene), 165
Tardive dyskinesia, 36, 137, 139, 163
Tegretol. *See* Carbamazepine
Temazepam (Restoril), 155, 157
Temporal lobe epilepsy, 213, 235–236
Temporomandibular joint syndrome, 281
Tenormin (atenolol), 188, 189
Thioridazine (Mellaril), 164, 251
Thiothixene, 138
Thioxanthene (Navane), 165
Thorazine (chlorpromazine), 126, 135, 151, 164, 250
Thyroid function tests, 290
Thyroid hormone, 131, 132
Thyrotropin releasing hormone response test (TRH), 293
Timolol (Blocadren), 189
Tindal (acetophenazine), 164
Toxic screens, 292
Trandate (labetalol), 189
Transference(s)
  during hospitalization, 37–38
  importance of, 79–80
  interpretation of, 112
  intertherapist conflict and, 105–106
  to medication, 91–94
  multiple, 80
  negative, 81–83, 85–87
  from patient to pharmacotherapist, 81–87
  positive, 81, 83–85
  between psychotherapist and pharmacotherapist, 88–91
Tranxene (chlorazepate), 155
Tranylcypromine (Parnate), 139, 176
Trazodone (Desyrel), 132, 138, 178, 179
Triazolam (Halcion), 155, 157
Tricyclic antidepressants
  dosages, 172
  for eating disorders, 138
  efficacy of, 170
  introduction of, 126, 169
  for mood disorders, 131
  panic disorders and, 127
  side effects, 171, 173
Trifluoperazine (Stelazine), 164
Trihexyphenidyl (Artane), 187
Triiodothyronine, 132
Trilafon (perphenazine), 164
Tryptophan, 131, 132, 149
"Twentieth-century disease," 280–281
Tyramine, 249–250

Valium (diazepam), 155
Valproic acid or valproate (Depakene), 133–134, 182, 185–186
Verapamil (Isoptin; Calan), 134, 182, 186
Veratrine, 124
Visken (pindolol), 189

Wernicke's encephalopathy, 219
Withdrawal dyskinesia, 36

Xanax (alprazolam), 127, 155, 156, 178, 179